Cardiovascular Molecular Morphogenesis

Books in the Series

Vascular Morphogenesis: in vivo, in vitro, in mente — *0-8176-3920-9*
C. D. Little, V. A. Mironov and E. H. Sage, editors

Living Morphogenesis of the Heart — *0-8176-4037-1*
M. V. de la Cruz and R. R. Markwald

Living Morphogenesis of the Heart

María Victoria de la Cruz
Roger R. Markwald
Editors

Springer Science+Business Media, LLC

Editors:
María V. de la Cruz, M.D.
Departamento de Biología del Desarrollo y Teratogénesis
Hospital Infantil de México "Federico Gómez"
México, D. F. C. P. 06720

Roger R. Markwald, Ph.D.
Department of Cell Biology and Anatomy
Medical University of South Carolina
Charleston, SC 29425

Library of Congress Cataloging-in-Publication Data

Cataloging in Process

Legend of cover design.
Three photographs of an in vivo labelling experiment in the chick embryo heart. They depict the appearance and the contribution of the primitive interventricular septum into the definitive interventricular septum. The first photograph shows the appearance of the primordium of the primitive interventricular septum in the ventral fusion line of both cardiac tubes in the straight-tube heart; the second photograph shows its first morphological expression in the apex of the first cardiac septum. The third photograph shows its contribution in the definitive interventricular septum of which it forms the middle and the apical thirds. See Chapter 5, figure 1.

ISBN 978-1-4612-7283-0 ISBN 978-1-4612-1788-6 (eBook)
DOI 10.1007/978-1-4612-1788-6
Typeset by Northeastern Graphic Services, Inc.

987654321

To the memory of my father, J. M. de la Cruz,
and my husband H. Losada.

Acknowledgments

Gracias al Dr. Jorge Espino-Vela, Editor en Jefe de Acta Pediátrica de México del Instituto Nacional de Pediatría, por su valiosa colaboración en la traducción del manuscrito del español al ingles. A la JEOL de México, S.A. de C.V. por su contribución económica en las ilustraciones del libro y Telefónos de México, S. A. de C. V. por su contribución económica. A Mario Jauregui por su asistencia fotográfica y a Marcela Salazar y a Laura Villavicencio por su colaboración técnica.

We would like to thank Dr. Jorge Espino-Vela, Editor in Chief of Acta Pediátrica de México at the Instituto Nacional de Pediatría de México, for his valuable collaboration in the translation of the original Spanish manuscript into English. We are also grateful to JEOL de México, S.A. de C.V. for the financial support of the illustrations of this book, and to Teléfonos de México, S.A. de C.V. for the financial support. Finally, we express gratitude to Mario Jauregui for the technical photography assistance, to Marcela Salazar and Laura Villavicencio for their expert technical assistance.

Contents

List of Contributors

Guillermo Anselmi, Instituto de Anatomía Patológica, Universidad Central de Venezuela, Caracas, Venezuela. Apartado 88120, Caracas 1084-A

María V. de la Cruz, Departamento de Biología del Desarrollo y Teratogénesis Experimental, Hospital Infantil de México "Federico Gómez", México D. F. C. P. 06720

Margaret L. Kirby, Institute of Molecular Medicine & Genetics (IMMAG), Developmental Biology Program, Medical College of Georgia, Augusta, GA 30912-2640

James W. Lash, Department of Cell and Developmental Biology, University of Pennsylvania, Philadelphia, PA 19104-6058

Kersti K. Linask, Department of Cell Biology, University of Medicine and Dentistry of New Jersey, Stratford, NJ 08084

Roger R. Markwald, Department of Cell Biology and Anatomy, Medical University of South Carolina, Charleston, SC 29425-2204

Ricardo Moreno-Rodríguez, Departamento de Biología del Desarrollo y Teratogénesis Experimental, Hospital Infantil de México "Federico Gómez", Dr. Marquez #162, Col. Doctores, México D. F. C. P. 06720

Concepción Sánchez-Gómez, Departamento de Biología del Desarrollo y Teratogénesis Experimental, Hospital Infantil de México, México D. F. C. P. 06720

Thomas Trusk, Department of Cell Biology and Anatomy, Medical University of South Carolina, Charleston, SC 29425-2204

Karen Waldo, Institute of Molecular Medicine and Genetics (IMMAG), Developmental Biology Program, Medical College of Georgia, Augusta, GA 30912-2640

Series Preface

The overall scope of this new series will be to evolve an understanding of the genetic basis of (1) how early mesoderm commits to cells of a heart lineage that progressively and irreversibly assemble into a segmented, primary heart tube that can be remodeled into a four-chambered organ, and (2) how blood vessels are derived and assembled both in the heart and in the body. Our central aim is to establish a four-dimensional, spatiotemporal foundation for the heart and blood vessels that can be genetically dissected for function and mechanism.

Since Robert DeHaan's seminal chapter "Morphogenesis of the Vertebrate Heart" published in *Organogenesis* (Holt Rinehart & Winston, NY) in 1965, there have been surprisingly few books devoted to the subject of cardiovascular morphogenesis, despite the enormous growth of interest that occurred nationally and internationally. Most writings on the subject have been scholarly compilations of the proceedings of major national or international symposia or multiauthored volumes, often without a specific theme. What is missing are the unifying concepts that can make sense out of a burgeoning database of facts. The Editorial Board of this new series believes the time has come for a book series dedicated to cardiovascular morphogenesis that will serve not only as an important archival and didactic reference source for those who have recently come into the field but also as a guide to the evolution of a field that is clearly coming of age. The advances in heart and vessel morphogenesis are not only serving to reveal general basic mechanisms of embryogenesis but are also now influencing clinical thinking in pediatric and adult cardiology.

Undoubtedly, the Human Genome Project and other genetic approaches will continue to reveal new genes or groups of genes that may be involved in heart development. A central goal of this series will be to extend the identification of these and other genes into their functional role at the molecular, cellular, and organ levels. The major issues in morphogenesis highlighted in the series will be the local (heart or vessel) regulation of cell growth and death, cell adhesion and migration, and gene expression responsible for the cardiovascular cellular phenotypes.

Specific topics will include the following:

- The roles of extracardiac populations of cells in heart development.
- Coronary angiogenesis.
- Vasculogenesis.
- Breaking symmetry, laterality genes, and patterning.

- Formation and integration of the conduction cell phenotypes.
- Growth factors and inductive interactions in cardiogenesis and vasculogenesis.
- Morphogenetic role of the extracellular matrix.
- Genetic regulation of heart development.
- Application of developmental principles to cardiovascular tissue engineering.

Roger R. Markwald
Medical University of South Carolina

Foreword

Another book on development of the heart? Do we really need another book on this area? And so goes the thoughts of publishers and book buyers alike. Yes, I believe we do need another book on development of the heart. There are three main reasons for this belief. First, as we approach the 21st century, developmental biology has entered a new era, an era that blends the findings of classic descriptive and experimental embryology with those of modern genetics, molecular biology, and the study of human birth defects. In this era, we are turning back to the morphological database acquired over the last century and rediscovering the necessity and value of comparative embryology. In this new era, we are layering onto the morphological, comparative database new information obtained utilizing in situ hybridization, which reveals the intricate, three-dimensional patterns of gene expression that underlie morphogenetic events. Thus, morphology and molecules are being studied hand-in-hand, and our understanding of embryonic development is growing exponentially. *Living Morphogenesis of the Heart* summarizes our vast knowledge on the morphology of heart development; provides a copious number of superb three-dimensional scanning electron micrographs, light micrographs of intact, living hearts, histological sections, and diagrams, the latter of which are the epitome of clarity; and uses a popular model system, the avian embryo, on which extensive experimental analyses have been conducted. In addition, two of the chapters deal with molecular embryology, emphasizing key molecules controlling embryogenesis and forming a bridge between anatomy and mechanism. Furthermore, one chapter expands on the theme of cardiac development, providing the latest information on development of the great vessels. Because of its extensive, multidisciplinary integrative coverage, *Living Morphogenesis of the Heart* will become a major, singular reference in the field of cardiac development.

Second, *Living Morphogenesis of the Heart* collates new data generated over the long and productive career of Dr. de la Cruz on dynamic changes in cardiac morphology over time, based on intensive analyses of living embryos. Standard anatomical procedures for studying morphology are limited. Fixed and processed embryos display a range of known, and possibly unknown, artifacts. Collections of a series of fixed embryos used to describe sequential developmental events require extrapolation between static stages, and assumptions must be made that such extrapolation adequately describes intermediate processes occurring between stages in the series. Finally, cell displacements and morphogenetic movements can only be inferred from fixed embryos, not directly observed, and such inferences may or may not be correct. The dynamic in vivo labeling technique employed by Dr. de la Cruz provides new information, impossible to obtain in any other fashion, and offers novel insight into the complexities of normal cardiac morphogenesis, as well as explanations of possible mechanisms of dysmorphogenesis underlying the formation of congenital cardiac anomalies.

Third, recent progress has made it possible to create at will birth defects in mouse embryos by generating gain-of-function and loss-of-function mutations using, respectively, transgenic techniques and gene knockouts through homologous recombination. Concomitantly, birth defects in humans are becoming tractable as the genetic basis of such disease and the molecular players become elucidated. *Living Morphogenesis of the Heart* provides a dynamic morphological and molecular database, essential for interpreting induced and spontaneous alterations of cardiogenesis.

In 10 chapters, the authors present a comprehensive body of information on cardiac development, which is foundational to our understanding of cardiogenesis. *Living Morphogenesis of the Heart* has an element of timelessness, assembling fundamental, detailed information that will endure for several years to come. Development of the heart is a fascinating process. *Living Morphogenesis of the Heart* shows the beauty of the process of cardiac development and reveals the exciting and interesting events that once assembled our own hearts. And like our own hearts, which continue to beat relentlessly throughout our lives, *Living Morphogenesis of the Heart* will remain at the center of the field, continuing to pump new insight and life into our understanding of cardiac development.

I have enjoyed immensely reading *Living Morphogenesis of the Heart* and I have learned much by doing so. The authors are to be congratulated for providing such an interesting, unique, and engaging contribution to the field.

Gary C. Schoenwolf, Ph.D.
University of Utah School of Medicine
Salt Lake City, Utah

Preface

Finding the molecular circuitry for routing undifferentiated precursor cells into a pair of heart-forming fields is only the beginning of a dynamic process that progressively, sequentially, and irreversibly leads first to the formation of a simple, straight, hollow tube that is transformed *over time* into a four-chambered organ.

The purpose of this book is not so much to describe the very latest genes that might regulate heart development, although Dr. Kirsti Linask reviews the most recent cellular and molecular concepts related to heart field formation. Rather, this book is mostly about how a heart becomes a heart, viz how primitive structures combine to form an organ that provides for one-way blood flow of two separate bloodstreams. It is written to show how the seemingly complex phenotype of the fully defined heart can be simplified and more fully grasped by studying living embryos using in vivo experimental approaches.

To our knowledge, this is the first book to present heart development from a living morphogenetic viewpoint. More than 20 years of in vivo labeling experiments performed in the laboratory of Dr. María Victoria de la Cruz form the core of this book. Many fundamental experiments are integrated conceptually here for the first time and include recent new work not previously published. For many, this book will contain information that will seem very new, particularly to those with a more molecular biology background. For those experienced in morphology, we attempt to integrate the dynamic changes in structure that occur over time with emerging molecular concepts. We believe the data presented here will prove to be a bridge between morphological and molecular studies that can serve as a lasting foundation on which new findings can be continually integrated and interpreted.

The recurring theme of the book is that the developing heart is a four-dimensional organ and that studies of fixed, postmortem tissues cannot provide the critical, temporal dimension required to correctly visualize the ephemeral, spatial connections that exist between a complex, mature anatomical structure and its developmental origins from primitive primordial structures. We show that the heart is put together from segments that form progressively along the caudo-cephalic axis. These segments, the grooves or folds that separate them, and the invaginations or expansions that form within them collectively integrate *over time* to ultimately form a complex final organ anatomy. When the fate of a primitive segmental sturcture is followed by in vivo labeling, we often find that the outcome is surprisingly different from what might have been expected after studying static images of fixed material.

In preparing this book, our goal was to expand the reader's vision of heart development by raising questions derived from the outcome of in vivo labeling experiments. We believe these questions can lead to new opportunities for seminal investigation. Some of these questions include:

(1) whether the future chambers of the fully defined heart are established all at once within the linear heart tube and whether each chamber has a single primordium;

(2) why mutations in laterality genes affect the two atria but not the two ventricles;

(3) whether there is a new segment of noncardiogenic origin that develops after looping is initiated and gives rise to the outlet region (the conus and truncus) of the heart;

(4) what the effect of looping and torsion is on the anatomical coordinates of the linear heart and the alignment of its segmental components;

(5) whether the origin of the major septum of the heart, the primitive ventricular septum, is from septal precursor cells derived from a ventral groove that is formed by the fusion of the paired heart fields or the junctional boundary that formed between ventricular segments;

(6) why the formation of the supraventricular crest correlates with the muscularization of the outlet septum and the alignment of the segmental precursors of the ventricular inlets and outlets;

(7) how the septal leaflet of the mitral valve comes to form the posterior wall of the left ventricular outlet;

(8) what is the origin of valve leaflets and why their initial formation is similar in some respects to limb development; and

(9) why the structures associated with the inner curvature of the looped, U-shaped heart seemingly disappear and what happens if they persist.

As might be expected, some of the observations made on living embryos will challenge existing dogma, particularly nomenclature derived from studies on postmortem tissues. For example, the term "bulbus cordis" is shown to be an obsolete concept whose existence cannot be supported in living embryos. We also show pitfalls of identifying a structure based only on its initial anatomical expression (e.g., shape).

The reasons why the chick embryo heart was chosen as the biological model are
(1) it is similar anatomically and embryologically to the human heart;
(2) it can be readily studied in vivo; and
(3) selective, site-directed labeling of specific segments or primitive structures can be made to determine final fate.

Finally, we also integrate our findings on normal embryos with abnormal heart development. A unifying hypothesis is proposed to explain why so many genes and environmental perturbations result in the same defective phenotype. Thus, this book should not only prove useful for the developmental and molecular biologist, but also should appeal to the teratologist, pathologist, pediatric cardiologist, and surgeon who specialize in congenital cardiopathies.

María V. de la Cruz
Hospital Infantil de México "Federico Goméz", México

Roger R. Markwald
Medical University of South Carolina

CHAPTER 1

Morphoregulatory Mechanisms Underlying Early Heart Development: Precardiac Stages to the Looping, Tubular Heart

Kersti K. Linask and James W. Lash

The formation of a single, beating, tubular heart in the embryo by the fusion of the two endocardial tubes is one of the early processes leading to normal heart development. Because of the prominence of this developmental event, there is often an underlying assumption that abnormalities that may lead to congenital heart disease arise during this fusion process and in the developmental events that follow during the later modeling of the chambers, septa, and valves. There is truth in this, but the developmental processes that take place before this are of equal or greater importance for cardiovascular development.

Whereas the avian heart begins to beat at approximately 33 hours of development, the 16 to 17 hours in the avian embryo before this encompass a period of paramount importance to normal heart development. Intricate cell–substratum processes will determine the directionality of precardiac cell migration to their final site of heart formation. Specific signaling occurring in this early period will determine the cells that differentiate into cardiomyocytes or endocardiocytes. These early processes specify where the lateral mesoderm will split to form the pericardial cavity, an event that results in delineating the cardiac population as a separate embryonic compartment. Regulation of the synthesis of molecules takes place that defines cardiac left-right asymmetry. These morphoregulatory molecules become necessary for subsequent normal heart looping that proceeds 10 hours later after their initial expression in the heart-forming areas. Slight alterations in these early developmental events may lead to serious consequences in later stages and may underlie aspects of heart disease seen in childhood and in the adult.

This chapter describes the current understanding of the early stages of normal heart development leading to the formation of a single, tubular heart that begins to loop. Emphasis in this chapter is placed primarily on the avian model. However, in a time when most developmental biologists do study a very select group of organisms, there is an awareness that there is a need to look also beyond our particular animal to determine the variation among the models in specific developmental processes. One should not assume that all processes will be identical among the different models. Differences in heart development are already reported among the different vertebrates. However, the molecules that are being described are conserved. Principal differences appear to relate to the timing of expression or pattern of modulation of the conserved molecules. Eventually it is by the integration of the differences that a greater understanding can be achieved of the basic developmental mechanisms involved (see also Bolker and Raff 1997).

PRECARDIAC CELL MOVEMENT

In the early part of the 19th century Pander crystallized the germ-layer concept for the chick embryo (cited in Oppenheimer 1967). He described for the first time the three germ layers in the embryo and used the term "blastoderm" for the embryonic form that they constituted. After gastrulation the upper layer, the epiblast, will become the ectoderm, and the lower layer, the hypoblast, will be replaced by the epiblast-derived endoderm. The process of gastrulation (ingression of the epiblast cells) creates the middle layer, the "mesoderm". Karl Ernst von Baer (1828–1837) extended the recognition of the germ layers of the chick embryo to vertebrate development in general. The fate of cells in the epiblast at the prestreak (before gastrulation) and early primitive streak (gastrulation) stages has been studied recently by injecting horseradish peroxidase into single cells at early stages and identifying the labeled descendants at midstreak to neural plate stages (Lawson et al 1991). The resulting fate map is essentially the same for the chick as for the mouse and urodeles, and indicates that topological fate relationships appear to be conserved among the vertebrates. An important observation from these studies is that clonal descendants of the epiblast cells were not necessarily confined to a single germ layer or to specific extraembryonic regions. This indicates that the fate of these cells is not determined at the beginning of gastrulation. The cells localized to the so-called heart region in the epiblast can migrate and localize to entirely different germ layers and embryonic regions and will differentiate according to their final location after migration.

The movement and origin of the avian cardiovascular system from the primitive streak to the lateral mesoderm plate has been mapped by the construction of quail/chick transplantation chimeras, by the use of QH-1 (an anti–quail endothelial/endocardial cell marker), and by injection of a vital fluorescent dye DiI into the primitive streak (Garcia-Martinez and Schoenwolf 1993). The results indicate that the cells that will form the myocardium and endocardium of the future heart are localized in the rostral half of the primitive streak at early stages of gastrulation and in a rostrocaudal sequence (i.e., cells that will form the future bulbus cordis are localized in a more rostral position in the streak than, for example, the cells that will form the future ventricle). Experiments addressing the state of determination of these cells within the primitive streak during ingression indicate that at this time the cells are quite labile as to their future fate (Inagaki et al 1993). These results based on chick/quail chimera transplantation experiments indicate that the presumptive cardiac and endothelial cells are not committed at the time of ingression; that the rostrocaudal patterning of the heart and blood vessels is determined through cell interactions after ingression; and that the pathway of cell migration from the primitive streak and into the mesodermal mantle is determined mainly by the rostrocaudal level of emigration of cells from the streak, and not by their original site of origin (Fig. 1). Thus cardiac, as well as endothelial, cell determination and ultimate patterning of the heart and blood vessels occurs at slightly later

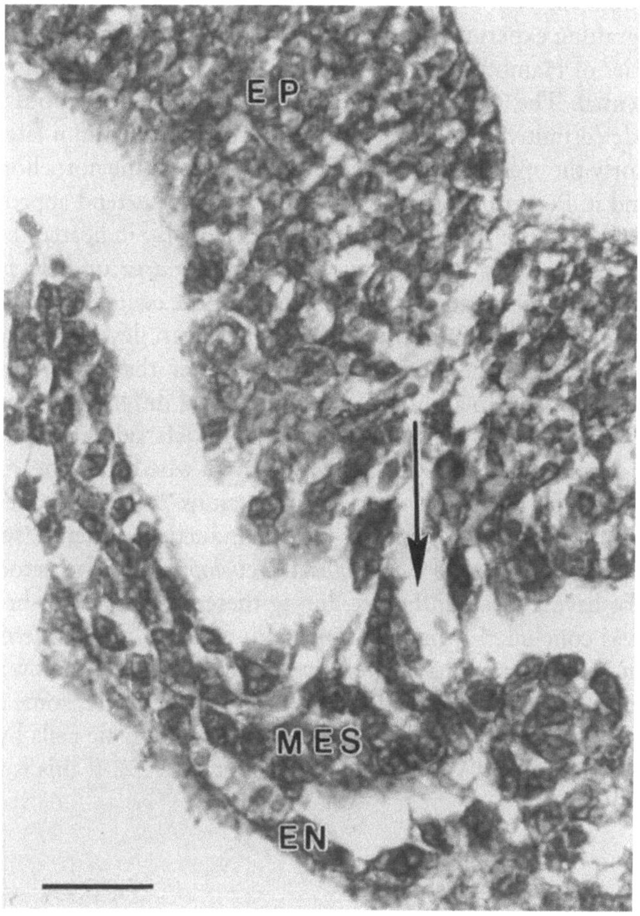

FIGURE 1. Cross-section through primitive streak area of a stage 3+ chick embryo. Cells from epiblast (EP) are migrating through the primitive groove (see arrow) to form the middle mesoderm (MES) layer. The endoderm (EN) underlies the emerging mesoderm. Magnification bar = 25 μm.

stages of development, apparently from local environmental influences in the lateral mesoderm. As the cells ingress and move toward the lateral regions, they may possibly use fibrillin fibrils in the extracellular matrix as guidance cues (Gallagher et al 1993). The Hensen's node region in the chick, which is homologous to the organizer region in the amphibian, has been reported to express a number of regulatory factors, e.g., *noggin*, *sonic hedgehog*, scatter factor, retinoic acid, *CWnt-8C*, *goosecoid*, and *nodal*, among others. Some of these factors, such as *nodal*, have been shown to be involved in the development of asymmetry. Hence, as the cardiac precursors pass in the vicinity of the Hensen's node region to form the mesoderm in the anterior bilateral, heart-forming regions, they already encounter signals that may provide competence for reception of subsequent signaling in the microenvironment of the bilateral mesoderm.

In a series of experiments, Rawles (1943) defined the bilateral heart-forming areas in the chick embryo by localizing the specific regions that are capable of producing cardiac muscle when grafted to the chorioallantoic membrane (see Fig. 2). By these grafting experiments, two large bilateral areas are defined at HH stage 5, staging series of Hamburger and Hamilton (1951), that specifically show heart-forming potential. The two heart-forming regions extend on both sides of the Hensen's node (primitive pit) from approximately 0.2 to 0.8 mm lateral from the node. Anteriorly the areas extend to the level of the tip of the notochord, but never extend beyond it. Posteriorly the heart-forming regions extend approximately 0.4 mm from the level of the primitive pit. Rawles (1943) also indicated that a gradient in developmental potency was observed within each area or field in which the capacity for heart differentiation was the highest at the center of the area.

Heart development illustrates the concept of the heart developmental field. This developmental field is generally found to be greater than the region that will actually form the organ. In addition, an asymmetrical difference between left and right heart-forming regions is noticeable with the left side apparently showing greater heart-forming potential. It is still not known whether the heart potential in the avian embryo is restricted to local interactions in the mesoderm only, or whether the underlying endoderm may have an inductive influence (see section on *Growth Factor Stimulation of Early Heart Development*). The ectoderm apparently does not have a direct influence during these early stages of heart development. This was concluded from experiments in which, after ectodermal removal, the precardiac cells migrate in a normal directional fashion (see below) and normal pulsating cardiac tissue was formed (DeHaan 1964). However, some studies indicate that there may be an inhibitory influence on cardiogenic cells by the neurogenic ectoderm (Arias and Villar 1986; Climent et al 1995). If this is the case, the

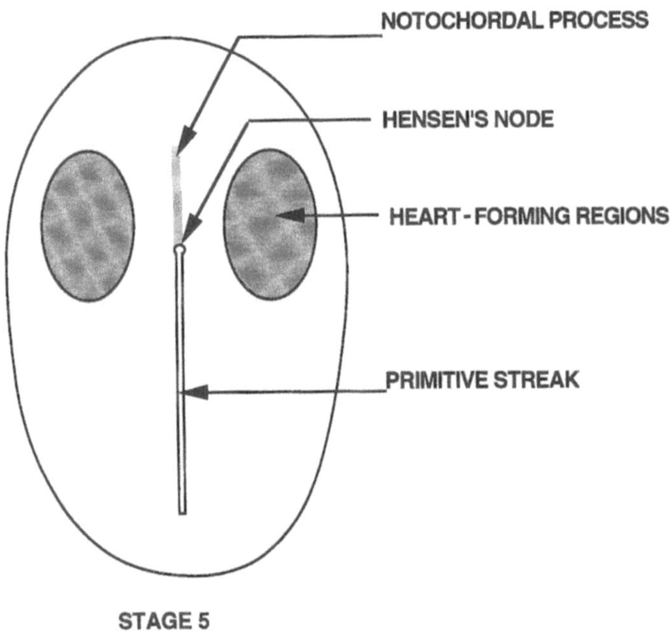

FIGURE 2. Heart developmental fields on anterior bilateral sides as described by Rawles (1943). The fields do not extend beyond the tip of the notochord.

inhibitory effect would be strongest on the dorsal mesoderm that lies closest to the ectoderm. These dorsal cells eventually form the somatic mesoderm. Possibly the inhibitory effect may prevent the dorsal mesoderm from forming cardiac tissue. The more ventral, precardiac mesoderm is further removed and can differentiate into the heart being inductively influenced by the endoderm. Eventually, by stage 7, the emerging pericardial coelom separates the ventral compartment even further from any possible inhibitory influence of the ectoderm.

Before HH stage 5 the mesoderm cells in the bilateral regions move in a random fashion, but at the end of stage 5, time-lapse studies show that the precardiac cells begin active directional movement anteriorly, as well as toward the midline (DeHaan 1963a). Concomitantly, the cells are also being passively moved toward the midline by the folding and formation of the lateral body walls and by the subsequent enclosure of the developing gut tube on the ventral side of the embryo.

The directionality of precardiac mesoderm movement depends on a fibrillar network of fibronectin that is being synthesized and deposited at the mesoderm–endoderm interface (Fig. 3) (Linask and Lash 1986). Fibronectin synthesis begins just before directional movement occurs in the more anterior regions and then progresses to form an anterior–posterior gradient across the heart-forming regions. If this gradient is perturbed by using either anti–fibronectin antibodies or synthetic peptides to the RGD (arginine-glycine-aspartic acid)-sequence in the cell-binding domain of integrin, cardiac tissue can differentiate, but migration is

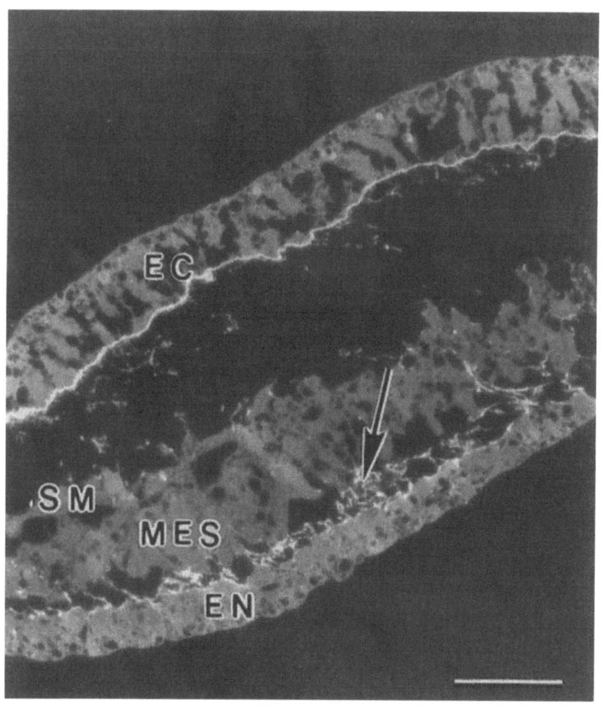

FIGURE 3. Immunohistochemical localization of fibronectin at the mesoderm (MES)–endoderm (EN) interface (arrow) of a stage 7 chick embryo. Precardiac mesoderm cells are elongating and making contact with fibronectin on their basal side. The ectoderm (EC) becomes separated from the precardiac mesoderm by the emerging coelom and somatic mesoderm (SM). Magnification bar = 30 μm.

perturbed and normal hearts cannot develop. Depending on the time of exposure during the migration period along the anterior–posterior axis within the heart-forming regions, the extent of abnormal development varies from cardia bifida (i.e., two bilateral hearts) to various extents of single cardiac tube development, indicating some migration and subsequent fusion of the endocardial tubes at the embryonic midline has taken place (Lash et al 1987; Linask and Lash 1988a 1990).

In a series of experiments perturbing fibronectin in the cardiac regions, the lateral heart-forming mesoderm and endoderm were microsurgically rotated 180°. The ectoderm was left intact. If these rotation experiments were carried out with HH stage 5 embryos, the formation of bilateral endocardial tubes and their ability to fuse cephalad to form a single tube appeared normal. When these same rotation experiments were carried out with HH stage 7 embryos, abnormal heart development followed. The abnormal heart tissue was localized to the lateral sides of the embryos, indicating no further migration to the midline and that the cardiac progenitor cells differentiated in place (Linask and Lash 1988b). At the time, the interpretation of the results dealt primarily with the perturbation of the normal precardiac cell–substratum interactions. From later experimentation, it became apparent that another important process is also occurring during these stages, i.e., between HH stages 5 through 7+, which leads to the stabilization of cardiac commitment and differentation. These initial results indicated that at stages 4 and 5 plasticity in cardiac cell commitment still exists (Linask and Lash 1988b). However, the results also suggest that some important signaling of early heart development occurs during the primitive streak stages just after HH stage 5. This signaling is activated progressively from anterior to posterior across the heart-forming region.

Pericardial Coelom Development, Precardiac Cell Epithelialization, and Cardiac Cell Differentiation

The important process of pericardial coelom formation begins to occur at the end of stage 5 (16 to 19 hours) in the bilateral heart-forming regions and extends to stage 8 (26 to 29 hours). This process proceeds rostrocaudad in wavelike progression, resulting in the mesoderm splitting to form two layers, the dorsal somatic mesoderm and ventral splanchnic precardiac mesoderm (Fig. 4). By the time of formation of the pericardial coelom the ectoderm becomes separated from the ventral precardiac mesoderm by the formation of the somatic mesoderm layer that lines the dorsal side of the emerging pericardial cavity on each lateral side of the embryo. The separation of the ectoderm from the precardiac mesoderm by the somatic mesoderm and coelomic cavity may contribute to the ectoderm having no known effect on heart development. From observations on the development of different animal species, von Baer stated that the middle (mesoderm) germ layer splits into an upper and lower layer of mesoderm (von Baer 1828–1837). Hence, in the mid-1800s von Baer may have been the first to recognize the splitting of the mesoderm being separated by the development of the coelomic cavity. Descriptions of the development of the pericardial coelom were later described in the rabbit embryo by Van der Stricht (1895) and in the chick by Sabin (1920).

Experiments are now beginning to define some of the events that precede the splitting of the mesoderm and that specify where the pericardial coelom forms in the heart-forming region. The formation of the pericardial coelom delineates the

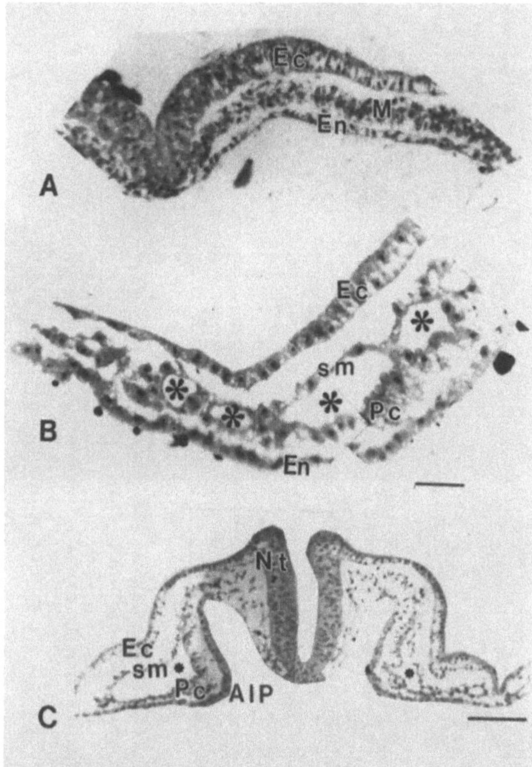

FIGURE 4. Development of the pericardial coelom delineates the precardiac population of cells as a separate compartment in the embryo. **A.** At stage 5 the mesoderm (M) remains as a single middle layer of cells. **B.** By stage 7 the precardiac mesoderm (Pc) is delineated as a result of the formation of the pericardial coelomic cavities (asterisks mark 4 cavities). This process results in the formation of the somatic mesoderm (sm) that now underlies the ectoderm (Ec). The ventral precardiac mesoderm forms a true epithelium and remains closely associated with the underlying endoderm (En). **C.** The coelomic cavities seen in (B) fuse and form two bilateral pericardial cavities (black asterisks) at stage 8 that eventually fuse as a tubular heart develops. The precardiac cells (Pc) remain closely associated with the lateral walls of the developing foregut. In this section the anterior intestinal portal is apparent (AIP). Magnification bar = 100 μm for (A) and (C); 35 μm for (B).

splanchnic cardiac compartment in the embryo for the first time (Linask et al 1997). This process appears to depend on the patterning of a calcium-dependent homotypic cell adhesion molecule, N-cadherin, and the intracellular protein, β-catenin, in the heart-forming region just before the separation process (Linask et al 1992; Linask 1992a, 1992b; Linask and Gui 1995; Linask et al 1997).

A spatiotemporal immunohistochemical localization of N-cadherin has been completed for the early stages of chick heart development, i.e., between HH stages 5 and 13 (18 to 52 hours of development). A complete description of this work has been published (Linask 1992a). N-cadherin is evenly distributed throughout the cell surfaces in the heart-forming mesoderm of a stage 5 embryo, often with an arrangement of brightly staining large central cells seen within the mesoderm. At stage 6 the N-cadherin immunostaining becomes restricted to the central areas of the mesoderm (Fig. 5). Similar staining is seen with α- and β-catenins (Linask et al

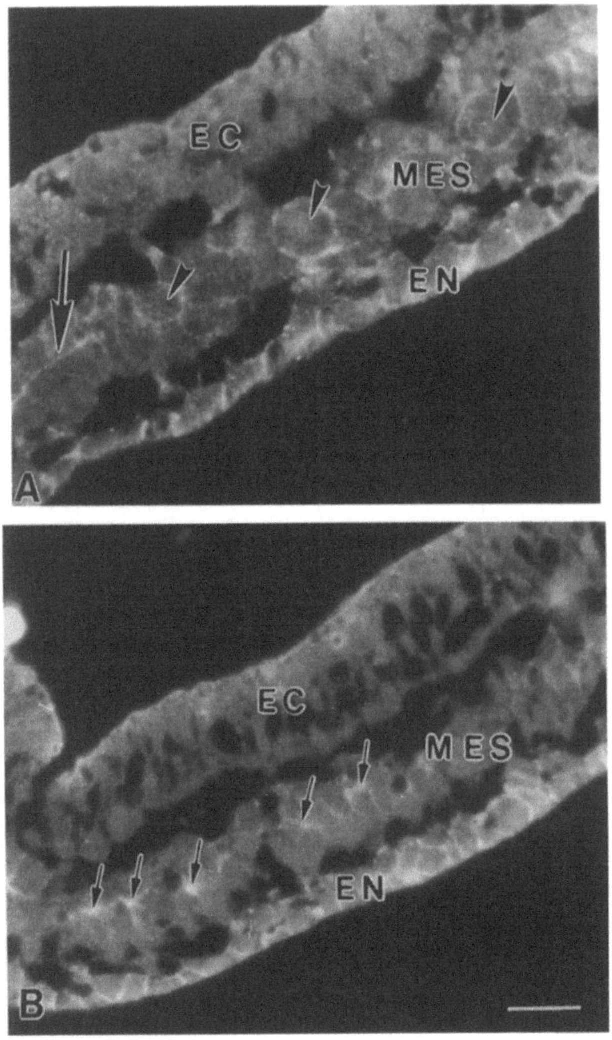

FIGURE 5. Immunohistochemical localization of N-cadherin in the heart-forming regions of two different stage embryos as seen in cross-section. **A.** Early stage 5 embryo: Large centrally localized cells (see arrowheads), possibly undergoing mitosis, are seen in the precardiac mesoderm (MES). These cells localize N-cadherin antibody and as a result appear to stand out in the mesoderm. On left side of photograph the N-cadherin localization (arrow) is beginning to be restricted to the midline of the mesoderm and is seen to form almost a line along the central cell boundaries. **B.** A stage 6 embryo: The N-cadherin now localizes to the midline of the mesoderm in patches (see small arrows). It is in these areas of N-cadherin localization where the pericardial coelomic cavities first begin to appear. Magnification bar = 10 μm.

1997). Confocal microscopy of N-cadherin localization indicates that it is within these regions of intense immunostaining for N-cadherin in the midline of the mesoderm where the first foci of small cavities appear. The periodicity of the small cavities is similar to the observed N-cadherin staining in patchlike areas within the mesoderm. These cavities enlarge and eventually coalesce to form the pericardial coelom (Fig. 6).

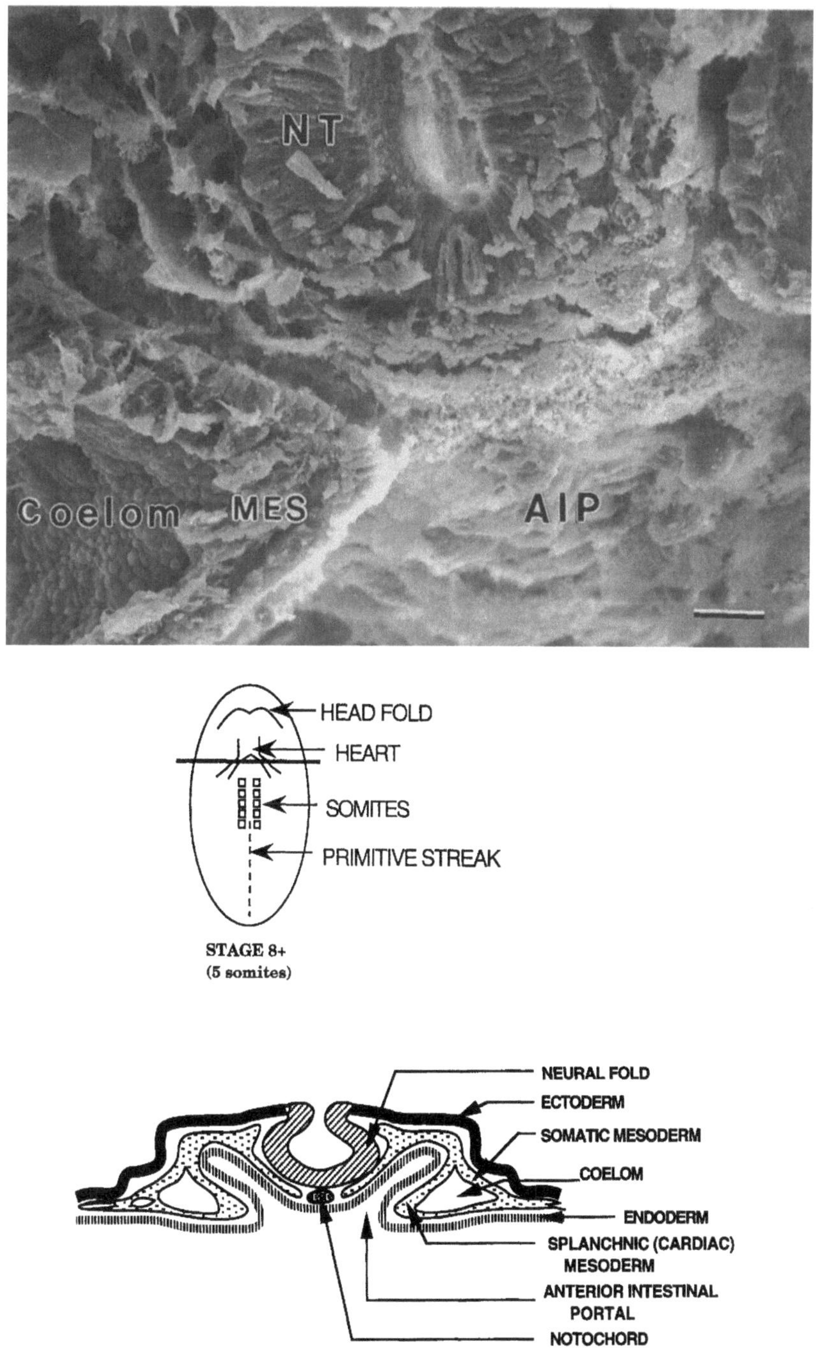

FIGURE 6. A scanning electron micrograph of a stage 8+ embryo fractured anteriorly at the level of the heart-forming regions and open foregut (AIP). The neural tube (NT) is apparent in the middle of the micrograph with the right heart-forming region seen on the left. The precardiac cells are elongated and are seen at the lateral wall of the anterior intestinal portal in the foregut region. The coelom is seen to the left of the precardiac cells. It can be seen that the apical regions of the precardiomyocytes are tightly packed to form a cobblestone appearance to face the cavity. The diagrams below the micrograph indicate the level of the fracture and a scheme of a typical cross-section through this region. Magnification bar = 50 μm.

Cadherins are known to associate with three intracellular proteins, α-, β-, and γ-catenins (McCrea et al 1991; Peifer et al 1991; Wheelock and Knudsen 1991; Peifer et al 1992). The catenins form a bridge linking the cytoplasmic domain of cadherins with the cytoskeleton. Evidence indicates that β-catenin, which is a homologue of the fruit fly *Drosophila* armadillo protein, interacts directly with the cytoplasmic domain of cadherins (Ozawa and Kemler 1992). Armadillo protein is a segment polarity gene product that is involved in rostrocaudal position specification within each segment of the insect embryo. α- and β-catenin protein localization during avian pericardial coelom development mimics that of N-cadherin in that it also shows a restricted expression to the boundary of the mesoderm preceding pericardial cavity development (Linask et al 1992a, 1997). Thus, in vertebrate heart development the N-cadherin–catenin interaction apparently plays a role in the specification of the position of the splitting of the mesoderm, which, as described above, results in the delineation and compartmentalization of the presumptive cardiac cell population. Thus, the somatic and splanchnic mesoderm precursors may be pluripotent before layer separation and cell commitment may occur as a consequence of mesoderm layer separation (Linask et al 1997). In addition, areas of catenin–N-cadherin interactions may serve subsequently as initial nucleating centers for myofibrillogenesis, which soon is observed in this region after precardiac epithelialization (see section below on *Cardiac Heart Beat and Myofibrillogenesis*). We hypothesize that the epithelialized N-cadherin-associated cells form the cardiomyocyte compartment. The more ventral cells that are excluded from the overlying epithelialized cells move ventrally into an instructive (or permissive) environment for endothelial-endocardial cell differentiation and downregulate N-cadherin expression.

The involvement of the armadillo homologue β-catenin in cardiac compartment boundary development indicates that a regulatory similarity may exist between segmental patterning in *Drosophila* and precardiac cell sorting and patterning during early vertebrate avian heart development. β-Catenin (armadillo) involvement in heart development may place some aspects of cardiogenesis in a regulatory pathway involving *wnt*-mediated cell–cell signaling. *Wnt-1* is the vertebrate counterpart of the *Drosophila* wingless (*wg*) gene, which normally functions in pattern regulation during segmentation, as well as during other periods of fly development (Nusse and Varmus 1992). Recently, evidence has been presented that shows a specific requirement for wingless function in *Drosophila* contractile vessel (heart) development (Wu et al 1995). *Wnt-1* protein associates with either cell surface or extracellular matrix molecules and is involved in signaling, including that of armadillo expression. The possible involvement of *Wnt* protein in heart development has been documented for *Wnt-11* in the avian model (Eisenberg et al 1997) and for *Wnt-2* in the mouse model (Monkely et al 1996).

Concomitant with N-cadherin's patterning role in positional specification of the pericardial coelom, it also appears to be involved in epithelialization of cardiac cell population (Linask 1992a, 1992b; Linask et al 1997). This latter role is indicated by (1) the restriction of N-cadherin to an apical expression where tight junctions form between precardiac cell surfaces lining the pericardial coelom, (2) the targeting of Na^+,K^+-ATPase to a primarily lateral cell surface expression in these cells after the precardiac mesenchymal-epithelial cell shape transformation has taken place, and (3) an enrichment of the fibronectin receptor, as shown by the detection of integrin (β1 subunit of the fibronectin receptor) on basal precardiac cell surfaces. In general cadherins appear to have a role in, and are characteristic of, epithelialization. It has been shown that expression of the epithelial cell adhesion molecule uvomorulin (E-cadherin) in transfected fibroblasts is sufficient to induce a polarized redistribution of Na^+,K^+-ATPase on formation of uvomorulin-mediated cell–cell contacts (McNeil et al 1990). This restriction of the distribution of Na^+,K^+-ATPase in fibroblasts, however, occurs in the absence of tight junctions, but coincides with the reorganization of the cytoskeleton. In the mouse, polar expression of Na^+,K^+-ATPase seems to be functionally involved in blastocoele development and cavitation (Wiley 1984). Experiments indicate chick pericardial coelom formation may mechanistically follow the same morphoregulatory events as occur in mouse blastocoele formation (Linask and Gui 1995).

A study was undertaken to determine whether epithelialization and compartmentalization of the precardiac mesoderm is a necessary prerequisite for heart formation and for cardiomyogenesis (Linask and Gui 1995). To perturb compartmentalization, ouabain was used to inhibit Na^+,K^+-ATPase activity. Results indicated that ouabain is effective in perturbing coelom development in a stage-dependent and dose-dependent manner. If coelom formation is inhibited by ouabain, precardiac cells do not epithelialize or form a tubular structure, nor do they undergo myogenesis. If treated after coelom formation and the cells have compartmentalized, a tubular structure can begin to develop in anterior regions, but cardiomyogenesis may not take place. The time between stage 5+ and stage 8, when one exposes the precardiac cells to ouabain, will determine the extent to which tubular structures will form and the degree of myogenesis that will occur. Ouabain inhibition is reversible by high extracellular K^+ concentration, as well as by removal of ouabain. Cells will recover from the arrest and begin to differentiate, even after a 20-hour exposure to ouabain. These results show that the three-dimensional aspect of heart tube development is apparently regulated independently and earlier than cardiomyogenesis. At stage 8 the signaling for both of these events has been completed across the heart-forming region and from stage 8 onward heart development is no longer affected by ouabain and will develop normally in its presence.

It is generally agreed that inhibition of the Na^+,K^+-ATPase pump elevates intracellular Na^+ levels, and as a result the Ca^{2+} levels increase by activation of the Na/Ca exchanger. An alteration in Ca^{2+} levels may affect cell-signaling transduction pathways, as well as cytoskeletal organization. Both of these cell-signaling processes have the ability to affect cell cycling and differentiation. Cell divisions and the timing of gene activation leading to differentiation are often linked. For example, in ouabain inhibition studies, intracellular Na^+ levels, phenotypic modulation of a nonmuscle myosin isoform, and entry of cells into the cell cycle are temporally related in cultured coronary artery smooth muscle cells (Seidel et al 1993). In a detailed study analyzing cell proliferation and cardiac development, Chacko and Joseph (1974) showed similar results regarding the staging of determination and differentiation of chick cardiac myocytes by inhibiting heart development using 5-bromodeoxyuridine. Another similar recent study using 5-bromodeoxyuridine (Montgomery et al 1994) confirmed these earlier results. All of these studies suggest that cell cycling is an important aspect of early steps leading to cardiac myogenic differentiation.

It is possible that the different regions of the heart are specified during the same window of time between stages 5 through 8. For example, as soon as sarcomeric myosin expression is detected in the heart, it is already ventricular specific (Linask and Gui 1995). Apparently this is also true for atrial region gene expression (Yutzey et al 1994). However, using in vivo labeling techniques, development of the atria has been placed at the looping heart stage 12 in the chick (see de la Cruz et al 1989). Thus, the timing and gene regulation of the specification of the different regions of the heart remain to be established.

Endothelial Cell Commitment and Formation of the Endocardium

The endocardium of the heart is composed of cells of endothelial cell lineage. There has been interest among vascular biologists in the question of the origin and differentiation of these cells. In light of the phenotypic diversity of the adult endothelia, it is of importance to understand the cellular biology of how the precursors of endothelial cells arise, and how they segregate from the mesoderm, migrate, and adhere to one another to form the cords and tubes that give rise to the lining of the entire vascular system, including the heart.

As the coelom enlarges, N-cadherin expression shows polarization and becomes localized to apical surfaces of the differentiating cardiac cells (Linask 1992a). The cardiomyocytes continue to express N-cadherin through the life of the organism. The somatic mesoderm downregulates N-cadherin expression during this time period. During this early time period the ventral population of endothelial cells that will form the endocardium continues to express N-cadherin initially and remains part of the precardiac mesoderm. They also begin to express endothelial-specific antigens as observed by QH-1 antibody localization. QH-1 antigen is specific for quail endothelial cells (Pardanaud et al 1987).

The sparsely localized QH-1-immunostaining cells are found within the lateral heart-forming mesoderm at stage 5. From our studies on explant cultures of precardiac mesoderm removed from stage 5 embryos, during 6 to 24 hours of incubation in vitro, endothelial cells that differentiate within the explant begin to coalesce to form cords of cells and eventually sheets (Linask and Lash 1993). As the endothelial cells continue to proliferate and differentiate they eventually downregulate N-cadherin (Linask and Lash 1993). After sorting out they form a sheet of cells underneath the cardiac mesoderm in vivo (Coffin and Poole 1988). The regulation of the cadherins apparently is involved in the sorting out of the endothelial population and, as discussed earlier, may be a consequence of being excluded from the epithelialized cardiac compartment. As the cells sort out, there may be a switchover from the expression of one cadherin to another. Lampugnani and associates (1992) have shown the expression of a cadherin specific for endothelial cells. These observations on the sorting out of the endocardial (endothelial) cells in the cardiac lateral plate mesoderm suggest that the precardiac mesoderm is a pluripotential (or bipotential) population of cells and that the endothelial cells and cardiac myocytes may have a common origin. Thus, the precardiac mesoderm is not a unipotential population of mesoderm cells that will form only cardiomyocytes (Mikawa et al 1992; Linask and Lash 1993; Cohen-Gould and Mikawa 1996; Sugi and Markwald 1996; Linask et al 1997).

A clonal cell line (QCE-6) has been developed from Japanese quail cardiogenic mesoderm (Eisenberg and Bader 1995). This cell line shares many properties with splanchnic mesodermal cells. Addition of retinoic acid and growth factors initiated cardiomyogenic differentiation in approximately 50% of QCE-6 cells as assessed by the expression of muscle- and cardiac-specific proteins. In addition, after cell differentiation these cultures also contain endothelial cells that express the QH-1 antigen. The QCE-6 cells appear to act as precursors to both the cardiomyocytes as well as endocardiocytes, confirming the above described observations of a possible common origin for the two cell populations.

In another study during the early morphogenetic period, Pardanaud and Dieterlen-Lievre, (1993) analyzed the hemangioblastic potential of primordial germ layers in the area pellucida. It was shown that the angioblastic (hemopoietic and endothelial) potential of mesoderm differs dramatically, depending on its association with ectoderm or endoderm. By means of interspecific grafts between quail and chick embryos, it was shown that splanchnopleural mesoderm (mesoderm associated with endoderm) gives rise to abundant endothelial cells and to numerous hemopoietic cells in a permissive microenvironment. On the other hand somatopleural mesoderm (mesoderm associated with the ectoderm) produces very few of these cells. The intraembryonic microenvironments permitting differentiation of hemopoietic cells appear to be more restricted than those permitting endothelial cell differentiation. Differentiation of the different cell types may depend on the presence of specific growth factors in the microenvironment of the mesoderm cells (see section below on *Growth Factor Stimulation of Early Heart Development*).

There appears to be a close relationship between the distributions of extracellular matrix (ECM) components and endothelial cell migration during the time of vessel formation (Drake et al 1990). Collagens type I and IV, fibronectin, and laminin are shown to be important ECM molecules for endothelial cell migration. Perturbation of cell–substratum interactions using CSAT antibody (a monoclonal antibody to the fibronectin receptor) to inhibit cell surface integrin (β-1 subunit) interaction with extracellular fibronectin or laminin molecules in the environment arrested vasculogenesis at the stage when assemblies of cordlike endothelial cells rearrange to form tubules (Drake et al 1992). These reports are consistent with studies indicating that embryonic capillaries develop in a fibronectin-rich matrix (Risau and Lemmon 1988; Risau et al 1988). Fibronectin appears to be required for early migratory events during embryonic vasculogenesis, as well as adult angiogenesis. The presence of specific growth factors, such as basic fibroblast growth factor, appears to be a necessary component of vasculogenesis, but possibly not for the initial induction of endothelial cell commitment (see *Growth Factor Stimulation of Heart Development* section). The extracellular matrix may act locally through its ability to selectively sequester growth factors that may support or inhibit cell migration and differentiation (Ingber et al 1987). The importance of fibronectin for normal development of the vasculature and the heart is apparent in transgenic mice in which homologous recombination technology has been used to inactivate the fibronectin gene and generate strains of mice deficient in fibronectin (George et al 1993). These mice show defects relating to heart development, vasculogenesis, and hemopoiesis.

RETINOIC ACID

The function of vitamin A in early embryonic development is an area of current widespread interest. During early avian embryogenesis recent studies have linked retinoic acid and retinoic acid receptors (RARs) to the specification of the vertebrate rostocaudal axis, to an influence of the Hensen's node region on early development, to limb polarity, and to early avian heart development (Heine et al 1985; Osmond et al 1991; Bryant and Gardiner 1992; Chen et al 1992; Chen and Solursh 1992; Dersch and Zile 1993; Smith 1994; Yutzey et al 1994).

The addition of exogenous retinoic acid (RA) to whole chick embryo cultures between stages 5 and 8 produces various anomalies (Osmond et al 1991). The retinoids are found to inhibit the craniomedial migration of precardiac mesoderm, resulting in a heart tube that is abnormal cranially and either normal or enlarged caudally. A local application of retinoic acid to the heart-forming areas disrupts the formation of the cardiogenic crescent and the subsequent development of a single midline heart tube resulting in various degrees of cardia bifida. It is suggested that many of the observed heart anomalies may be related to a disruption of normal precardiac cell–matrix interactions that could then lead to abnormal precardiac cell migration during early heart development. The heart anomalies described are similar to results obtained with perturbation of cell–fibronectin interactions during early heart development (Linask and Lash 1988a 1988b 1990). Addition of exogenous retinoic acid to whole avian embryo cultures also has been shown to affect the rostrocaudal polarity in the developing chick heart and the expression of the atrial-specific myosin heavy chain AMHC1 (Yutzey et al 1994). The latter study indicates that RA treatment produces an expansion of the caudal (atrial) domain of the heart and suggests that diversified fates of cardiomyogenic progenitors can be altered by RA. In a similar study adding exogenous RA during zebrafish embryo incubation also showed rostrocaudal heart tube effects (Stainier and Fishman 1992). Concentrations of 10^{-8} and 10^{-7} mol/L RA caused a progressive truncation of the heart tube beginning with the arterial (ventricular) end. In retinoic acid-deficient quail embryos the posterior region (sinoatrial region) does not develop, and large, dilated, nonlooping hearts are obtained (Heine et al 1985; Dersch and Zile 1993). The condition is lethal at approximately 3.5 days of development (Linask, unpublished observations). It is interesting to note that RA deficiency, as well as addition of exogenous RA, can produce truncation of the heart tube. This suggests that the maintenance of a critical concentration range of RA is necessary for normal heart development and this may differ for different developmental periods. In all of the above studies rostrocaudal regions of the heart are affected, with a predominance of effects on the more posterior areas (i.e., sinoatrial regions). Significantly, during cardiogenesis it is predominantly the posterior part of the normal heart, the sinus venosus region, where the highest level of the retinoic acid receptor RARβ2 is expressed; it is also this region that is most perturbed in the vitamin A-deficient embryo (Kostetskii et al 1995).

Abnormal heart development in the retinoic acid-deficient quail model can be rescued by the addition of all-*trans*-retinoic acid. Treatment of embryos with doses of 0.1 μg of all-*trans*-retrinoic acid at the beginning of incubation results in normal cardiovascular development (Dersch and Zile 1993). There is a critical time point within the first 22 to 28 hours of RA-deficient quail embryogenesis at which all-*trans*-RA is effective at stimulating normal cardiogenesis. Blocking experiments with anti–retinoic acid monoclonal antibody produced embryos with similar cardiovascular anomalies as seen in the retinoic acid-deficient embryos (Twal et al 1995). Mice whose genes for various retinoic acid receptors have been mutated display myocardial and ocular malformations that belong to the fetal vitamin A deficiency syndrome (Chambon 1994; Kastner et al 1994; Mendelsohn et al 1994; Lampron et al 1995). From recent analyses of the modulation of RARs in the

RA-deficient quail embryo, it was found that the vitamin A status primarily regulates the expression of RARβ2 during early embryogenesis and early heart organogenesis (Kostetskii et al 1995). RAR α and RAR γ expression remain relatively constant during quail development in both normal and deficient models.

The cell biology of retinoic acid effects on differentiation and development clearly involves the modulation of the various known receptors that bind either all-*trans*- or 9-*cis*-RA. These receptors belong to a larger superfamily of receptors for steroids and steroidlike molecules, such as vitamin D and thyroid hormone, and thus the function of the retinoids is interwoven with that of many other regulatory molecules (see review by Gudas et al 1994). Retinoids are known to control the expression of genes for many cytokines and their receptors, as well as the expression of proto-oncogenes and other regulatory factors. It is apparent that the ability of cytokines or retinoids to elicit specific cellular responses may also depend to a great extent on the local extracellular matrix (Nathan and Sporn 1991). Thus, the function of retinoids in heart development must be considered in a specific biologic context, as well as in a spatiotemporal and concentration-dependent manner. Retinoids and growth factors are of apparent importance in providing information relating to the specification of differentiation and proliferation of specific cell populations.

GROWTH FACTOR STIMULATION OF EARLY HEART DEVELOPMENT

Throughout the history of experimental embryology there has been a quest for the mechanisms of development and the signals that are generated by one group of cels that control the fate of neighboring cells. This process is referred to as embryonic induction (Spemann 1901; Spemann and Mangold 1924; Gurdon 1987; Melton 1991; Jessel and Melton 1992). There is ample evidence in the literature that growth factors are intercellular signals mediating growth, determination, and differentiation of specific tissues during embryogenesis and organogenesis in the early embryo. One of the most extensively studied examples of embryonic induction in vertebrates is that of mesodermal induction in the frog *Xenopus laevis*. Much of the work indicates that a surprisingly wide range of growth factors can induce mesoderm (Jessel and Melton 1992; Kessler and Melton 1994). Several classes of growth factors can mimic different aspects of mesodermal induction. These include members of the fibroblast growth factor (FGF) family including both basic and acidic FGF. Members of the transforming growth factor-β family (TGF-β) are known potent mesoderm inducers, including activins A and B, TGF-β2 and TGF-β3, and bone morphogenetic protein (BMP-2 and BMP-4). Studies also show that members of the *Wnt* family can induce mesoderm (Nusse and Varmus 1992). Interestingly, different cell types can be induced from the same responding cells in a dose-dependent manner (Green and Smith 1990). It is also becoming apparent that identical concentrations of specific growth factors can induce different types of mesoderm, indicating that there are regional differences in the competence of cells to respond to growth factors (Sokol and Melton 1991). Preliminary evidence suggests that there are molecular agents, termed competence modifiers, that may modify the response of tissues to growth factors (Moon and Christian 1992). These factors in the heart region remain unidentified, although some of the identified growth factors in this region may act as competence modifiers.

It has been suggested that mesoderm with the capacity to form heart muscle arises in response to an inductive influence of the anterior endoderm (reviewed by Jacobson and Sater 1988). The evidence for this seems to be the strongest in the urodeles. More recently there has been a renewed interest in heart mesoderm induction in the avian model and the signaling molecules that may be involved. Early experiments indicated that when anterior endoderm was removed from stage 4 to 5 chick embryos, heart formation was inhibited (Orts-Llorca 1963; Orts-Llorca and Gil 1965). But more recently, in studies in which the endoderm was removed from stage 3 (Inagaki et al 1993) or stage 4 to 5 embryos (Antin et al 1994), it was shown that isolated precardiac mesoderm alone can differentiate into cardiac tissue. In experiments in which precardiac mesoderm explants were cultured in medium containing serum or embryo extract, it was also shown that explants taken from stage 4 to 7 avian embryos can differentiate in vitro into cardiac tissue that is often beating (Lash et al 1987; Yamazaki and Hirakow 1991; Linask and Lash 1993).

The differentiation of cardiac precursor cells has been studied by single cell analysis in vitro in serum-containing medium (Gonzalez-Sanchez and Bader 1990; Montgomery et al 1994). These studies established that single mesodermal cells from stage 4 embryos are capable of myocyte differentiation, although heart region-specific, i.e., ventricular or atrial, cardiac, heavy myosin was not detected. If these same cells are grown at high clonal density or in organ culture, then atrial- or ventricular-specific myosin heavy chains were detected, indicating that cell–cell contacts are important for differential myosin expression. This is similar to the in vivo situation in which a role for N-cadherin is seen in establishing tight junctions during precardiac epithelialization that precedes phenotypic differentiation (Linask 1992a). N-cadherin-associated cell junctions appear to be necessary for myofibrillogenesis (Goncharova et al 1992; Soler and Knudsen 1994; Linask et al 1997; Imanaka-Yoshida et al, 1998). In addition, if epithelialization is inhibited by ouabain, cardiac myogenesis does not occur (Linask and Gui 1995). Another study indicated that in vitro stage 4+ cells are capable of differentiating into heart tissue without the presence of anterior endoderm (Antin et al 1994). The authors also indicated that explants incubated with endoderm showed an increased amount of myocyte differentiation and a shortened interval between the expression of myosin heavy chain and the onset of beating. In these latter experiments, however, explants were obtained from embryos at different stages between stages 4+ and as late as 6−. Staging of embryos during these early time periods of development is of critical importance. It has been our experience that even two experienced researchers may not always agree on the exact staging of young avian embroys. Significantly, during the early stages, 1 or 2 hours can make a difference in the percentage of cells that may have already become committed along the anterior–posterior axis within the heart region, and this becomes important in the interpretation of the results on explants taken from the various staged embryos (see Fig. 7 schematic diagram of heart commitment; also Linask and Gui 1995). Other investigations of the cardiogenic potential of anterior endoderm in comparison to posterior endoderm indicated that only anterior endoderm has the potential to regulate terminal differentiation of presumptive cardiac myocytes (Sugi and Lough 1994). Growth, however, occurred regardless of the source of endoderm, whereas mesoderm did not survive if cultured in the absence of endoderm. In addition only anterior mesoderm in the heart-forming region was competent to respond to the influence of the endoderm. One of the cardiac muscle markers that is induced by anterior

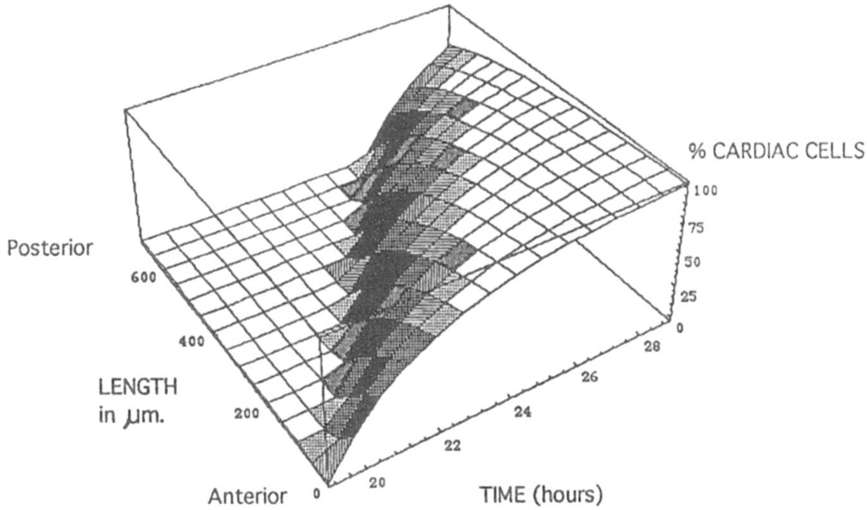

FIGURE 7. A diagram depicting the wavelike progression of differentiation across the heart-forming region between stages 5 and 8 in the avian embryo. The X-axis depicts the time scale between 16 hours (beginning of HH stage 5) to approximately 30 hours when the heart is forming a tube and just beginning to show contractions. The Y-axis depicts the approximate percentage of cells that have differentiated to form cardiomyocytes as based on MF-20 staining and ouabain perturbation experiments (see Linask and Gui 1995). The Z-axis shows the approximate length of the heart-forming area, as based on calculations from Rawles (1943). The progression of cardiomyocyte differentiation follows closely epithelialization of the precardiomyocyte.

endoderm is cNkx-2.5 (Schultheiss et al 1995). Therefore, as was shown earlier (see section on *Precardiac Cell Movement*), there apparently are local factors in the bilateral heart-forming regions that provide the proper milieu and signaling for cardiac cell determination and differentiation. Possibly the initial signal may be caused by a paracrine stimulation of the anterior bilateral mesoderm arising from signals from the anterior endoderm. Possible mechanisms by which inducing signals can control the pattern of cells is described in a review on vertebrate embryonic induction (Jessel and Melton 1992). In precardiac mesoderm induction the initial signal may be the endodermal signal, which in turn may induce the responsive anterior mesoderm cells. Subsequently the mesoderm cells may spread the inducing signal within the mesoderm from cell to cell caudad, with the subsequent responsive mesoderm cells each acquiring inducing properties. As Jessel and Melton (1992) point out, the attenuation of inducing activity may result from the cells adopting specific cell fates. As indicated earlier, this may coincide with the epithelialization of the cardiomyocyte compartment. These events take place between stages 5 and 8 in the heart-forming region. The initial activation signal initiating differentiation apparently occurs approximately at stage 5+ or 6, because at early stage 5 normal cephalocaudad signaling can still take place even if the heart-forming regions are rotated 180° (Linask and Lash 1988b).

Initial characterization of endoderm-secreted proteins from stage 5 or 6 to stage 8 embryos demonstrates that conditioned medium from endoderm explants contains proteins that include fibronectin and inhibin β_A, which is a homologue of activin A that has been shown to induce the formation of axial and mesodermal structures (Mitrani et al 1990; Kokan-Moore et al 1991). In *Xenopus*, activin A has been shown to induce the expression of the myosin heavy chain (MHC) α-isoform gene in isolated animal pole explants (Logan and Mohun 1993). This induction may involve the regulation of *GATA-4* gene expression, which is also known to modulate α-MHC (Molkentin et al 1994) (see section below on *Molecular Biology of Early Heart Development*). This induction is dose-dependent, requiring higher doses of the growth factor, as compared with the lower concentrations necessary for skeletal muscle differentiation.

In the axolotl, when precardiac mesoderm explants are incubated in the presence of TGF-β1 or platelet-derived growth factor BB (PDGF-BB), an increase in the frequency of heart tissue formation is noted (Muslin and Williams 1991). Immunocytochemical studies have revealed that basic fibroblast growth factor (bFGF) also appears in the heart-forming region between stages 6 and 15 (Parlow et al 1991). At stage 6 there is only a faint antibody reaction in the endoderm underneath the precardiac mesoderm. At stage 9+, during heart tube fusion, bFGF is first detected in the myocardium. FGF receptors are widely distributed in the embryo and are also localized to the endothelial and myocardial cells at stage 9. By stage 15 the expression decreased in the myocardium, but not in the endothelium. Expression of bFGF in the myocardium appearing at stage 9+ suggests that it is not an inducing molecule, but rather that it may be involved in maintenance of the differentiated state of the cardiomyocyte in possibly an autocrine fashion in which the cells are synthesizing a molecule that maintains its own differentiated state. Basic FGF also localizes in the myocardium of the adult heart (Kardami and Fandrich 1989). Perturbation of FGF-2 by incubation of stage 6 embryos in the presence of antisense oligodeoxynucleotides complementary to FGF-2 mRNA in defined medium demonstrated that there was a 50% inhibition in the cells' proliferative ability and subsequent contractility. The inhibitory effects were prevented by including recombinant FGF-2 protein in the medium. Thus FGF-2 may be involved in regulation of precardiomyocyte proliferation and, as a result, possibly differentiation, as measured by an effect on contractility. Further studies have indicated that there is also the concomitant developmental expression of fibroblast growth factor receptor-1 (cek-1; flg) during heart development. Expression begins in the endoderm at stage 6, then in the foregut endoderm and precardiac mesoderm at stage 8, and finally in the myocardium of the single heart tube at stages 9 to 10 (Sugi et al 1995).

Members of the transforming growth factor-β (TGF-β family, specifically TGF-β2, localize to the precardiac region in mouse embryos, as shown by studies on mRNA and protein expression (Dickson et al 1993). TGF-β3 does not appear to be expressed during the early stages of cardiogenesis. In the mouse embryo, TGF-β2 mRNA is expressed at high levels in all cells that have the potential to differentiate into cardiomyocytes. In addition, the underlying endoderm also expresses high levels of TGF-β. As cardiomyogenesis begins, TGF-β2 mRNA expression decreases with a concomitant increase in TGF-β2 protein expression in the differentiating cardiomyocyte population. The expression of this protein persists throughout development and continues in the adult. A similar detailed study of TGF-β2 in the avian model during cardiogenesis has not been carried out. There is, however, a localization of TGF-β2 to the cell surfaces surrounding the developing pericardial cavity at stages 7 and 8 (Linask 1992b). A similar localization has also been noted in the mouse embryo. TGF-β1 has been localized to the later stages of the embryonic chick heart beginning with stage 11 (Choy et al 1991). TGF-β1 was found to be localized to the endocardial surface and epicardial surface of the stage 11 heart, but its expression decreased from these locations in later stages. The cardiac jelly, endocardial cushions (stages 18, 23, and 26), and later the heart valve leaflets (stage 36) intensely express TGF-β1. Additional studies by Potts and colleagues (1991) suggest that TGF-β3 is an important myocardial induction signal during epithelial-mesenchymal transformation of endocardial cells during endocardial cushion development. The mesenchymal cells that arise in the primordial valve regions are produced by the transformation of endothelial cells lining the atrioventricular canal. Once formed, the mesenchymal cells invade the extracellular matrix and become precursors of the valves and septa of the heart (Potts et al 1991). Thus, the different isoforms of TGF-β have a differential spatiotemporal pattern of expression during early heart development, possibly indicating specific roles for these growth factors. During the stages of precardiac cell commitment and early differentiation, TGF-β2 appears to be the predominant form. With its high level of expression in the endoderm underlying the precardiac mesoderm, this suggests a possible early inductive, paracrine function. Later as the precardiac mesoderm differentiates, an autocrine mechanism appears to be established as the protein expression increases in the myocardium.

Recently, receptor tyrosine kinases (RTKs) have been characterized that are specific to endothelial cells and label endothelial cell precursors as early as the primitive streak stage in mouse embryos (Yamaguchi et al 1993). RTKs form a large family of transmembrane receptors for polypeptide growth factors with diverse biological activities. The tyrosine kinase function is activated on binding of the ligand, which results in phosphorylation of the receptor and multiple cellular substrates. This can lead to the regulation of a number of different cellular reseponses. One such RTK is *flk*-1, an *flt*-related gene, that is a high-affinity receptor for vascular endothelial growth factor (VEGF) (Millauer et al 1993). VEGF has been reported to be an endothelial cell-specific mitogen (Ferrara and Henzel 1989). *Flk*-1 is first expressed in the embryonic precardiac mesoderm (Yamaguchi et al 1993). By the head fold stage it is observed in the endocardial cells of the heart primordia, as well as in the blood islands of the yolk sac and the developing allantois. It then is detected in the endothelium of all the major embryonic and extraembryonic blood vessels as they form. It appears to be a very early marker of endothelial cell differentiation and is expressed one day earlier than *tek* (Dumont et al 1992), another RTK that is expressed in differentiating endothelial cells. What the inductive interactions are that are involved in the specification of the endocardium and endothelial precursors and what determines the organization of the vascular channels in precise areas within the embryo remain unknown. A number of growth factors have been shown to be angiogenic (Folkman and Klagsbrun 1987), including fibroblast growth factors (acidic and basic), which were the first to be so reported. Chick/quail transplantation experiments suggest that assembly of blood vessels by endothelial cells is controlled by environmental cues that reside within the mesenchyme (Noden 1990).

MOLECULAR BIOLOGY OF EARLY HEART DEVELOPMENT

The molecular regulation of determination of the mesoderm toward the cardiac lineages of endocardium and myocardium and of the subsequent differentiation of the terminally differentiated cell types is poorly understood. One common theme beginning to emerge is that transcription factors that regulate basic developmental processes in *Drosophila* embryos have homologous counterparts in vertebrate embryos. This appears to be true for *Xenopus*, mouse, and avian embryos. Much of the information known about transcription factors involved in early cardiogenesis is based on genes involved in *Drosophila* mesoderm formation and patterning and in the restriction of various differentiated cell types to visceral and skeletal muscle. A second theme is that concentrations of the involved factors are important for induction of different types of cells that are competent to respond. One concentration may affect one cell population to differentiate in a particular pathway, and another concentration may invoke a different pathway. A third theme is that factors serving as competence modifiers in the microenvironment of cells can have a negative, as well as a positive, effect on neighboring cells. Some factors, for example, may inhibit differentiation and by their presence prevent the premature differentiation of cells. Such factors in vivo may also serve as boundaries of developmental fields. Dilutions of specific concentrations of such inhibitoy factors may occur when explants of undifferentiated tissue are put into culture either as explants or as dissociated cells. In vitro these cells, after the establishment of proper cell–cell interactions, may be released from the inhibitory effect and can begin to express phenotypic differentiation markers. Thus, a potentially significant difference should be taken into consideration when using in vitro culture to elucidate in vivo events.

In *Drosophila* the dorsal–ventral polarity in the early embryo is under the control of a cascade of maternally active genes. This cascade ends with a gradient of the transport of *dorsal* morphogen from the cytoplasm to the nucleus. The dorsal protein is uniformly distributed in the egg and is activated in a gradient fashion on which *dorsal* migrates into the nuclei on the ventral side of the egg (Melton 1991). Because of the high nuclear concentration of dorsal protein in the ventral embryonic region, two zygotic genes, *twist* and *snail*, are activated to direct mesoderm formation. Both *twist* and *snail* are required for the initial steps of mesoderm differentiation. In the absence of these genes, the mesoderm does not develop and normal gastrulation does not occur. Such genes that function during mesoderm development in the chick have yet to be identified. The molecular basis for most of the subsequent events of mesoderm development that are involved in the subdivisions of the mesoderm into specific compartments and the functional requirements of these regulatory genes are also unknown. This is also true for most genes involved in regulating pericardial coelom development and the concomitant delineation of the cardiac mesoderm described above (see *Pericardial Coelom Development, Precardiac Cell Epithelialization, and Cardiac Cell Differentiation* section).

Some genes involved in the vertebrate heart-forming mesoderm have been recently identified. One such homeobox gene that is downstream from *twist* and *snail*, expressed very early in the *Drosophila* mesoderm, and required for the formation of the contractile vessels (*Drosophila* "heart") and visceral muscle, is the *tinman* gene (Bodmer 1993). Genes with significant homology to *tinman* have also been characterized in the mouse (*Nkx-2.5* Lints et al 1993), in *Xenopus* (*Xnkx-2.5* Tonissen et al 1994), and in the chick (*cNkx-2.5*, Schultheiss et al 1995). In situ hybridization localization of *Nkx-2.5* mRNA pattern in the mouse, chick, and frog embryos indicates that this gene is expressed in precardiac cells during head fold stages. The expression precedes the onset of myogenesis and continues in cardiomyocytes of embryonic, fetal, and adult hearts. The *Nkx 2.5* transcripts are also detected in the bilateral endoderm underneath the heart-forming mesoderm, as well as in the presumptive thyroid region at the floor of the foregut, in close association with the developing heart. The expression pattern suggests that homologues of *tinman* may function in commitment or differentiation of the myocardial lineage (Lints et al 1993). Interestingly, TGF-β2 mRNA is expressed in tissues similar to those expressing *Nkx-2.5*, including the bilateral anterior regions of late primitive streak embryos, the precardiac mesoderm and its associated endoderm, the floor of the foregut, and the presumptive thyroid area (Dickson et al 1993). Lints and coworkers (1993) suggest that possibly *Nkx-2.5* expression may be an early result of TGF-β2 induction in the region of the developing heart.

Interestingly, the targeted interruption of *Nkx-2.5* in mouse embryos resulted in normal heart tube formation (Harvey et al 1994; Lyons et al 1995). The primary defect appeared to be on heart looping, which was not initiated at its normal period between embryonic day (ED) 8.25 and 8.5. Commitment to the cardiac muscle lineage, expression of most myofilament genes, and myofibrillogenesis were not perturbed. *Nkx-2.5*-null mutants die at approximately 9 to 10 days of gestation. The details of the function of this regulatory factor need further investigation.

Other possible candidates for important early regulatory genes in early heart development encompass the GATA binding factors. Each protein in this family is highly conserved in a central DNA-binding domain, which specifically recognizes a core WGATAR or closely related sequence (Evans et al 1990). GATA-1 is an important determinant of erythroid gene expression (Evans and Felsenfeld 1989). GATA-2 has been shown to be expressed in vascular endothelial cells and has also been implicated in regulating endothelial cell gene expression (Wilson et al 1990). GATA-3 is abundantly expressed in the T-lymphocyte cell lineage (Ko et al 1991). GATA-4, -5, and -6 are transcribed in the developing heart and gut (Kelley et al 1993; Laverriere et al 1994). The chick GATA-5 is transcribed in the cardiogenic crescent region as early as stage 7 (Laverriere et al 1994). After formation of the tubular heart, GATA-5 transcripts are present in both endocardium and myocardium. It is absent from the paraxial mesoderm (somites) and the intermediate mesoderm (nephric tissue). This GATA gene is also transcribed in the embryonic gut and in later stages is sequentially upregulated in distinct areas of the gastrointestinal epithelia as the cells terminally differentiate. Chick GATA-4 is also found abundantly in the chick early heart and is differentially regulated in a spatiotemporal manner similar to the expression pattern in *Xenopus* (Kelley et al 1993; Laverriere et al 1994). α-Cardiac myosin heavy chain has been shown to be a target for GATA-4 (Molkentin et al 1994). The presence of GATA-4 and -5 in the cardiogenic region before tubular heart formation and the apparent involvement of GATA-4 in cardiac muscle-specific gene expression of the α-MHC suggest that these genes play a role in early heart development, specifically in the myogenic pathway. Thus, the GATA gene family is implicated in the regulation of several developmental processes that are involved in coordinating the completion of a functional cardiovascular system. Specifically, these processes include erythropoiesis, vasculogenesis via its effect on endothelial cell gene expression, and early heart development both of the endocardium and myocardium.

In situ hybridization studies and transgenic mouse models based on targeted disruption of some of the GATA genes have provided more information in relation to their possible function. In situ hybridization and immunohistochemical studies indicate an association of GATA-4 with heart development as early as day 7 of gestation. GATA-4 is expressed during looping stages and in the endocardium, endocardial cushion tissue, and myocardium of a day 9 embryo (Heikinheimo et al 1994). Mice homozygous for a GATA-4-null allele arrested in development between ED 7.0 and ED 9.5 (Kuo et al 1997; Molkentin et al 1997). Notably two bilaterally symmetric myocardial tubes failed to migrate ventrally and resulted in cardia bifida. This most likely resulted from a general loss in lateral to ventral folding throughout the embryo (Kuo et al 1997). Differentiated cardiomyocytes were observed comprising the heart tube. Thus, organ formation was disrupted, but not phenotypic differentiation of cardiomyocytes. Ventral morphogenesis was specifically disrupted, as seen by the presence of a defective foregut and anterior intestinal pore formation and lack of a ventral pericardial cavity and a single heart tube. It thus appears that GATA-4 is not essential, as was also the case for *Nkx-2.5*, for the specification of cardiac cell lineages. GATA-5, a member of the family of zinc finger transcription factors, is detectable early in the mouse in the precardiac mesoderm, followed by expression within atrial and ventricular regions at ED 9.5, and by ED 12.5 it becomes restricted to the atrial endocardium (Morrisey et al 1997). Subsequently, it is not expressed in the heart during late fetal and postnatal development. GATA-5 is also expressed during early lung development. Studies of mice homozygous for the GATA-5-null allele have not been reported. GATA-6, like GATA-4, is abundantly expressed throughout mouse development in the myocardium, stomach epithelium, and small intestinal epithelium (Narita et al 1996). Only GATA-6 was expressed in vascular smooth muscle. Overlapping distributions of GATA-4 and -6 in the heart support the possibility that one gene may functionally compensate for the other if one has been "knocked out". GATA-6 may, however, have a specific role in vascular smooth muscle. Overexpression of GATA-6 in *Xenopus* inhibits expression of cardiac actin and heart-specific myosin light chain (Gove et al 1997). This inhibitory effect is heart-specific. As seen in our earlier described ouabain studies, in the GATA transgenics morphogenesis of a tubular heart forms independently of the effects on contractile protein expression.

Other transcription factors have been reported to be involved in the regulation of myogenesis. Activation of skeletal muscle gene expression is controlled by a small family of muscle-specific transcription factors that share homology within a basic-helix-loop-helix (bHLH) motif. Four members of this muscle regulatory gene family, *MyoD*, *myogenin*, *myf5*, and *MRF4*, are implicated in skeletal muscle differentiation in vertebrates (Lyons and Buckingham 1992). These myogenic bHLH proteins are expressed exclusively in skeletal muscle and have not been detected in the heart, despite the fact that many of the genes that are regulated by these factors are expressed in both skeletal and cardiac muscle. DNA-binding assays with cardiac muscle nuclear extracts have suggested the existence of specific bHLH proteins in the heart (Litvin et al 1993). It is hypothesized that myogenic bHLH proteins act through intermediate myogenic regulators to activate muscle-specific genes.

One regulator of muscle-specific genes is myocyte enhancer factor 2 (MEF2), which is a member of a family of transcription factors that bind a conserved. A/T-rich sequence in the control regions of many skeletal and cardiac muscle genes. The in situ hybridization patterns of *MEF2C* in the mouse indicate that it is also present in the mesoderm of the cardiogenic crescent that represents the precursor population of the cardiomyocytes (Edmondson et al 1994). It is found to be expressed before α-cardiac actin and α-myosin heavy chain transcripts are detected in the heart region Edmonson et al 1994. The β-myosin heavy chain contains an MEF2 site in its promoter that is important for expression in cardiac muscle. Elsewhere in the embryo during these early stages, *MEF2C* mRNA is not detected above background levels. Although *MEF2* transcripts are predominantly associated with the myogenic lineages during early embryogenesis, *MEF2* becomes more widespread as development continues. *MEF2* also becomes expressed in cartilaginous prevertebrae, developing ribs, the developing gut, neural crest cells, and the developing brain (Edmondson et al 1994). In mice homozygous for a null mutation of MEF2C, the heart tube did not undergo looping morphogenesis, the future right ventricle did not form, and a subset of cardiac muscle genes was not expressed (Lin et al 1997). Thus, *MEF2C* is apparently essential for regulating cardiac myogenesis and apparently right ventricular development.

Exciting progress has been made in understanding the families of regulatory genes and growth factors that regulate early heart development and myogenesis. The appearance of the homeobox gene *tinman*, and the genes for GATA-4 and -5 and MEF2 appear to coincide in a spatiotemporal fashion. It will be interesting to determine how these genes are expressed in relation to the process of compartmentalization and pericardial coelom formation, and whether these genes are primarily involved in the regulation of myogenesis or in the regulation of the formation of the three-dimensional heart tube. It remains to be determined how these factors relate to the early processes ongoing in the embryo that set aside a distinct compartment of cardiac cells. From our earlier work, as well as a number of the more recently cited studies, the formation of a three-dimensional heart tube and myogenic differentiation appear to involve independently regulated, but parallel, pathways (see Linask and Gui 1995). These parallel pathways may be coordinated by the expression and modulation of cell adhesion molecules during heart morphogenesis.

CARDIAC HEART BEAT AND MYOFIBRILLOGENESIS

The embryonic chick heart reaches a functional state at around HH stage 10 (approximately at 33 hours), i.e., the 9- to 10-somite stage. During this period (around 29 hours of development) the single cardiac tube comprising the fused ventricular region begins to show feeble contractions. By 33 hours, as the atrial region develops, the rate and the amplitude of contractions are increased. The atrial region establishes the rate of the heart at this time. Later, as the sinus venosus is established from the most posterior part of the heart-forming region, it establishes the rate of the entire tube. Blood circulation with a functioning heart is established around stage 12, or the 16 to 17-somite stage.

The observed rostrocaudal gradient of beat rate has been confirmed experimentally. DeHaan and coworkers (DeHaan 1963b; Rosenquist and DeHaan 1966) initially determined that the rostromedial part of each cardiogenic crescent-shaped region in the stage 5 to 7 chick embryo forms conus arteriosus, the middle part predominantly forms ventricular tissue, and the caudolateral portion forms sinoatrial tissue. If these three regions are microsurgically separated and the embryo incubated, each separated part will differentiate into a spontaneously beating vesicle of heart tissue that expresses left-right differences and rostrocaudal beat rate gradients (Satin et al 1988). The left presinoatrial tissue showed the fastest rate, and the right preconus tissue the slowest. In cardia bifida embryos, the left heart-forming area beat faster than the right, confirming the left-right asymmetry in beat rate. In exchange experiments of left presinoatrial tissue transplanted into right preconus region, the local region surrounding the explant determined the beat rate of the explanted tissue, suggesting that local regional cues can alter the intrinsic beat rate of the differentiating precardiac cells. The first signs of electrical activity in the heart-forming region have also been determined at approximately stage 7 (Kamino 1991). What these local regional cues that affect beat rate are remain unknown. Inductive modulation in the number or properties of pump or channel proteins, as a cause for beat rate change, is a possibility. The rostrocaudal polarization of Na, K^+-ATPase during epithelialization of the precardiac mesoderm between stages 5 and 8 may be involved in the electrical activity that is first detected in this region on the basis of Na^+ and K^+ exchange (Linask 1992b). Ion fluxes may also affect cardiomyocyte differentiation (Linask and Gui 1995).

Precardiac cells in the bilateral heart-forming regions become committed to myogenesis between stages 5 and 8 of chick development (Linask and Lash 1988a, 1988b; Gonzalez-Sanchez and Bader 1990; Linask et al 1992; Linask 1992a, 1992b; Linask and Gui 1995; Linask et al 1997). Sarcomeric myosin heavy chain can be detected by stage 7. It is found in some cells of the presumptive heart-forming mesoderm that borders the lateral and cranial borders of the anterior intestinal portal (Han et al 1992). The myosin appears to be distributed in a nonstriated pattern along the apical surfaces of the polarized cardiomyocyte precursor. This is the region where N-cadherin and catenins initially localize at the adherens junctions (Linask et al 1992; Linask 1992a). In later stages 12 and 13 in the chick myocardium, sarcomeric myosin heavy chain continues to be organized at regions of N-cadherin and catenin localization (Linask et al 1997). In the normal embryonic mouse myocardium, β-catenin is especially noticeable at the outer curvature of the heart where initial contractions are first discernible in the embryonic heart (Fig. 8).

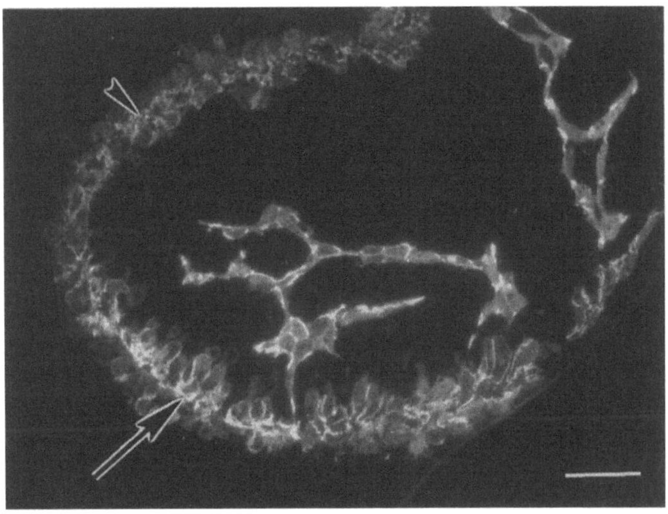

FIGURE 8. β-Catenin immunostaining is present primarily at regions of cell to cell contacts (arrowhead) and not on the outer surfaces of the cardiomyocytes forming the tubular mouse heart at ED 8.5. Note prevalence of β-catenin expression on outer curvature of the looping heart (arrow). This is the region where the first signs of contractility are discernible. Magnification bar = 25 μm.

The assembly of the contractile apparatus of cardiac muscle involves several developmental stages, including the interaction between neighboring myoblasts via junctional complexes, progressive assembly of thin and thick filaments into cytoplasmic arrays, and the subsequent appearance of aligned sarcomeric structures with characteristic and uniformly spaced Z-disks and M-lines. In a recent study analyzing the initial steps of myofibrillogenesis in precardiac mesoderm cultures (Imanaka-Yoshida et al 1998), the following observations have been made. Explants of heart-forming mesoderm isolated from stage 6 to 7 chick embryos do not have any sarcomeric structures at the beginning of culture. Before myofibrillogenesis, precardiomyocytes have N-cadherin and α-catenin around the periphery of the cell. After 9 hours in culture, sarcomeric α-actinin appears as tiny dots; after 48 hours α-actinin shows periodicity in its localization within the cell (Fig. 9, courtesy of Dr. Kyoko Imanka-Yoshida, Mie University, Japan). Z-lines formed around 20 hours as myocytes first begin to contract in vitro. This sequence of events is similar to that seen in vivo (see below). The patterns are also similar to what is observed when differentiated cardiomyocytes are dissociated and myofibrillogenesis is monitored as myofibrils are reassembled during incubation in vitro. Nascent myofibrils assemble in close proximity to the sarcolemma and then expand until they occupy most of the cell volume (Holtzer et al 1959; Sanger et al 1984, 1986). Antibodies directed against the nonmuscle myosin isoforms, IIB, react with the premyofibrils at the cell periphery and with nascent myofibrils, revealing short bands of myosin between closely spaced bands of α-actinin (Rhee et al 1994). Nonmuscle myosin IIB antibodies do not react with mature myofibrils in spreading myocytes. Recently it has been re-

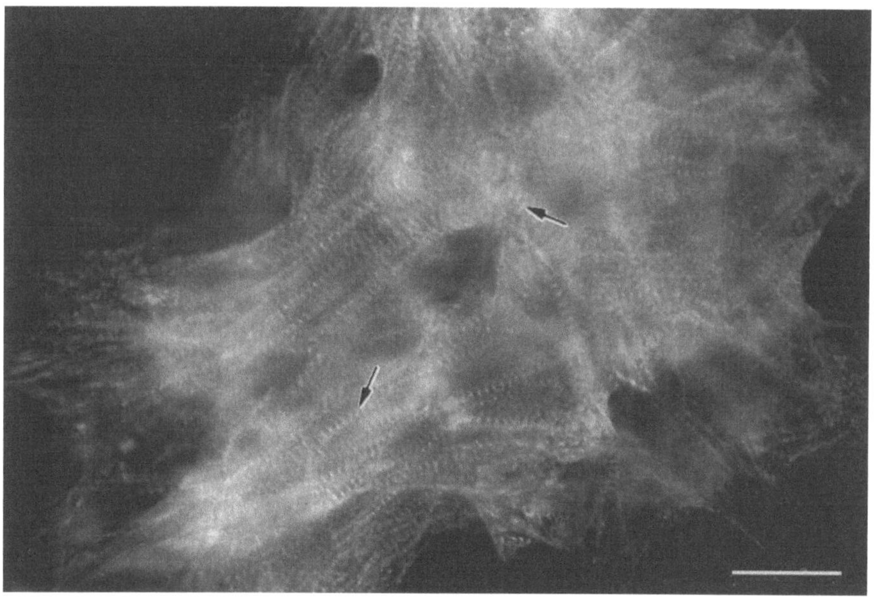

FIGURE 9. Stage 5 precardiac mesoderm explants were put in culture and incubated for 20 to 24 hours and are shown here immunostained for α-actinin. Two spread-out cells can be seen showing sarcomere assembly and α-actinin present in Z-bands (see small arrows). The appearance of nascent sarcomeres follows a similar pattern as has been described for differentiated cardiomyocytes in culture after cell dissociation and incubation. Magnification bar = 1 μm.

ported that N-cadherin localization becomes associated with myofibrillar structures in differentiating cardiomyocytes (Goncharova et al 1992; Soler and Knudsen 1994). Antibodies to N-cadherin, which are able to block adherens junction formation in culture, also have an inhibitory effect on the development and alignment of myofibrils (Goncharova et al 1992; Soler and Knudsen 1994).

In mice homozygous for an *N-cadherin*-null allele, a tubular heart structure forms (Radice et al 1997). This indicates possible compensation by another cadherin or involvement of other adhesion systems in the earlier noted cell-sorting process leading to pericardial coelom formation. A primary effect of N-cadherin loss in these null mutants appears to be on cardiac myofibrillogenesis in that the cardiomyocytes can only weakly contract and cells are loosely associated with each other. The possibility that another cadherin is upregulated in these transgenic mice cannot be ruled out at present. At a time point when myocardial integrity is essential for embryonic survival, the embryos die at approximately 9.5 to 10 days of gestation.

In the embryo in the 4- to 7-somite cardiac primordia (stage 8 to early stage 9), myosin and actin show only a uniform labeling throughout the cytoplasm of the myocytes (Tokuyasu and Maher 1987; Goncharova et al 1992; Han et al 1992; Soler and Knudsen 1994). By the 9- to 10-somite stage, myosin-positive cells completely encircle the heart tube. Between the 8- to 11-somite stage, the number of myofibrils rapidly increases, and they begin to show striations and periodicity (Tokuyasu and Maher 1987; Han et al 1992). Growth of the myocardium largely reflects results from mitotic activity of differentiated myocytes, as all new myocytes appear to result from the mitotic division of other myofibril-containing myocytes (Jeter and Cameron 1971). Using replication-defective retroviral vectors, Mikawa and colleagues (1992) showed that clonally related myocytes form vertically arrayed, cone-shaped colonies, which often extend through the entire thickness of the ventricular wall of hatched chick hearts.

In recent years it has been found that differences in the types of contractile proteins expressed in the adult myocardium play a major role in determining contractile function. The expression of different myosin isoforms has been correlated with aspects of functional performance in all animals that have been examined (Schwartz et al 1981; Wilman-Coffelt et al 1982). The differences in contractile properties of the atria and ventricles are consistent with their different functional loads and are paralleled by differences in myosin composition of the myocardia of these chambers. There is evidence from several laboratories that the initial stages of cardiac myogenesis include the expression of tissue-specific myosin heavy chains (Gonzalez-Sanchez and Bader 1984; Sweeney et al 1987; Gonzalez-Sanchez and Bader 1990; Yutzey et al 1994; Linask and Gui 1995). Evidence at both the mRNA and protein level suggests that transitions in myosin gene expression occur relatively early in avian cardiac development. As early as embryonic day 6, the distribution of myosin isoforms becomes similar to that of the adult myocardium (Sweeney et al 1987). This has occurred at a stage when the embryonic heart has become a 4-chambered organ.

LEFT-RIGHT ASYMMETRY AND HEART LOOPING

To place the observations on heart looping in context, a brief background of this developmental period follows. Between stages 8 and 10 in a rostrocaudal manner two endocardial tubelike structures form from the left and right epithelial cardiac mesoderm. Shortly, as soon as they have formed, the myocardial-endocardial tubes begin to fuse anteriorly to establish a single tubular structure. Subsequently, the right lateral margin of the heart tube begins to bend, forming a C-shaped tubular structure (see Fig. 10). This event is termed "looping". Looping of the heart begins at stage 10 and normally occurs to the right (Castro-Quezada et al 1972). The mechanisms underlying the looping process remain unknown, though it is generally agreed that multiple factors are involved.

The apical surface of the myocardium is free and faces the pericardial cavity; the basal surface is in contact with an extended basal lamina extracellular matrix called the cardiac jelly (Manasek et al 1972; Nakamura and Manasek 1978). Cardiac jelly thus lies between the relatively thick developing myocardium and the thin endocardium. Initially the heart is a midline structure. It then undergoes a transformation to form a C-shaped structure that continues to deepen to eventually place the initially posterior atrial region cephalad of the ventricular region. In a study on cell movements during looping, iron oxide particles were placed directly on the ventral myocardial surface of explanted embryos (Manasek et al 1972). These iron particles were carried around the side of the heart during looping. Accordingly, the left myocardial surface of the tubular heart becomes the right surface of the C-shaped heart as looping continues. Thus, there are two components to the looping process: bending of the right side of the myocardium (C-formation) and a rotation of the tubular heart around on an anterior–posterior axis. Concomitant with these proc-

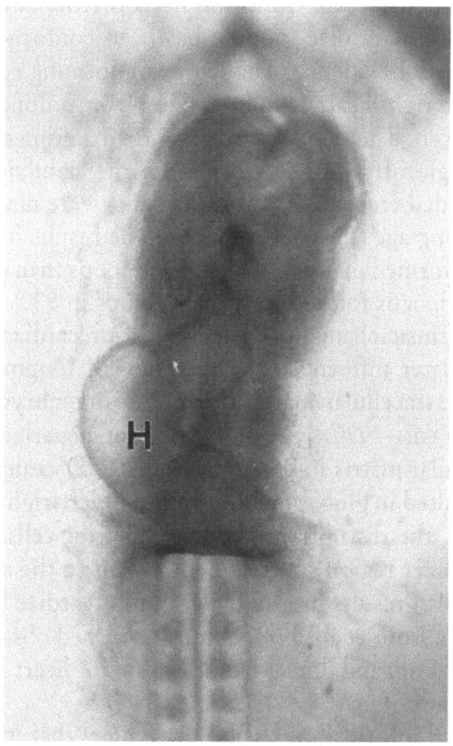

FIGURE 10. A stage 11 embryo as seen from its ventral side. The heart (H) is in the process of bending to the right (C-formation) or "looping".

esses, changes in myocardial cell shape and alignment are also discernible (Manasek et al 1972).

Experimental evidence supports the contention that the ventricular bending and looping is intrinsic to the heart itself. If isolated hearts are grown either in culture or ectopically, C-shaped hearts and looping still occur, even though the hearts are freed from their normal surrounding tissue (Butler 1952; Orts Llorca and Gil 1967). It has also been shown that cardiac function (hemodynamics and contractility) is not necessary for looping, since hearts arrested by high concentrations of potassium still loop normally (Manasek and Monroe 1972). Extracardiac factors, such as an interrelationship between direction of cranial and cervical flexure and heart looping, apparently are not involved in normal positional changes of the heart during looping (Manner et al 1995). Degradation of hyaluronic acid, which makes up a large component of the cardiac jelly, does not prevent normal looping in rat embryos (Baldwin and Solursh 1989). This further supports the hypothesis that looping is inherent to the myocardium. An important role appears to be played by actin bundles. When embryos were cultured with cytochalasin B dissolved in the medium, the heart remained a symmetrical structure, but continued to grow in size. If a small crystal of cytochalasin B is applied to the caudal part of the heart tube on either the left or right side, looping is affected (Itasaki et al 1991). Disorganization of actin on the left side results in right-blending of the heart; disorganization on the right side, in left-bending. These authors conclude that the actin bundles on both sides of the straight heart tube produce tension in a circular direction and the heart is pulled toward the dorsal mesocardium. When tension on one side becomes greater than on the other side, this results in heart rotation and bending.

The intrinsic nature of cardiac looping has been confirmed more recently by several additional lines of evidence. The left heart-forming region of one embryo was replaced with the right heart-forming region from a donor embryo forming a two-right-sided embryo. The same transplantation experiment was made with the left heart-forming region from one embryo into the right side of a host embryo forming a two-left-sided embryo. These transplants were made between embryos of the same or differing age (Hoyle et al 1992). The results indicated that double-right-sided embryos formed many more left-hand loops than did double-left-sided embryos. Control embryos formed right-hand loops in 97% of cases. The results suggested that an intrinsic change occurred in the precardiac mesoderm between stages 5 and 6 that later influenced the direction of looping of the heart tube. Perturbation of the extracellular matrix of amphibian embryos by inhibiting proteoglycan synthesis (Yost 1990) with β-xyloside or heparinase or by perturbing normal cell–extracellular matrix interactions using RGD-containing synthetic peptides (Yost 1992) resulted in global randomization of left-right asymmetry of heart looping. In *Xenopus*, the disruption of dorsal–anterior cells, including cells that give rise to the organizer region (*Xenopus* equivalent to the avian Hensen's node) and the notochord, also results in randomization of cardiac left-right asymmetry (Danos and Yost 1995; Lohr et al 1997). Our unpublished observations also suggest a role for the endocardium and dorsal mesocardium for heart looping (Linask et al, manuscript in preparation).

Recently, additional information has been obtained that may be a factor in the looping of the heart. The expression of the protein flectin (F-22) has been described during heart development. It is expressed early at the 3-somite stage in the avian embryo in the heart-forming regions in a bilaterally asymmetric fashion (Tsuda et al 1996). Flectin is an extracellular matrix (ECM) protein that was extracted from 18-day chick embryo retinal pigment epithelial cells and has been initially characterized in ocular (Mieziewska et al 1994a 1994b) and somite development (Lash et al 1992). It is an evolutionarily highly conserved molecule. Flectin apparently is also closely associated with other extracellular matrix molecules, e.g., chondroitin sulfate during eye development and fibronectin during heart looping (Linask et al, manuscript in preparation).

Antibody immunohistochemical localization of flectin using F-22 antibody during various stages of heart development in chick embryos (White Leghorn embryos; stages 7 to 22) has been carried out (Tsuda et al 1996). Flectin is expressed in the precardiac mesoderm as early as stage 7+ and persists throughout the process of looping. Localization of F-22 antibody is first detected in the precardiac mesoderm primarily in the ECM of the left heart-forming region. As development continues, flectin begins to be expressed in the developing myocardium of the right heart-forming region. This delay in synthesis in the right side leads to an asymmetric distribution that is maintained during heart looping and development. In general flectin seems to be associated with epithelia that are undergoing bending, i.e., it is associated with contractility of epithelial cells to cause invagination. In addition, at these early stages flectin localizes to the lining of the foregut and areas of initial neural crest migration near the dorsal neural tube. By stage 14, flectin localizes to the myocardium. It is significantly enriched on the basal side of the myocardium and extends in a gradient as an organized fibrillar scaffolding within the cardiac jelly to the endothelium (Fig. 11). At this time period the localization at the basal side of the myocardium is similar to results from an earlier report on fibronectin localization (Icardo and Manasek 1983). An asymmetric localization of flectin continues to be apparent in that more is present on the basal side of the myocar-

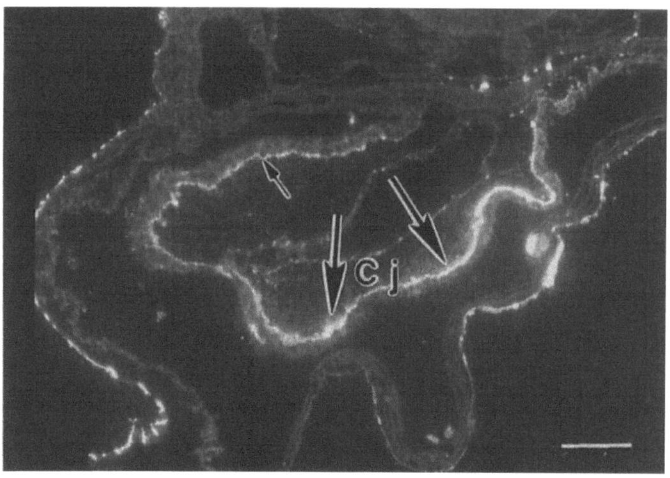

FIGURE 11. Immunohistochemical localization of flectin, a recently characterized extracellular matrix protein, that shows an asymmetrical localization in the chick heart before and during the looping process. Initially flectin is predominately expressed in the left heart-forming region and as seen in a similar stage embryo (see Fig. 10) becomes primarily localized to the outer, convex side of the looping heart. Enhanced expression of flectin is seen on the basal surface of the myocardium (large arrows) and extends through the cardiac jelly (cj) to the endocardial layer. Magnification bar = 100 μm.

dium on the bulging, convex side of the rotating and looping heart than is present on the other side. By stage 22, after looping has finished, localization of flectin expression is significantly decreased and asymmetry is no longer discernible. In day 4 hearts, flectin localization is seen primarily in the perivascular trabecular region of the myocardium, and reduced levels continue to be expressed by the myocardium. Preliminary observations of flectin antibody perturbation experiments indicate that looping is inhibited in chick embryos treated at early time periods (i.e., treated at stage 5).

In a similar study on flectin localization during mouse heart looping a different pattern emerges relative to that seen in the chick embryonic heart (Tsuda and Linask, manuscript in preparation). In the prelooping heart at ED 8 flectin localizes in a specific fibrillar pattern, but not asymmetrically (Fig. 12 A). It then localizes transiently to the left side of the bulbus cordis and is present in the inner curvature of the looping heart and within the left side of the distal heart tube. During looping at ED 9.0 flectin now shows a specific asymmetric, differential expression in both the cardiac jelly and the myocardial extracellular matrix (Fig. 12B). Flectin is also expressed in the cephalic neural crest pathway. After ED 11, flectin expression decreases and is no longer detectable at ED 15.

Flectin expression appears to be modulated by retinoic acid in that vitamin A-deficient quail embryos express little flectin and show reduced amounts of cardiac jelly and hearts that do not loop. These embryos also exhibit increased *situs inversus* in that the location of the heart tube with respect to the midline is randomized and often on the left. It is interesting to note that retinoic acid is normally enriched in the Hensen's node region of the chick during the early periods of gastrulation (Chen et al 1992).

Recently, another extracellular matrix molecule, JB3, has been reported to also have asymmetric distribution in the precardiac regions (Smith et al 1997). Of potential importance is that its distribution is the mirror image of flectin, i.e., there is more JB3 signal in the right than in the left heart-forming fields, as measured by confocal microscopy. Exogenous RA treatment using RA-soaked beads placed on the embryo's right side lateral to Hensen's node causes inverse looping in a dose-dependent manner. Placement of RA-soaked beads on the left side does not change normal looping, except at the highest concentrations used. Exogenous retinoic acid treatment results in decreased JB3 expression on the treated side. Significantly, both with flectin and JB3, the expression of these molecules is altered by retinoic acid concentrations, suggesting that retinoids are an important component of specifying asymmetry in the heart-forming areas. It cannot be ruled out that the retinoic acid effect may be a general effect on matrix synthesis (see also Tsuda et al 1996). However, these two molecules, flectin and JB3, are two candidates for which the genes, once cloned, may provide more information regarding establishment of asymmetry in the heart-forming region and the looping process.

Some recent progress has been made in finding specific genes involved in right-left determination. One of the earliest asymmetrically expressed genes that has been reported in the chick is the activin receptor-IIa (cAct-RIIa), which seems to mediate local suppression of sonic hedgehog (*shh*). By stage 4+ it becomes restricted to the left side of the Hensen's node (Levin et al 1995). *Shh* subsequently activates the expression of the nodal-related gene, *cNR-1*, in the lateral plate mesoderm. Heart looping is randomized if *shh* is misexpressed on the right side. In perhaps a parallel manner, a snail-related zinc finger gene *cSNR* may also be involved in controlling

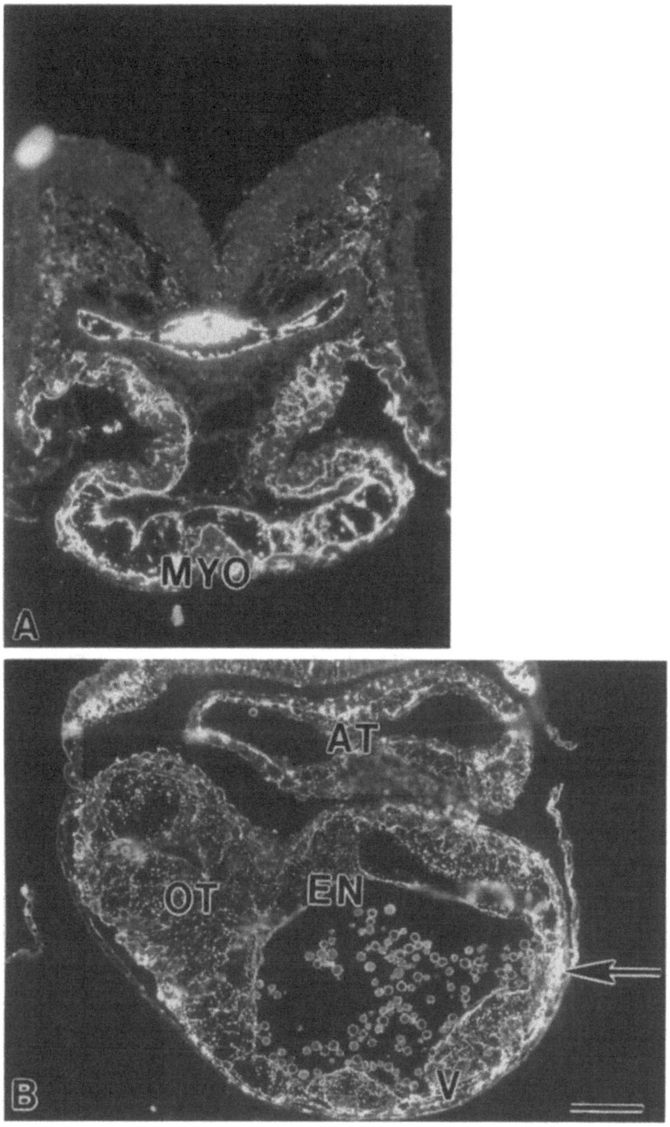

FIGURE 12. Flectin localization in the mouse heart before (A) and during (B) looping. **A.** Flectin expression in ED 8.0 mouse embryonic heart (cross-section). Flectin is expressed in the extracellular matrix of the tubular heart, dorsal mesocardium, and foregut. Within the tubular heart, flectin expression is specifically localized at the basal side of the myocardium in a fibrillar pattern within the cardiac jelly, which interconnects the myocardium and endothelium-endocardium. Flectin expression pattern appears to be symmetrical. The bright material in the foregut is nonspecifically stained.
B. Flectin expression in ED 9.0 mouse embryonic heart (cross-section). Flectin is now predominantly localized in the left side of the heart (arrow), both in the myocardium and cardiac jelly. Flectin is also expressed in the cardiac jelly of the outflow tract in a specific fashion and in the endocardium of the atrium. There is no apparent asymmetry in the atrial endocardium. At this stage of the tubular heart, flectin expression pattern is slightly different in each cardiac compartment. OT, outflow tract; AT, atrium; V, ventricle; MYO, myocardium; and EN, endocardium. Magnification bar = 100 μm.

heart looping (Isaac et al 1997). Another set of genes, *eHAND* and *dHAND*, appear to be involved in heart looping (Srivastava et al 1995). *eHAND* and *dHAND* may, however, also be associated with ventricle specification. *Lefty*, another gene also involved in asymmetry, is believed to act at a relatively late stage of left-right determination (Meno et al 1996). The protein is transiently expressed at ED 8.0 in the anterior left side of the ventral floor of the neural tube and in the left side of the splanchnopleura.

An insertional mutation mouse model identifies a gene, the *inv* gene, that is apparently involved in embryonic left-right asymmetry (Yokoyama et al 1993). This *inv* gene remains uncharacterized. Another previously identified mouse gene, *iv* gene, is also involved in controlling left-right asymmetry of the heart and viscera (Brueckner and Horwich 1989). These two genes, *inv* and *iv*, have been determined to be nonallelelic. It is noteworthy that randomization of looping is also detected in patients with heterotaxy syndrome, in which the usual organized visceral laterality is perturbed (i.e., *situs inversus*) (Britz-Cunningham et al 1995). These patients are reported to have connexin 43 gap junction gene, *Cx 43*, mutations. Observations of transgenic *Cx 43* mouse lines also indicate that gap junctions may mediate cell-signaling events important in the specification of laterality in several systems, including early cardiovascular development (Ewart et al 1997). The possibility thus exists that signaling involved in establishment of asymmetry (laterality) may also be modulated by gap junction-mediated information exchange. This suggests a link between retinoic acid and gap junction signaling in determining laterality. Effects of retinoids on gap-junctional communication have been shown in several systems to be closely correlated with the expression of the mRNA and protein for connexin 43 (Rogers et al 1990; Guo et al 1992).

Regulation of heart looping is apparently very complex and will involve the coordination of multiple pathways. From our observations, any gene that will disrupt pathways associated with the cytoskeleton, cell adhesion, or formation of a highly organized, extracellular matrix during organ formation has the potential of perturbing normal heart looping, as well as the formation of a single heart tube. In addition, if there are perturbations resulting in endocardial changes and in the dorsal mesocardium, these also will have adverse effects on looping.

SUMMARY

The embryonic stages leading from early gastrulation to the formation of a beating, looping, tubular heart have received considerable attention during the last 10 years. New technologies and application of molecular biology promise to advance our knowledge of these early stages even further. These are stages that are not be be discounted in their importance for later events of heart development. Indeed certain disease states of the adult myocardium and aspects of congenital heart disease may have had their origins in these early heart developmental processes (Clark 1986; Ferencz 1990). Severe alterations of normal processes most likely would lead to embryonic lethality or fetal wastage. Subtle changes can lead to alterations that may be amplified during subsequent heart development. All of the above mentioned work has been done on lower animals. Very little is known about heart development in human embryos during the stages described. Integration and transfer of knowledge from the basic research on developmental processes relating to heart development as observed in avians, rodents, and the fruit fly may yield useful clues for understanding these processes during human development. In the context of the human embryo, the events described in this chapter take place primarily during the first 21 days of development (Larsen 1993; Moore 1993). The endocardial tubes begin to fuse on day 19 of gestation; looping begins on day 23 (Larsen 1993). The result of looping is to bring the four presumptive chambers of the future heart into the correct spatial orientation for future modeling of the heart. Much of subsequent stages of heart development involve processes that remodel the developing chambers and that control the development of the heart septa and valves.

REFERENCES

Antin PB, Taylor RG, Yatskievych T. 1994. Precardiac mesoderm is specified during gastrulation in quail. Dev Dyn 200:144–54.

Arias M, Villar JM. 1986. Differentiation of chick embryo cardiomyocytes in cellular cultures: influence of the neurogenic ectoderm. Cytobios 47:7–18.

Baldwin HS, Solursh M. 1989. Degradation of hyaluronic acid does not prevent looping of the mammalian heart in situ. Dev Biol 136:555–9.

Bodmer R. 1993. The gene *tinman* is required for specification of the heart and visceral muscles in *Drosophila*. Development (Camb) 118:719–29.

Bolker JA, Raff RA. 1997. Beyond worms, flies, and mice: it's time to widen the scope of developmental biology. J NIH Res 9:35–9.

Britz-Cunningham SH, Suppan CW, Fletcher WH. 1995. Connexin 43 (alpha 1) gap junction gene mutations associated with heart malformations and laterality defects. N Engl J Med 332:1323–9.

Brueckner M, D'Eustachio P, Horwich AL. 1989. Linkage mapping of a mouse gene, *iv*, that controls left-right asymmetry of the heart and viscera. Proc Natl Acad Sci USA 86:5035–.

Bryant SV, Gardiner, DM. 1992. Retinoic acid local cell-cell interactions and pattern formation in vertebrate limbs. Dev Biol 152:1–25.

Butler JK. 1952. An experimental analysis of cardiac loop formation in the chick. MA Thesis. The University of Texas, Austin.

Castro-Quezada A, Nadal-Ginard B, de la Cruz M. 1972. Experimental study of the formation of the bulbo-ventricular loop in the chick. J Embryol Exp Morphol 27:623–37.

Chacko S, Joseph X. 1974. The effect of 5-bromodeoxyuridine (Brdu) on cardiac muscle differentiation. Dev Biol 40:340–54.

Chambon P. 1994. The retinoid signaling pathway: molecular and genetic analyses. Semin Cell Biol 5:115–25.

Chen Y, Huang L, Russo AF, Solursh M. 1992. Retinoic acid is enriched in Hensen's node and is developmentally regulated in the early chicken embryo. Proc Natl Acad Sci USA 89:10056–9.

Chen Y, Solursh M. 1992. Comparison of Hensen's node and retinoic acid in secondary axis induction in the early chick embryo. Dev Dyn 195:142–51.

Choy M, Armstrong MT, Armstrong PB. 1991. Transforming growth factor-β1 localised within the heart of the chick embryo. Anat Embryol 183:345–52.

Clark EB. 1986. Cardiac embryology. Its relevance to congenital heart disease. Am J Dis Child 140:41–4.

Climent S, Sarasa M, Villar JM, Murillo-Ferrol NL. 1995. Neurogenic cells inhibit the differentiation of cardiogenic cells. Dev Biol 171:130–48.

Coffin JD, Poole TJ. 1988. Embryonic vascular development: immunohistochemical identification of the origin and subsequent morphogenesis of the major vessel primordia in quail embryos. Development (Camb) 102:735–48.

Cohen-Gould L, Mikawa T. 1996. The fate diversity of mesodermal cells within the heart field during chicken early embryogenesis. Dev Biol 177:265–73.

Danos MC, Yost J. 1995. Linkage of cardiac left-right asymmetry and dorsal-anterior development in Xenopus. Development (Camb) 121:1467–74.
DeHaan RL. 1963a. Organization of the cardiogenic plate in the early chick embryo. Acta Embryol Morphol Exp 6:26–38.
DeHaan RL. 1963b. Regional organization of pre-pacemaker cells in the cardiac primordia of the early chick embryo. J Embryol Exp Morphol 11:65–76.
DeHaan RL. 1964. Cell interactions and oriented movements during development. J Exp Zool 157:127–138.
de la Cruz MV, Sanchez-Gomez C, Palomina MA. 1989. The primitive cardiac regions in the straight tube heart (stage 9−) and their anatomical expression in the mature heart: an experimental study in the chick embryo. J Anat 165:121–31.
Dersch H, Zile MH. 1993. Induction of normal cardiovascular development in the vitamin A-deprived quail embryo by natural retinoids. Dev Biol 160:424–33.
Dickson MC, Slager HG, Duffie E, Mummery CL, Akhurst RJ. 1993. RNA and protein localisations of TGF-β2 in the early mouse embryo suggest an involvement in cardiac development. Development (Camb) 117:625–39.
Drake CJ, Davis LA, Little CD. 1992. Antibodies to β1 integrins cause alterations of aortic vasculogenesis in vivo. Dev Dyn 193:83–91.
Drake CJ, Davis LA, Walters L, Little CD. 1990. Avian vasculogenesis and the distribution of collagens I, IV, lamimin, and fibronectin in the heart primordia. J Exp Zool 255:309–22.
Dumont DJ, Yamaguchi TP, Conlon RA, Rossant J, Breitman ML. 1992. *tek*, a novel tyrosine kinase gene located on mouse chromosome 4, is expressed in endothelial celss and their presumptive precursors. Oncogene 7:1471–80.
Edmondson DG, Lyons GE, Martin JF, Olson EN. 1994. *Mef2* gene expression marks the cardiac and skeletal muscle lineages during mouse embryogenesis. Development (Camb) 120:1251–63.
Eisenberg CA, Bader D. 1995. QCE-6: a clonal cell line with cardiac myogenic and endothelial cell potentials. Dev Biol 167:469–81.
Eisenberg CA, Gourdie RG, Eisenberg LM. 1997. Wnt-11 is expresed in early avian mesoderm and required for the differentiation of the quail mesoderm cell line QCE-6. Development (Camb) 124:525–36.
Evans T, Felsenfeld G. 1989. The erythroid-specific transcription factor Eryf1: a new finger protein. Cell 58:877–85.
Evans T, Felsenfeld G, Reitman M. 1990. Control of globin gene transcription. Annu Rev Cell Biol 6:95–124.
Ewart JL, Cohen MF, Meyer RA, Huang GY, Wessels A, Gourdie RG, Chin AJ, Park SMJ, Lazatin BO, Villabon S, Lo CW. 1997. Heart and neural tube defects in transgenic mice overexpressing the Cx43 gap junction gene. Development (Camb) 124:1281–92.
Ferencz C. 1990. A case-control study of cardiovascular malformations in liveborn infants: the morphogenetic relevance of epidemiologic findings. In: Clark EB, Takao A, editors. Developmental cardiology: morphogenesis and function. Mount Kisco, NY: Futura. 523–39.
Ferrara N, Henzel WJ. 1989. Pituitary follicular cells secrete a novel heparin-binding growth factor specific for vascular endothelial cells. Biochem Biophys Res Commun 161:851–8.
Folkman J, Klagsbrun M. 1987. A family of angiogenic peptides. Nature (Lond) 329:671–2.
Gallagher BC, Sakai LY, Little CD. 1993. Fibrillin delineates the primary axis of the early avian embryo. Dev Dyn 196:70–8.
Garcia-Martinez V, Schoenwolf GC. 1993. Primitive-streak origin of the cardiovascular system in avian embryos. Dev Biol 159:706–19.
George EL, Georges-Labouesse EN, et al. 1993. Defects in mesoderm, neural tube and vascular development in mouse embryos lacking fibronectin. Development (Camb) 119:1079–91.
Goncharova EJ, Kam Z, Geiger B. 1992. The involvement of adherens junction components in myofibrillogenesis in cultured cardiac myocytes. Development (Camb) 114:173–83.

Gonzalez-Sanchez A, Bader D. 1984. Immunochemical analysis of myosin heavy chains in the development chicken heart. Dev Biol 103:151–8.

Gonzalez-Sanchez A, Bader D. 1990. In vitro analysis of cardiac progenitor cell differentiation. Dev Biol 139:197–209.

Gove C, Walmsley M, Nijjar S, Bertwistle D, Guille M, Partington G, Bomford A, Patient R. 1997. Over-expression of GATA-6 in *Xenopus* embryos blocks differentiation of heart precursors. EMBO (Eur Mol Biol Organ) J 16:355–68.

Green JBA, Smith JC. 1990. Graded changes in dose of a xenopus activin a homologue elicit stepwise transitions in embryonic fate. Nature (Lond) 347:391–470.

Gudas LJ, Sporn MB, Roberts AB. 1994. Cellular biology and biochemistry of the retinoids. In: Sporn MB, Roberts AB, Goodman DS, editors. The retinoids: biology, chemistry, and medicine. New York: Raven, pp 443–520.

Guo H, Acevedo P, Parsa FD, Bertram JS. 1992. Gap-junctional protein connexin 43 is expressed in dermis and epidermis of human skin: differential modulation by retinoids. J Investig Dermatol 99:460–7.

Gurdon JB. 1987. Embryonic induction-molecular prospects. Development (Camb) 99:285–306.

Hamburger V, Hamilton HL. 1951. A series of normal stages in the development of the chick embryo. J Morphol 88:49–92.

Han Y, Dennis JE, Cohen-Gould L, Bader DM, Fischman DA. 1992. Expression of sarcomeric myosin in the presumptive myocardium of chicken embryos occurs within six hours of myocyte commitment. Dev Dyn 193:257–65.

Harvey RP, Lyons I, Li R, Parsons LM, Hartley L, Andrews J, Smith M. 1994. Targeted mutagenesis of the heart-expressed homeobox gene *Nkx-2.5* results in abnormal heart development and embryonic lethality. J Cell Biochem Suppl 18D:477a.

Heikinheimo M, Scandrett JM, Wilson DB. 1994. Localization of transcription factor GATA-4 to regions of the mouse embryo involved in cardiac development. Dev Biol 164:361–73.

Heine UI, Roberts AB, Munoz EF, Roche NS, Sporn MB. 1985. Effects of retinoid deficiency on the development of the heart and vascular system of the quail embryo. Virchows Arch B Cell Pathol 50:135–52.

Holtzer H, Abbott J, Cavanaugh MW. 1959. Some properties of embryonic cardiac myoblasts. Exp Cell Res 16:595–601.

Hoyle C, Brown NA, Wolpert L. 1992. Development of left/right handedness in the chick heart. Development (Camb) 115:1071–8.

Icardo JM, Manasek FJ. 1983. Fibronectin distribution during early chick embryo heart development. Dev Biol 95:19–30.

Imanaka-Yoshida K, Knudsen K, Linask KK 1998. N-cadherin is required for the differentiation and initial myofibrillogenesis of chick cardiomyocytes. Cell Motility Cytoskel 39:52–62.

Inagaki T, Garcia-Martinez V, Schoenwolf GC. 1993. Regulative ability of the prospective cardiogenic and vasculogenic areas of the primitive streak during avian gastrulation. Dev Dyn 197:57–68.

Ingber DE, Madri JA, Folkman J. 1987. Endothelial growth factors and extracellular matrix regulate DNA synthesis through modulation of cell and nuclear expansion. In Vitro Cell Dev Biol 23:387–94.

Isaac A, Sargent MG, Cooke J. 1997. Control of vertebrate left-right asymmetry by a smail-related zinc finger gene. Science (Wash DC) 275:1301–4.

Itasaki N, Nakamura H, et al. 1991. Actin bundles on the right side in the caudal part of the heart tube play a role in dextro-looping in the embryonic chick heart. Anat Embryol 183:29–39.

Jacobson AG, Sater AK. 1988. Features of embryonic induction. Development (Camb) 104:341–59.

Jessel TM, Melton DA. 1992. Diffusible factors in vertebrate embryonic induction. Cell 68:257–70.

Jeter JR, Cameron IL. 1971. Cell proliferation patterns during cytodifferentiation in embryonic chick tissues: liver, heart and erythrocytes. J Embryol Exp Morphol 23:403–22.

Kamino K. 1991. Optical approaches to ontogeny of electrical activity and related functional organization during early heart development. Physiol Rev 71:53–91.

Kardami E, Fandrich RR. (1989). Basic fibroblast growth factor in atria and ventricles of the vetebrate heart. J Cell Biol 109:1865–75.

Kastner P, Grondona JM, Mark M, Gansmuller A, LeMeur M, Decimo D, Vonesch JL, Dolle P, Chambon P. 1994. Genetic analysis of RXR developmental function: convergence of RXR and RAR signaling pathways in heart and eye morphogenesis. Cell 78:987–1003.

Kelley C, Blumber H, Zon LI, Evans T. 1993. GATA-4 is a novel transcription factor expressed in endocardium of the developing heart. Development (Camb) 118:817–27.

Kessler DS, Melton DA. 1994. Vertebrate embryonic induction: mesodermal and neural patterning. Science (Wash DC) 266:596–604.

Ko LJ, Yamamoto M, Leonard MW, George KM, Ting P, Engel JD. 1991. Murine and human T lymphocyte GATA-3 factors mediate transcription through a cis-regulatory element within the human T-cell receptor delta gene enhancer. Mol Cell Biol 11:2778–84.

Kokan-Moore NP, Bolender DL, Lough J. 1991. Secretion of inhibin β by endoderm cultured from early embryonic chicken. Dev Biol 146:242–5.

Kostetskii I, Linask KK, Zile MH. 1995. Vitamin A deficiency and the expression of retinoic acid receptors (RARs) in early quail embryo. Roux's Arch Dev Biol 205:260–71.

Kuo CT, Morrisey EE, Anandappa R, Sigrist K, Lu MM, Parmacek MS, Soudais C, Leiden JM. 1997. GATA 4 transcription factor is required for ventral morphogenesis and heart tube formation. Genes Dev 11:1048–60.

Lampron C, Rochette-Egly C, Gorry P, Dolle P, Mark M, Lufkin T, LeMeur M, Chambon P. 1995. Mice deficient in cellular retinoic acid binding protein II (CRABPII) or in both CRABPI and CRABPII are essentially normal. Development (Camb) 121:539–48.

Lampugnani MG, Resnati M, Raiteri M, Pigott R, Pisacane A, Houen G, Ruco LP, Dejane E. 1992. A novel endothelial-specific membrane protein is a marker of cell-cell contacts. J Cell Biol 118:1511–22.

Larsen WJ. 1993. Human Embryology. New York: Churchill Livingstone.

Lash JW, Linask KK, Yamada KM. 1987. Synthetic peptides that mimic the adhesive recognition signal of fibronectin: differential effects on cell-cell and cell-substratum adhesion in embryonic chick cells. Dev Biol 123:411–20.

Lash JW, Rhee D, Zibrida JT, Philip N. 1992. A monoclonal antibody that reacts with the ventro-caudal quadrant of newly formed somites. In: Bellairs R, Sanders EJ, Lash JW, editors. Formation and differentiation of early embryonic mesoderm. New York: Plenum Press. 169–80.

Laverriere AC, MacNeill C, Mueller C, Poelmann RE, Burch JB, Evans T. 1994. GATA-4/5/6, a subfamily of three transcription factors transcribed in developing heart and gut. J Biol Chem 269:23177–84.

Lawson KA, Meneses JJ, Pedersen RA. 1991. Clonal analysis of epiblast fate during germ layer formation in the mouse embryo. Development (Camb) 113:891–911.

Levin M, Johnson RL, Stern CD, Kuehn M, Tabin C. 1995. A molecular pathway determining left-right asymmetry in chick embryogenesis. Cell 82:803–14.

Lin Q, Schwarz J, Bucana C, Olson EN. 1997. Control of mouse cardiac morphogenesis and myogenesis by transcription factor MEF2C. Science (Wash DC) 276:1404–7.

Linask K, Gui YH, Rasheed R, Kwon L. 1992. Pattern development during pericardial coelom formation and specification of the cardiomyocyte cell population by N-cadherin and the *Drosophila* armadillo protein homologue in the early chick embryo. Mol Biol Cell 3 (Suppl):206A.

Linask KK. 1992a. N-cadherin localization in early heart development and polar expression of Na, K-ATPase, and integrin during pericardial coelom formation and epithelialization of the differentiating myocardium. Dev Biol 151:213–24.

Linask KK. 1992b. Regulatory role of cell adhesion molecules in early heart development. In: Bellairs R, Sanders EJ, Lash JW, editors. Formation and differentiation of early embryonic mesoderm. New York: Plenum. p 301–13.
Linask KK, Gui YH. 1995. Inhibitory effects of ouabain on early heart development and cardiomyogenesis in the chick embryo. Dev Dyn 203:93–105.
Linask KK, Knudsen KA, Gui YH. 1997. N-cadherin–catenin interaction: necessary component of cardiac cell compartmentalization during early vertebrate heart development. Dev Biol 185:148–64.
Linask KK, Lash JW. 1986. Precardiac cell migration: fibronectin localization at mesoderm–endoderm interface during directional movement. Dev Biol 144:87–101.
Linask KK, Lash JW. 1988a. A role for fibronectin in the migration of avian precardiac cells. I. Dose dependent effects of fibronectin antibody. Dev Biol 129:315–23.
Linask KK, Lash JW. 1988b. A role for fibronectin in the migration of avian precardiac cells. II. Rotation of the heart-forming region during different stages and its effects. Dev Biol 129:324–29.
Linask KK, Lash JW. 1990. Fibronectin and integrin distribution on migrating precardiac mesoderm cells. Ann NY Acad Sci 588:417–20.
Linask KK, Lash JW. 1993. Early heart development: dynamics of endocardial cell sorting suggests a common origin with cardiomyocytes. Dev Dyn 195:62–9.
Lints TJ, Parsons LM, Hartley L, Lyons I, Harvey RP. 1993. *Nkx-2.5*: a novel murine homeobox gene expressed in early heart progenitor cells and their myogenic descendants. Development (Camb) 119:419–31.
Litvin J, Montgomery MO, Goldhamer DJ, Emerson CP, Bader DM. 1993. Identification of DNA-binding protein(s) in the developing heart. Dev Biol 156:409–17.
Logan M, Mohun T. 1993. Induction of cardiac muscle differentiation in isolated animal pole explants of *Xenopus laevis* embryos. Development (Camb) 118:865–75.
Lohr JL, Danos MC, Yost HJ. 1997. Left-right asymmetry of a nodal-related gene is regulated by dorsoanterior midline structures during *Xenopus* development. Development (Camb) 124:1465–72.
Lyons G, Buckingham ME. 1992. Developmental regulation of myogenesis in the mouse. Semin Dev Biol 3:243–53.
Lyons I, Parsons LM, Hartley L, Li R, Andrews JE, Robb I, RP H. 1995. Myogenic and morphogenetic defects in the heart tubes of murine embryos lacking the homeo box gene *Nkx 2.5*. Genes Dev 9:1654–66.
Manasek FJ, Burnside MB, Waterman RE. 1972. Myocardial cell shape change as a mechanism of embryonic looping. Dev Biol 29:349–71.
Manasek FJ, Monroe RG. 1972. Early cardiac morphogenesis is independent of function. Dev Biol 27:584–8.
Manner J, Seidl W, Steding G. 1995. The role of extracardiac factors in normal and abnormal development of the chick embryo heart: cranial and ventral thoracic wall. Anat Embryol 191:61–72.
McCrea PD, Turck CW, Gumbiner B. 1991. A homolog of the armadillo protein in drosophila (plakoglobin) associated with E-cadherin. Science (Wash DC) 254:1359–61.
McNeil H, Ozawa M, Kemier R, Nelson WJ. 1990. Novel function of the cell adhesion molecule uvomorulin as an inducer of cell surface polarity. Cell 62:309–16.
Melton DA. 1991. Pattern formation during animal development. Science (Wash DC) 252:234–41.
Mendelsohn C, Lohnes D, Decimo D, Lufkin T, LeMeur M, Chambon P, Mark M. 1994. Function of the retinoic acid receptors (RARs) during development. Development (Camb) 120:2749–71.
Meno C, Saijoh Y, Fujii H, Ikeda M, Yokoyama T, Yokoyama M, Toyoda Y, Hamada H. 1996. Left-right asymmetric expression of the TGF-β-family member lefty in mouse embryos. Nature (Land) 381:151–5.

Mieziewska K, Szel A, Van Veen T, Aguirre GD, Philp N. 1994a. Redistribution of insoluble interphotoreceptor matrix components during photoreceptor differentiation in the mouse retina. J Comp Neurol 345:115–124.
Mieziewska KE, Devenny J, van Veen T, Aguirre GD, Philp N. 1994b. Characterization of a developmentally regulated component of ocular extracellular matrix that is evolutionarily conserved. Investing Ophthalmol Vis Sci 35:1608a.
Mikawa T, Borisov A, Brown AMC, Fischman DA. 1992. Clonal analysis of cardiac morphogenesis in the chicken embryo using a replication defective retrovirus: 1 Formation of the ventricular myocardium. Dev Dyn 193:11–23.
Millauer B, Wizigmann-Voos S, Schnurch H, Martinez R, Moller NPH, Risau W, Ullrich A. 1993. High affinity VEGF binding and developmental expression suggest flk-1 as a major regulator of vasculogenesis and angiogenesis. Cell 72:835–46.
Mitrani E, Ziv T, Thomsen G, Shimoni Y, Melton DA. 1990. Activin can induce the formation of axial structures and is expressed in the hypoblast of the chick. Cell 63:495–501.
Molkentin JD, Kalvakolanu DV, Markham BE, 1994. Transcription factor GATA-4 regulates cardiac muscle-specific expression of the alpha-myosin heavy-chain gene. Mol Cell Biol 14:4947–57.
Molkentin JD, Lin Q, Duncan sA, Olson EN. 1997. Requirement of the transcription factor GATA 4 for heart tube formation and ventral morphogenesis. Genes Dev 11:1061–72.
Monkley SJ, Delaney SJ, Pennisi DJ, Christiansen JH. 1996. Targeted disruption of the *Wnt2* gene results in placentation defects. Development (Camb) 122:3343–53.
Montgomery MO, Litvin J, Gonzalez-Sanchez A, Bader D. 1994. Staging of commitment and differentiation of avian cardiac myocytes. Dev Biol 164:63–71.
Moon R, Christian JL. 1992. Competence modifiers synergize with growth factors during mesoderm induction and patterning in *Xenopus*. Cell 71:709–12.
Morrisey EE, Ip HS, Tang Z, Lu MM, Parmacek MS. 1997. GATA-5: a transcriptional activator expressed in a novel temporally and spatially-restricted pattern during embryonic development. Dev Biol 183:21–36.
Moore KL. 1993. The Developing Human: Clinically Oriented Embryology. Philadelphia: WB Saunders.
Muslin AJ, Williams LT. 1991. Well-defined growth factors promote cardiac development in axolotl mesodermal explants. Development (Camb) 112:1095–101.
Nakamura A, Manasek FJ. 1978. Experimental studies of the shape and structure of isolated cardiac jelly. J Embryol Exp Morphol 43:167–183.
Narita N, Heikinheimo M, et al. 1996. The gene for transcription factor GATA-6 resides on mouse chromosome 18 and is expressed in myocardium and vascular smooth muscle. Genomics 36:345–8.
Nathan C, Sporn M. 1991. Cytokines in context. J Cell Biol 113:981–6.
Noden DM. 1990. Origins and assembly of avian embryonic blood vessels. Ann N Y Acad Sci 558:236–49.
Nusse R, Varmus HE. 1992. *Wnt* genes. A review. Cell 69:1073–87.
Oppenheimer JM. 1967. Essays in the History of Embryology and Biology. Cambridge, MA: The M.I.T. Press.
Orts Llorca F, Gil DR. 1967. A causal analysis of the heart curvatures in the chick embryo. Wilhelm Roux, Arch Entwicklungsmech Org 158:52–63.
Orts-Llorca F. 1963. Influence of the endoderm on heart differentiation during the early stages of development of the chick embryo. Wilhelm Roux' Arch Entwicklungsmech Org 154:533–51.
Orts-Llorca F, Gil DR. 1965. Influence of the endoderm on heart differentiation. Wilhelm Roux' Arch Entwicklungsmech Org 156:368–70.
Osmond MK, Butler AJ, Voon, FCT, Bellairs, R. 1991. The effects of retinoic acid on heart formation in the early chick embryo. Development (Camb) 113:1405–17.

Ozawa M, Kemler R. 1992. Molecular organization of the uvomorulin-catenin complex. J Cell Biol 116:989–96.

Pardanaud L, Atlmann C, Kitos P, Dieterlen-Lievre F, Buck CA. 1987. Vasculogenesis in the early quail blastodisc as studied with a monoclonal antibody recognizing endothelial cells. Development (Camb) 100:339–49.

Pardanaud L, Dieterlen-Lievre F. 1993. Emergence of endothelial and hemopoietic cells in the avian embryo. Anat Embryol 187:107–14.

Parlow MH, Bolender DL, Kokan-Moore NP, Lough J. 1991. Localization of bFGF-like proteins as punctate inclusions in the preseptation myocardium of the chicken embryo. Dev Biol 146:139–47.

Peifer M, McCrea PD, Green KJ, Wieschaus E, Gumbiner BM. 1992. The vertebrate adhesive junction proteins β-catenin and plakoglobin and the *Drosophila* segment polarity gene *armadillo* form a multigene family with similar properties. J Cell Biol 118:681–91.

Peifer M, Rauskolb C, Williams M, Riggleman B, Wieschaus E. 1991. The segment polarity gene armadillo interacts with the wingless signaling pathway in both embryonic and adult pattern formation. Development (Camb) 111:1029–43.

Potts JD, Dagle JM, Walder JA, Weeks DL, Runyan RB. 1991. Epithelial-mesenchymal transformation of embryonic cardiac endothelial cells is inhibited by a modified antisense oligodeoxynucleotide to transforming growth factor beta 3. Proc Natl Acad Sci USA 88:1516–20.

Radice GL, Rayburn H, Matsunami H, Knudsen KA, Takeichi M, Hynes RO. 1997. Developmental defects in mouse embryos lacking N-cadherin. Dev Biol 181:64–78.

Rawles ME. 1943. The heart-forming areas of the early chick blastoderm. Physiol Zool 16:22–44.

Rhee D, Sanger JM, Sanger JW. 1994. The premyofibril: evidence for its role in myofibrillogenesis. Cell Motil Cytoskeleton 28:1–24.

Risau W, Lemmon V. 1988. Changes in the vascular extracellular matrix during embryonic vasculogenesis and angiogenesis. Dev Biol 125:441–50.

Risau W, Sariola H, Zerwes H-G, Sasse J, Ekblom P, Kemler R, Doetschman T. 1988. Vasculogenesis and angiogenesis in embryonic-stem-cell-derived embryoid bodies. Development (Camb) 102:471–8.

Rogers MB, Berestecky JM, Hossain MZ, Guo HM, Kadle R, Nicholson BJ, Bertram JS. 1990. Retinoid-enhanced gap junctional communication is achieved by increased levels of connexin 43 mRNA and protein. Mol Carcinog 3: 335–43.

Rosenquist GC, DeHaan RL. 1966. Migration of precardiac cells in the chick embryo: a radioautographic study. Carnegie Inst Washington, Contrib Embryo 38:111–21.

Sabin FR. 1920. Studies on the origin of blood-vessels and of red blood corpuscles as seen in the living blastoderm of chicks during the second day of incubation. Carnegie Contrib Embryol 9:213–62.

Sanger JM, Mittal B, Pochapin MB, Sanger JW. 1986. Myofibrillogenesis in living cells microinjected with fluorescently labeled alpha-actinin. J Cell Biol 102:2053–66.

Sanger JW, Mittal B, Sanger JM. 1984. Formation of myofibrils in spreading chick cardiac myocytes. J Cell Motil 4:405–16.

Satin J, Fujii S, DeHaan RL. 1988. Development of cardiac beat rate in early chick embryos is regulated by regional cues. Dev Biol 129:103–13.

Schultheiss TM, Xydas S, Lassar AB. 1995. Induction of avian cardiac myogenesis my anterior endoderm. Development (Camb) 121:4203–14.

Schwartz K, LeCarpentier Y, Martin JL, Lompre AM, Mercadier JJ, Swynghedauw B. 1981. Myosin ioenzymic distribution correlates with speed of myocardial contraction. J Mol Cell Cardiol 13:1074–5.

Seidel CL, Dennison DK, Amick S, Allen JC. 1993. Relationship between functional Na pumps and mitogenesis in cultured coronary artery smooth muscle cells. Am J Physiol 264:C169–78.

Smith SM 1994. Retinoic acid receptor isoform β2 is an early marker for alimentary tract and central nervous system positional specification in the chicken. Dev Dyn 200:14–25.
Smith SM, Dickman ED, Thompson B, Sinning A, Wunsch A, Marwald R. 1997. Retinoic acid directs cardiac laterality and the expression of early markers of precardiac asymmetry. Dev Biol 182:162–71.
Sokol S, Melton DA. 1991. Pre-existent pattern in *Xenopus* animal pole cells revealed by induction with activin. Nature (Lond) 351:409–11.
Soler AP, Knudsen KA. 1994. N-cadherin involvement in cardiac myocyte interaction and myofibrillogenesis. Dev Biol 162:9–17.
Spermann H. 1901. Uber Korrelationen in der Entwicklung des Auges. Verh Anat Ges 15:61–79.
Spemann H, Mangold H. 1924. Uber Induktion von Embryonalanlagen durch Implantation artfremder Organisatoren. Arch Mikrosk Anat Entw Mech 100:599–638.
Srivastava D, Cserjesi P, Olson EN. 1995. A subclass of bHLH proteins required for cardiac morphogenesis. Science (Wash DC) 270:1995–9.
Stainier DYR, Fishman MC. 1992. Patterning the zebrafish heart tube: acquisition of antero-posterior polarity. Dev Biol 153:91–101.
Sugi YJS, Barron M, Lough J. 1995. Developmental expression of fibroblast growth factor receptor-1 (cek-1; flg) during heart development. Dev Dyn 202:115–25.
Sugi Y, Lough J. 1994. Anterior endoderm is a specific effector of terminal cardiac myocyte differentiation of cells from the embryonic heart forming region. Dev Dyn 200:155–62.
Sugi Y, Markwald RR. 1996. Formation and early morphogenesis of endocardial endothelial precursor cells and the role of endoderm. Dev Biol 175:66–83.
Sweeney LJ, Zak R, Manasek FJ. 1987. Transitions in cardiac isomyosin expression during differentiation of the embryonic chick heart. Circ Res 61:287–95.
Tokuyasu KT, Maher PA. 1987. Immunocytochemical studies of cardiac myofibrillogenesis in early chick embryos. I. Presence of immunofloresence titin spots in premyofibril stages. J Cell Biol 105:2781–93.
Tonissen KF, Drysdale TA, Lints TJ, Harvey RP, Krieg PA. 1994. *XNkx-2.5*, a *Xenopus* gene related to *Nkx-2.5* and *tinman*: evidence of a conserved role in cardiac development. Dev Biol 162:325–8.
Tsuda T, Philp N, Zile MH, Linask KK. 1996. Left-right asymmetric localization of flectin in the extracellular matrix during heart looping. Dev Biol 173:39–50.
Twal W, Roze L, Zile MH. 1995. Anti-retinoic acid monoclonal antibody localizes all-trans-retinoic acid in target cells and blocks normal development in early quail embryo. Dev Biol 168:225–34.
Van der Stricht O. 1895. La premiere apparition de la cavite coelomique dans l'aire embryonnaire du lapin. C Seances Soc Biol Ses 10. 12:207–11.
von Baer KE. 1828–1837. Uber Entwicklungsgeschichte der Theire. Beobachtung und Reflexion. Konigsberg.
Wheelock MJ, Knudsen KA. 1991. N-cadherin-associated proteins in chicken muscle. Differentiation. 46:35–42.
Wiley LM. 1984. Cavitation in the mouse preimplantation embryo: Na/K-ATPase and the origin of nascent blastocoele fluid. Dev Biol 105:330–42.
Wilman-Coffelt J, Refsum H, Hollosi G, Rouleau L, Chuck L, Parmley WW. 1982. Comparative force-velocity relation and analyses of myosin of dog atria and ventricles. Am J Physiol 243:H391–7.
Wilson DB, Dorfman DM, Orkin SH. 1990. A nonerythroid GATA-binding protein is required for function of the human preproendothelin-1 promoter in endothelial cells. Mol Cell Biol 10:4854–62.
Wu X, Golden K, Bodmer R. 1995. Heart development in *Drosophila* requires the segment polarity gene *wingless*. Dev Biol 169:619–28.
Yamaguchi TP, Dumont DJ, Conion RA, Breitman ML. 1993. *flk-1*, an flt-related receptor

tyrosine kinase is an early marker for endothelial cell precursors. Development (Camb) 118:489–98.

Yamazaki Y, Hirakow R. 1991. Factors required for differentiation of chick precardiac mesoderm cultured in vitro. Proc Jpn Acad Ser B Phys Biol Sci 67:165–9.

Yokoyama T, Copeland NG, Jenkins NA, Montgomery CA, Elder FFB, Overbeek PA. 1993. Reversal of left-right asymmetry: a situs inversus mutation. Science (Wash DC) 260:679–82.

Yost HJ. 1990. Inhibition of proteoglycan synthesis eliminates left-right asymmetry in *Xenopus laevis* cardiac looping. Development (Camb) 110:865–74.

Yost HJ. 1992. Regulation of vertebrate left-right asymmetries by extracellular matrix. Nature (Lond) 357:158–61.

Yutzey KE, Rhee JT, Bader D. 1994. Expression of the atrial-specific myosin heavy chain AMHC1 and the establishment of anteroposterior polarity in the developing chicken heart. Development (Camb) 120:871–83.

CHAPTER **2**

Formation and Septation of the Tubular Heart: Integrating the Dynamics of Morphology With Emerging Molecular Concepts

Roger R. Markwald, Thomas Trusk, and
Ricardo Moreno-Rodriguez

FORMATION OF THE PRIMITIVE SEGMENTS OF THE TUBULAR HEART

Segments Arise Sequentially From the Heart-Forming Fields

In the present chapter, we seek to integrate the progressive and dynamic changes in structure that transform a bent, hollow tube into a mature, fully defined, four-chambered heart with emerging concepts of molecular regulation.

Among the most fundamental of the dynamic processes of early heart development are those that produce a linear series of hollow compartments or segments that collectively, over time, will establish the primitive heart tube (de la Cruz et al 1989). In other words, the heart tube is formed one piece at a time. Some developmental biologists may object to our calling these pieces "segments", reserving that term for more traditional repeating units like somites or somitomeres. However, as shown throughout this book, the segments of the tubular heart, like the somites, form progressively along an anterior to posterior (A-P) axis with each segment being an undifferentiated, morphogenetic unit separated by boundary interfaces. Studies in living embryos reveal that these fundamental cardiac building units will integrate and differentiate to form the mature chambers of the heart (chapter IV).

Each segment is defined by two epithelia, the premyocardium and endocardium (Fig. 1). A continuous sleeve of extracellular matrix, historically termed cardiac jelly, separates the two epithelia of each segment. The myocardium secretes most of this matrix and includes proteins characteristic of basement membranes (Rongish and Little 1995). This has prompted us to propose that the cardiac jelly is the basement membrane of the myocardium (Kitten et al. 1987). Although found in each segment, the myocardial basement membrane–cardiac jelly varies segmentally in structure and composition in a manner that correlates with diversity of fate and final form (Mjaatvedt et al 1987).

Beginning at stage 9− in the chick and continuing until stage 14, four segments of the future heart tube emerge progressively from the crescent of cardiogenic cells

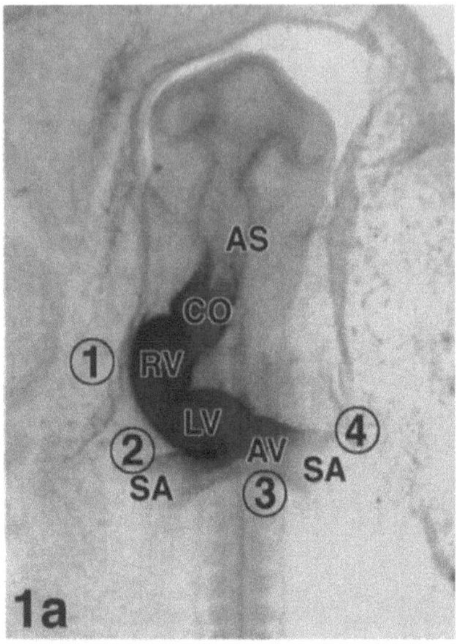

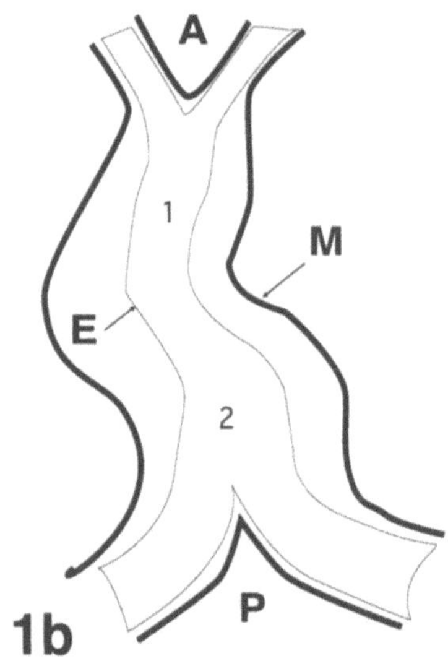

FIGURE 1. The primitive heart tube of a chick embryo after the onset of looping and torsion. **a.** The primative cardiac segments are shown in a stage 13 embryo immunostained as a whole mount for α-smooth muscle actin (courtesy of Dr. Robert Poelmann). The antigen is one of the first to be expressed in cells that have become committed to a myocardial lineage (Ruzicka and Schwartz 1988). As summarized in Table 1, at stage 13, the AV segment (#3) is being formed at the fusion point or crescent of the paired heart fields. The future fourth or sinoatrial (SA) segment is still within the unfused regions of each heart field and exhibits little or no α-smooth muscle actin expression. The formation of the conus (CO) has also begun. It extends anteriorly from the first segment, the future trabeculated region of the right ventricle (RV). Note expression of the antigen progressively diminishes in the area where the conus approaches the aortic sac (AS), consistent with the hypothesis that the conus is a fifth segment recruited from undifferentiated mesenchyme of this area. Finally, note that in this C-shaped heart, the loop or bend forms between the first two segments and defines the inner curvature and the two limbs of the heart. **b.** Diagram of the histology of the looped heart at approximately stage 11. Each of the two segments is formed of two epithelia, the outer myocardium (M) and endocardial endothelium (E), which blend imperceptibly between segments. The intervening space contains the extracellular matrix of the cardiac jelly (Davis 1924) Anterior/cephalic (A); posterior/caudal (P).

formed by the union of the two heart-forming fields (chapters III and IV). In the chick, at the point of fusion each segment of the tubular heart arises as the future myocardium and associated cardiac jelly from each heart field encircle a three-dimensional tubular framework of anastomizing, endocardial cells (Fig. 2). A distinct fusion line is seen ventrally on the straight heart tube, which ultimately will come to mark the site at which the interventricular septum will take origin (de la Cruz et al 1997). From in vivo marking studies, the linear heart tube has only two segments. The first segment is the most anterior and clearly defined. It forms the bulk of the so-called straight heart tube (chapter III) because the posterior portion of the second segment is still within the heart fields. When the second segment has become clearly separated from the heart fields, looping begins at stages 10 and 11.

A common perception is that the cells that will give rise to all future cardiac chambers exist within the straight heart tube. If this were true, transgenes having promoter constructs that were engineered to be expressed in specific segments or

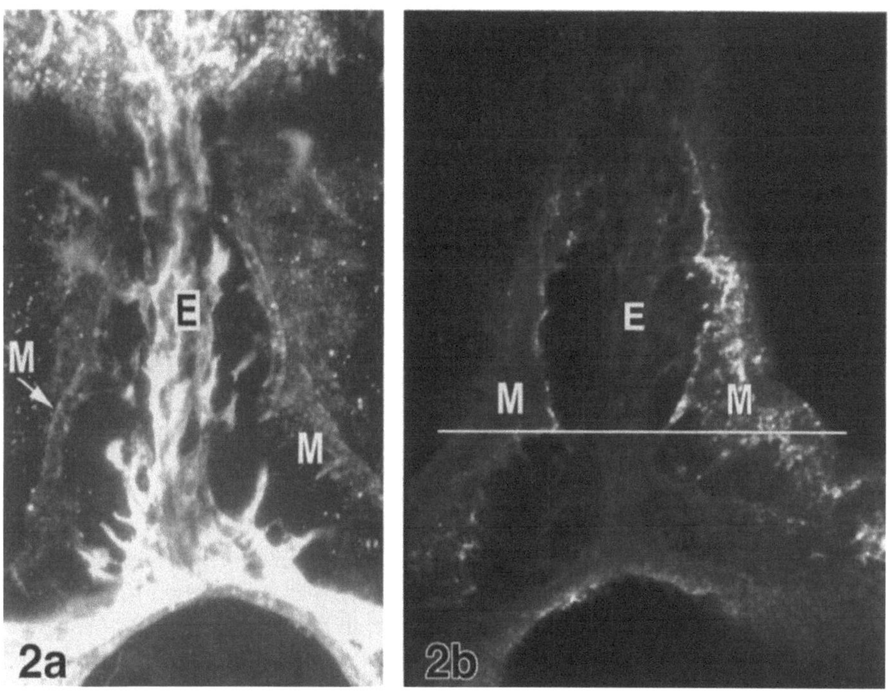

FIGURE 2. The linear or straight heart tube of a stage 9+ quail embryo. The line indicates the junction between the two segments of the straight heart tube. The first segment is a tubular structure separated from the paired heart fields. The second segment is in the process of formation; it is represented by the two, unfused hollow primordia associated with the anterior ends of the heart fields. As shown in 2a, at the point of fusion of the heart fields, vasculogenic mesenchymal cells integrate to form the endocardium (E) as revealed by immunostaining with an antibody (QH1) specific for endothelial cells. As shown in 2a and 2b (each 800×), the developing endocardium extends anterior-cranial to the fused heart fields to form a three-dimensional scaffolding around which the two myocardial precursors (M) will fuse to form the definitive outer epithelial mantle. The molecular asymmetry of the two segments is revealed in 2b by immunostaining with flectin antibodies, which primarily stain left-side structures (Tsuda et al 1996). Figure 2a, courtesy of Yukiko Sugi; Figure 2b, courtesy of Kirsti Linask and Robert Thompson.

compartments might be expected to be visualized as stripes within the linear tube. However, this was never observed by Franco and associates (1997); rather, regionalized expression occurred later, after looping had begun. This would support the concept of a tubular heart formed by the progressive addition of segments during and after the looping process (de la Cruz et al 1989) (chapter IV).

From the elegant grafting experiments of Schoenwolf and collegues (Garcia-Martinez and Schoenwolf 1993), we know that the future segments of the heart tube have anterior to posterior polarity as they leave the primitive streak to form the heart fields; however, the polarity of the cardiogenic precursors within the streak is not yet fixed or irreversible. From the beat rate, polarity along the A-P axis remains plastic even within the heart fields and appears to be regulated by the environment (Satin et al 1988). We have obtained data that suggests the heart fields are dynamic in the sense that the fate of the cells at any given position along the A-P axis of the field may vary with time. As shown in Fig. 3, based on established fate maps, five 10-μm beads were equally spaced along the A-P axis of the left heart field of several late stage 6 embryos (Ricardo Moreno, unpublished observations). If the same embryos were then maintained in shell-less, whole embryo culture until stage 12, most (3 to 5) of the beads eventually ended up in the developing primitive inlet (atrioventricular canals, AVC) segment (segment #3). The most anterior bead was often, but not always, found in the trabeculated region of the right ventricle, and occasionally, the left. Similarly, in another experiment, we endeavored to label the heart fields of 10 stage 5 embryos by a single 10-uL injection of a high titer (10^7) of spleen necrosis retrovirus carrying a LacZ reporter (kindly provided by Takashi Mikawa). If incubation was continued until stage 15, the apical trabeculated region of the right ventricle contained most of the labeled cells. A few labeled cells were found also in the left ventricle, but none elsewhere. We interpret these preliminary findings to be consistent with the notion that the heart tube is assembled from segments that arise within the heart fields at different time points or "conception dates". At any specific time point, the heart fields may have more cells of one segmental identity than another along the A-P axis.

One hypothesis as to how this might occur is that new cells are being "recruited" into a cardiogenic lineage at the posterior boundaries of the heart fields while more differentiated cells move anteriorly. Consistent with this hypothesis, mesodermal cells immediately posterior (caudal) to the heart fields can be induced (recruited) into a cardiomyogenic lineage by bone morphogenetic protein (BMP), a member of the transforming growth factor-β (TGF-β) gene family that is expressed in the heart-forming fields (Lough et al 1996; Schulteiss et al 1997). Preliminary correlative observations in zebrafish (Fishman and Chien 1997) suggest that a downstream target of BMP may be *Nkx-2.5*. As discussed in chapter I, *Nkx* genes are the mammalian homeodomain homologues of the *Drosophila tinman*, which is required for heart development (Lyons et al 1995). Thus, one possible scenario, consistent with the in vivo labeling experiments, is that, over time, posterior uncommitted, mesodermal cells in the immediate vicinity of the heart fields come under the environmental influence of secreted BMP, or some other morphogen expressed at the same time and place like cerberus (Bouwmeester et al. 1996), and commit to a cardiogenic fate.

Birth Dates of the Primitive Segments

Table 1 lists the stages at which the cardiac segments of the chick first appear cranial to the fused heart fields. Their fate can be determined with in vivo labeling tech-

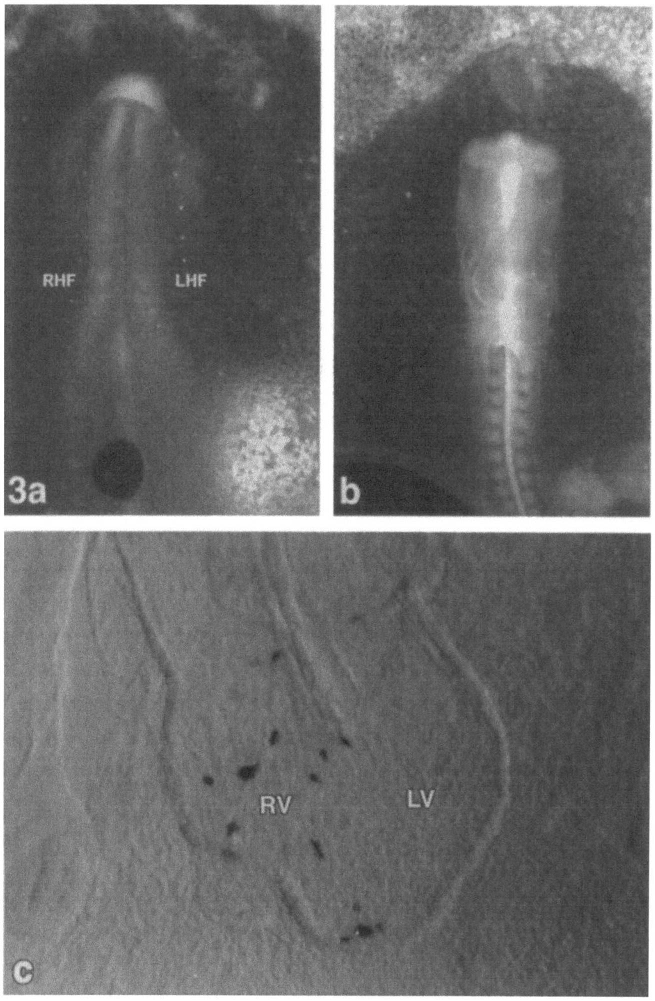

FIGURE 3. Segmental dynamics within the heart fields. In 3a, based on fate maps (Rawles 1943), five 10-μm beads were positioned along the anterior–posterior axis of left heart field of an HH stage 6 embryo (40×, bright-field). Incubation in shell-less culture was continued until stage 12 (3b, 40×) whereupon 3–4 beads, on average, were found in the developing third segment (AV canal). Usually, the most anterior bead was associated with the second segment (apical trabeculated region of the left ventricle). In 2c (Nomarski optics, 200×), a stage 15 embryo is seen in which the right heart field had been labelled *in ovo* at stage 5 by microinjection with a lacZ-retrovirus. Note that most of the viral label (dark spots) has integrated into the trabeculated region of the right ventricle with lesser labeling evident in the left ventricle but none in any other segment including the conus.

niques described in more detail in chapters III and IV. We also include predicted conception dates within the heart fields. These are based on the two series of labeling experiments, one with the 10-μm beads, the other with retroviruses, and should be regarded as preliminary and hypothetical. The first two segments form the future apical trabeculated regions of the right and left ventricles, respectively. The third segment, the AVC (or primitive ventricular inlet) is established during looping and forms the ventricular inlets. The last segment to be formed from the

TABLE 1. Birth Dates of the Primitive Cardiac Segments Along the Anterior–Posterior Axis

Segment No.	"Birth"	Predicted "Conception" HH Stage[a]	Fate
1	9–	4/5	RV[b]
2	9–/10	5/6	LV[c]
3	12	6/7–	AVC[d]
4	13–14	8/9	Sinoatrial[e]
5[f]	12–17	unknown	Conus (truncus)[g]

[a] Hamilton and Hamburger (1951).
[b] Apical trabeculated region of the right ventricle (RV).
[c] Apical trabeculated region of the left ventricle (LV).
[d] Atrioventricular canal (AVC), the future inlet region of each ventricle.
[e] Possibly two closely spaced individual segments.
[f] Proposed as a segment arising from non–heart field mesoderm.
[g] Truncus develops after stage 17, origin uncertain.

fused heart fields is the primordium of the sinus venosus and common atrium. Like the AVC inlet segment, it appears after looping and torsion have begun. The sinatrial segment may represent two individual segments that are closely spaced or even partially fused. If true, the sinatrial folds would be the boundary between the two putative, primordial segments (Wenink 1987). The origin of the pulmonary veins in the chick (DeRuiter et al 1995) and mouse (Tasaka et al 1996) supports the notion of two separate segments at the caudal, venous end of the heart tube.

Looping Follows Segmentation

Perhaps only coincidental, the first indication of a bend or loop in the heart does not occur until stage 11, at a time when both of the first two segments have been "cleared" from the fused heart fields. The crease or bend develops at the junction of the two future trabeculated ventricular segments, not within the confines of a specific segment. Thus, although the process and direction of looping may be linked to laterality genes (see chapter's I and IX), it is as if progressive sequestration of the segments promotes bending or looping, perhaps merely by providing a weak seam or hinge point or possibly for reasons more causal to the process than presently understood. However, there is general consensus that looping is probably the most central defining event of cardiac morphogenesis (chapter's III and IV; Manasek 1976) and should be considered more carefully than as merely providing a readout for the expression of laterality genes (Levin et al 1995). In this regard, it is important to remember that the primitive straight tube heart "twists" to the right (clockwise) as it bends to the right. Accordingly, what was the original right–left axis in the linear heart tube becomes the new dorsal–ventral axis in the looped C-shaped or U-shaped heart (chapter's III and IV). Therefore torsion and looping go hand-in-hand, and together they establish a working blueprint for all future segmental interactions that will define the fully mature, four-chambered heart (chapter III; Manasek 1976). Also, it is necessary to remember that looping is an ongoing process that only begins with the formation of the crease between the first two segments. It will continue until the two limbs created by the loop are eventually brought together along their hinge point, the inner (or lesser) curvature.

Gittenberger-de Groot and colleagues (Bouman et al 1995) describe looping as having two phases: the first begins at stage 10+ and ends at stage 17 with formation of the U-shaped heart; the second phase begins with the onset of septation at stage 17 and ends at stage's 35 to 39 with a fully defined heart. This critical second phase of looping primarily involves a progressive "deepening" of the inner curvature (ventricular-infundibular fold). When this phase of looping is completed, the inlet and outlet segments will have aligned such that each ventricle has balanced inlet and outlet orifices. If correctly accomplished, the aortic portion of the arterial pole will have literally "wedged" itself into the atrial portion of the posterior limb. A comparable period for all this to occur in man would be approximately weeks 3 through 10. In the mouse, it is from day 8 through day 15.

Is There a Segment for the Outflow or Outlet of the Tubular Heart?

The term "outflow tract" is commonly used by embryologists to describe the vascular conduit between the right ventricle and the aortic arches (Thompson and Fitzharris 1985). It is a term with many definitions and obfuscating descriptions. In general, most definitions include two or more of the possible anatomical regions. In their normal proximal to distal sequence, these are the conus, truncus, and aortic sac (see Pexieder 1995 for a discussion of nomenclature). Because of the imprecision of these terms and their different meanings to different investigators, many developmental anatomists, pathologists, and pediatric surgeons prefer not to use the term outflow tract. As described in chapter VII, the conus is the ventricular outlet that becomes the infundibulum and aortic vestibule of the mature heart. The truncus and aortic sac collectively are designated the arterial pole of the heart, forming in the mature heart the semilunar valves and trunks of the great arteries, respectively.

From in vivo labeling data (chapter VII), the conus develops between stages 12 and 17 as a cephalic extension from the right ventricle that connects directly to the aortic sac. Between stage's 17 and 22, yet another new structure, the truncus, develops between the conus and aortic sac (Fig. 4) (de la Cruz et al 1977). The aortic sac is the "pharyngeal basket" (chapter IX) that feeds the aortic arch arteries. The origin, septation, and integration of the conus and truncus with the two ventricles proximally and the aortic sac distally are among the most challenging and important unanswered questions in all of heart development.

Regarding the origin of the conus, new in vivo labeling experiments (chapter IV) raise the possibility that the conus (and maybe the truncus) arise from a developmentally late-appearing, fifth segment of non–heart field origin. Specifically, when a label is placed immediately cranial to segment #1 (future apical region of the right ventricle) of a stage 9+ embryo, the label invariably ends up at stage 22 at the boundary interface between right ventricle and conus (the conoventricular junction). These data suggested to us that the conus might be formed from mesenchyme located anterior or cephalic to the first segment (de la Cruz et al 1977). The splanchnic mesoderm anterior to the first segment is not normally considered to be of heart field origin. If, as suggested, the conus is derived from extracardiac mesoderm, how do we account for it having a myocardial wall when, traditionally, only precardiac mesoderm of the heart fields is thought to be in a myocardial lineage. One possibility suggested by the experiments of Lough and coworkers (1996) and Schulteiss and associates (1997) indicated that morphogens normally secreted by the heart fields, like BMP or cerberus can induce undifferentiated mesenchyme to

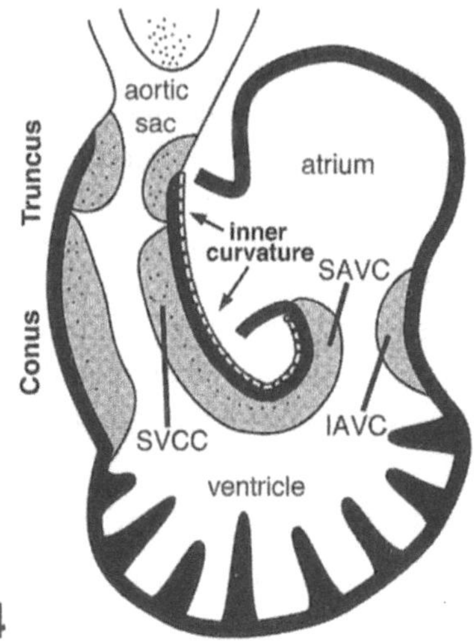

4

FIGURE 4. Diagram of a U-shaped heart tube, similar in stage and orientation to that of Figs. 5 and 6a. The inner curvature is the hinge-point of the looped heart and extends from the truncus to the anterior portion of the atrioventricular canal. It is lined by a continuous sleeve of mesenchyme formed by the union of the sinistroventral conal cushion (SV, CC) and the superior AV cushion (SAVC). In the inlet limb, the SAVC and the inferior atrioventricular cushion (IAVC) fuse to form separate inlets for each ventricle. The outlet limb is formed from the right ventricle, conus, and truncus (up to the point where the myocardium ends). The arterial pole or aortic sac connects the outlet to the arteries of the pharyngeal arches. The migratory pathway and relative quantitative distribution of neural crest cells are shown as black dots.

enter a myocardial lineage when normally they were not fated to do so. Thus, as with the heart fields, perhaps some cardiogenic signaling cells persist within the future right apical trabecular ventricular segment that recruit a conus from non-heart mesenchyme.

In mice, the expression of the *hdf* segmental gene in myocardial cells of both the right ventricle and conus (Fig. 5) seemingly argues for a common origin (the first segment). However, it cannot be ruled out that segmental interactions, over time through cell–cell communications or secretion of morphogens, may lead to the expansion of gene expression across boundaries as suggested by Yamamura and colleagues (1997) for the *hdf* gene. Although there is broad consensus that the aortic sac is most likely of branchial origin (Noden et al 1995), the derivation of the truncus remains a mystery. Like the conus, the truncus is encircled by a myocardial mantle (Fig. 4, 6; Thompson and Fitzharris 1979), and as suggested for the conus, possibly there may be two options for its origin: recruitment from extracardiac mesenchyme versus a direct outgrowth of a preexisting structure, in this case, the conus. To date, in vivo labeling has failed to reveal an origin for the myocardial cells of the truncus, although grafting experiments (Noden 1991) indicate the truncal endocardium is a derivative of extracardiac mesoderm. The weaker expression of the *hdf* gene at day 11 in the truncus compared with the conus does not really prove or disprove a common origin, but a single gene mutation in the Keeshond dog that affects the conus, but not the truncus, indicates that these regions of the outflow limb may not necessarily be two halves of the same coin (Patterson et al 1993).

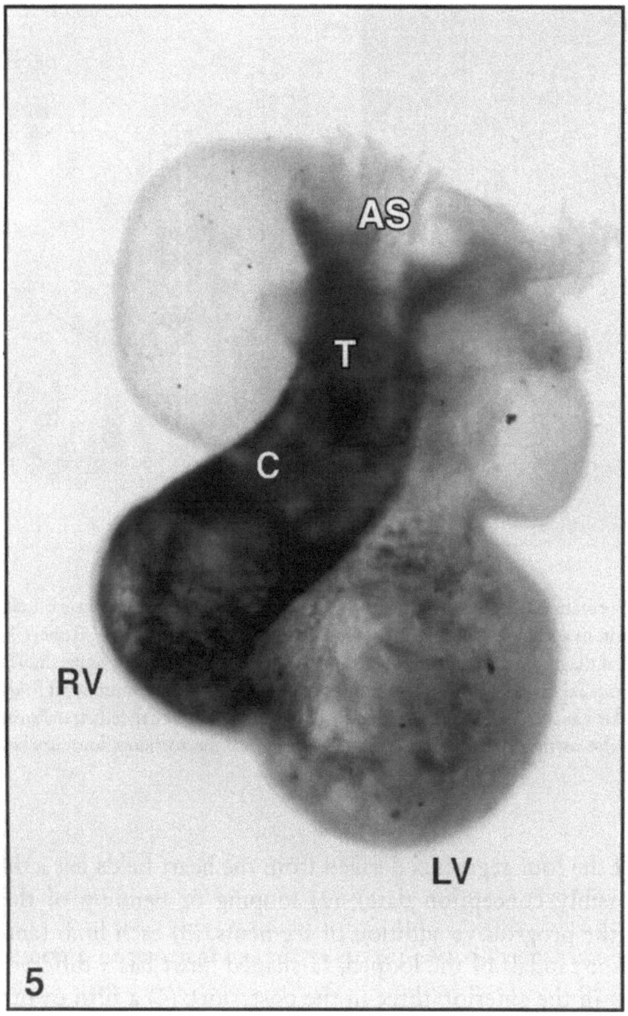

FIGURE 5. Segmental pattern of expression of the *hdf-lacZ* gene (Yamamura et al 1997) in 11.5 day +/− mouse embryonic heart. The *hdf* gene is expressed in the right ventricle (RV) and conus (C); weak expression in the truncus (T) ends abruptly in the aortic sac (AS). Left ventricle (LV) (180×).

Thus, in response to the question of an outflow segment, for the moment we propose there is a fifth cardiogenic segment that (1) forms the conus (and possibly the truncus), (2) is derived or recruited from extracardiac mesoderm, and (3) integrates with the ventricular segments to form the outlet of each ventricle. Until in vivo labeling can be combined with segmental markers, this will remain an open question but one with significant relevance for future molecular studies of regulation.

Summary of Cardiac Segment Formation

Six points are pertinent to the sequential formation of the cardiac segments by the fusion of the heart fields: (1) from studies in living embryos (de la Cruz et al

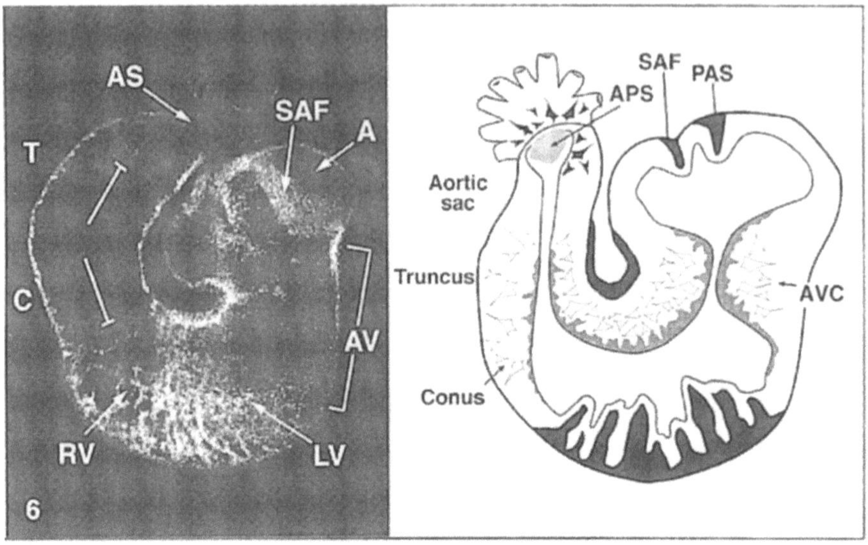

FIGURE 6. Formation of septal primordia in the segments of the tubular heart. **Left**, phallocidin staining for α-actin in a stage 19 chick heart (saggital section, 60× courtesy of Robert Thompson). **Right**, histological diagram of a similarly staged heart. In the right and left ventricles (RV, LV) and atrium (A), myocardial invaginations or infoldings are formed (e.g., the sinuoatrial folds [SAF]. In the atrioventricular canal (AVC), conus (C), and truncus (T), endothelial cells transform into cushion mesenchyme. In the aortic sac, neural crest cells give origin to the aorticopulmonary septum (APS).

1989), each of the four segments derived from the heart fields has a different birth date (and possibly conception date), (2) looping or bending of the heart tube accompanies the progressive addition of segments, (3) each limb (anterior-cranial versus posterior-caudal) of the looped, U-shaped heart has a different number of segments (one in the anterior, three in the posterior), (4) a fifth or outlet segment may form outside the heart fields, (5) the segments have different developmental fates, and (6) none of the segments are directly equivalent anatomically to a specific chamber of the adult heart; instead, they integrate to form the definitive heart chambers.

What is the Significance of Segmentation?

Because the segments of the primitive heart tube have different birth dates (and possibly conception dates), each may come under different gene regulation as the temporal and spatial patterns of expression for potential transcriptional regulators change during early heart development. This could account for the variation in developmental fates, particularly as to the role of segments in septation. The expression pattern of *hdf* (Yamamura et al 1997) and three genes that encode transcription factors—*MEF-2* (Lin et al 1997), *dHAND*, and *eHAND* (Srivastava et al 1997)—are consistent with the concept of candidate "segmental genes". *hdf* and *dHAND* are both expressed in the right ventricle whereas *hdf* is also expressed in the conus. Mutations in either of these genes inhibits development of the right ventricle and in *hdf* −/− mice also the conus. Interestingly, the knockout of the

MEF2-C gene, although expressed in all segments, phenocopies mutations of *dHAND*, indicating that the latter might be a downstream target of *MEF* genes (Lin et al 1997; Srivastava et al 1997). In mice (but not chick), *eHAND*, although highly homologous to *dHAND*, is expressed in the left ventricle, aortic sac, and pharyngeal arches. Other genes (*BMP-2,-4*) (Wall and Hogan 1994) and the homeobox gene *Msx-2* (Chan-Thomas et al 1993) are expressed in the primitive inlet or AVC (segment #3) and the conus (putative segment #5).

How segmentally expressed genes regulate the fate of a segment has received little investigative attention. In the case of *hdf*, the gene appears to directly or indirectly regulate formation of extracellular macromolecules associated with the transdifferentiation of endocardium into cushion mesenchyme. Some, like *BMP-2* and *-4*, encode morphogens related to the TGF supergene family that directly affect differentiation or lineage progression (Winnier et al 1995; Zhang and Bradley 1996). Others may act to site-direct gene expression of structural and functional proteins to a particular segment or future chamber. For example, all segments initially express both atrial and ventricular isoforms of myosin heavy chains, but with time, their expression becomes restricted to atrium or ventricle (Wessels et al 1991). Specific combinations of *cis*-acting promoter elements in myosin or desmin genes, perhaps in response to *trans*-acting factors, like MEF-2 proteins or CARP (cardiac-specific ankyrin repeat protein; Zou et al 1997), direct expression to a particular heart segment (Ross et al 1996; Franco et al 1997).

Thus, even though the histological components of each segment appear to blend homogeneously during formation of the primitive heart tube, it is clear by molecular imaging of gene or protein expression, that there is molecular diversity in potential regulatory genes, consistent with their acquisition of different segmental phenotypes. However, as initially observed by Yutzey and associates (1994), boundaries of restricted gene expression can be crossed, as seen after treatment with retinoids in *hdf* mutants (Yamamura et al 1997). Results from *hdf* −/− mice raise the interesting prospect that segments may interact normally across boundaries to stabilize phenotype.

FATE OF THE PRIMITIVE SEGMENTS IN RELATIONSHIP TO SEPTATION

Each primitive segment contributes to septation of the tubular heart (Fig. 6). In the atrium and ventricles, myocardial ingrowths into the lumen form the primary interventricular and ventricular muscular septum, respectively. In the primitive inlet (AVC) segment, conus, and truncus, mesenchymal expansions or "cushions", which project into the lumen of these segments, develop. The fusion of the major AVC cushions creates the mesenchymal AV septum that knits or glues together the atrial and ventricular muscular septa and helps to partially seal off direct communication between the ventricles. The conal cushions fuse to form a septum that forms a separate outlet and arterial connection for each ventricle. Thus, even when two segments or regions give rise to similar type structures, e.g., cushions, as occurs in the AVC, conus, and truncus, important differences may still exist that reflect either variable segmental gene expression (e.g., *Mox-1* Msx-1 or *Msx-2*) or cellular contributions, e.g., neural crest, epicardium, or branchial arch mesoderm (Noden et al 1995).

Sinoatrial Segment

This segment is the last to be formed by the heart fields, has the shortest half-life, and is probably the least understood, particularly in mammals. Partly, this is because few, if any, genes or markers have been identified that might be used to trace origins of the cells or their relationships, especially during formation of the pulmonary veins and later as the sinus and its horns are asymmetrically absorbed into the posterior wall of the atrium.

The atrium is the only segment that becomes composed of two halves, one right and the other left, from its first appearance. For this reason, the atrium is the only mature chamber to have relevance to laterality genes, e.g., the *iv* gene (Layton 1978; Brueckner and Horwich 1989). In man, each side of the atrium has a marker (isoforms of creatine kinase; Wessels et al 1991, 1998) that can be used to confirm molecular phenotype. Thus, mutations or environmental perturbations may result in atrial isomerisms (two anatomically right or left atria). However, one never sees a laterality counterpart in the ventricles because, consistent with the concept of segmentation, the ventricles form in series (not parallel) as separate segments along the A-P axis.

The primary atrial septum (septum primum) is but one of several myocardial infoldings or ingrowths into the lumen of the common atrium (Fig. 6). Formation

---

FIGURE 9. **a.** A computerized, confocal reconstruction of the outlet (conus [C] and truncus [T]) and the arterial pole or aortic sac (As) of a human stage 17 embryonic heart (front and back) with and without the ensheathing myocardium (magenta). The aortic (A) and pulmonary (P) blood streams are shown in red and pink, respectively. The yellow asterisk denotes where neural crest mesenchyme emerges from aortic arches 4 and 6 to form the green-colored, aorticopulmonary septum. The white line is the boundary between the conus (C) and truncus (T). Note that the aorticopulmonary septum septates not only the aortic sac but also impales the truncus as well. It does not penetrate below the white line where, in vivo, the conal ridges fuse to form the future muscular outlet septum. (Courtesy of Robert Thompson). **b.** The aortic outlet or posterior regions of the conus (C) and truncus (T) are shown in relation to the inner curvature of a stage 30 chick. Cardiac myosin heavy chain is labeled red, proliferating cells are green (16 hours after sinlge injection of bromodeoxyuridine [BrdU]) and TUNEL-positive, apoptotic cells are yellow. Note that myocardialization (arrowheads) occur within the cushions of the conus but not in the truncus. Myocardial cells that are invading (muscularizing) the dextrodorsal conal cushion are neither BrdU nor TUNEL positive. Clusters of dividing cells are seen within the cushion while apoptotic cells are present (arrows) in the myocardium of the conus up to its junction with the truncus.

FIGURE 10. Anti–myosin heavy chain peroxidase immunostaining of normal human embryonic hearts (a, 35–38 days; b, 56 days), a day 14 trisomy 16 mouse heart (c) and a stage 30 (d) chick truncus region. **a.** the mesenchymalized endocardial cushions (EC) of the conus region normally become muscularized by the invasion of myocardial tissue (arrowheads) resembling trabeculae. Myocardialization occurs during and after fusion of the cushions to form an outlet septum, 600×. **b.** a transverse section immediately below the level of the forming valves to show that myocardialization of the original mesenchymalized outlet septum results in the latter becoming a muscularized septum (arrowhead), 60×. This muscularized septum creates a separate outlet for each ventricle. **c.** In the trisomy 16 mouse (day 14), the outlet septum remains mesenchymalized (or incompletely myocardialized) and the right ventricle has a double outlet (arrows) leading to the aorta (A) and pulmonary trunk (P), 80×. **d.** a transverse section at the level where the aorticopulmonary septum (APS) contacts the truncal ridges. Note that the myocardium of the truncus bordering the inner curvature appears to either be lost or has failed to express muscle antigens. (Figures 10a, b, and c were provided by Dr. Andy Wessels, 10d from A. Gittenberger-deGroot).

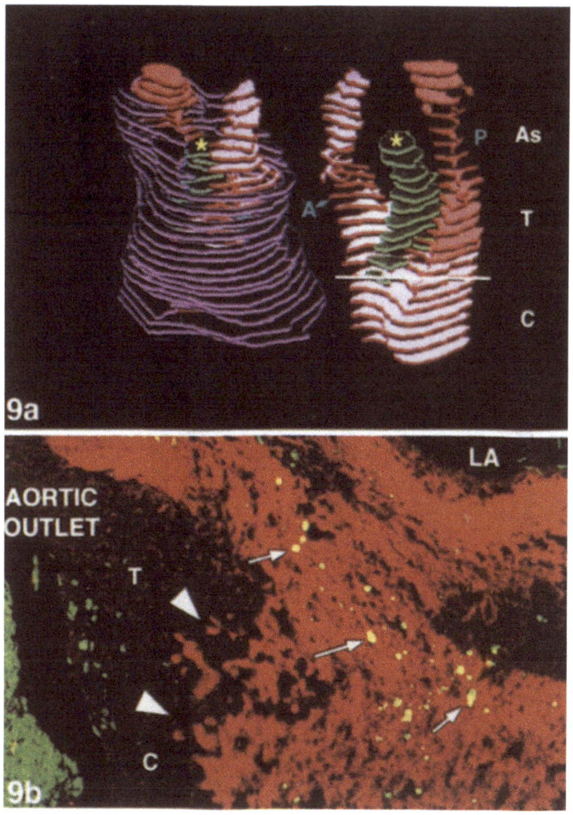

FIGURE 9.

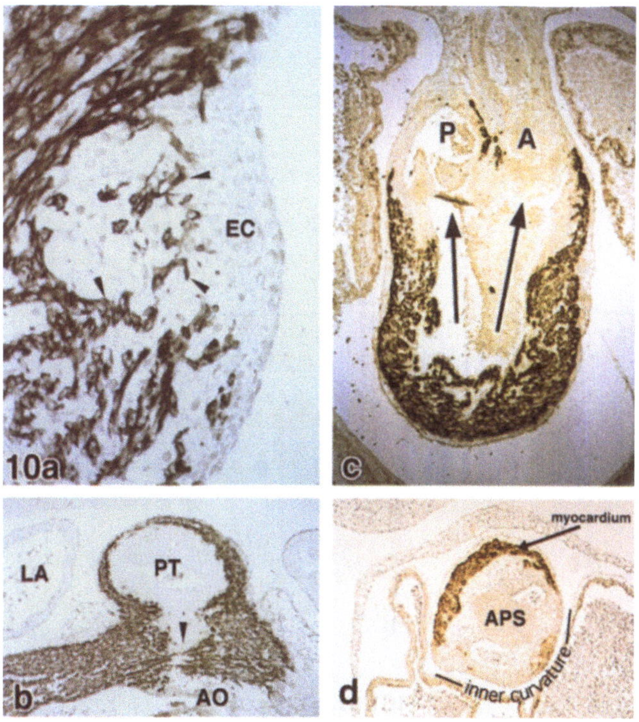

FIGURE 10.

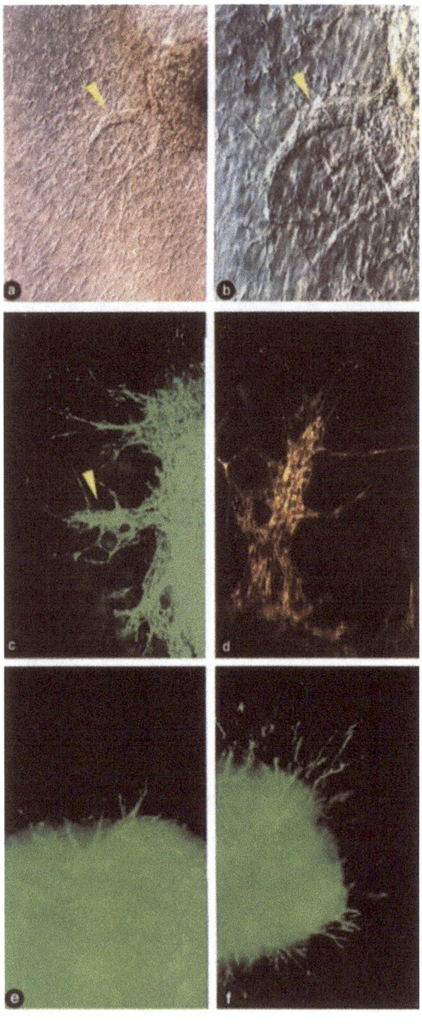

FIGURE 16.

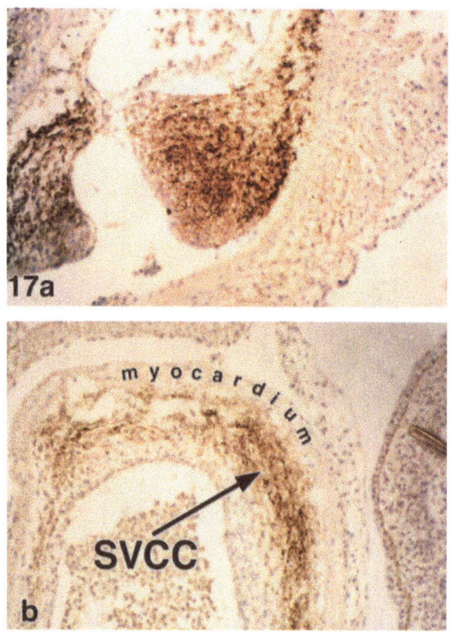

FIGURE 17.

of these multiple invaginations of myocardial origin largely define the atrial phenotype. These include the sinoatrial folds or "venous valves", pulmonary ridges, and the primary and secondary atrial septa (Webb et al 1997a, b). As shown in Fig. 7, the primary atrial septum develops from two parts, a muscular infolding from the posterior aspect of the atrial wall and extracardiac mesenchyme termed the spina vestibuli (Asami and Koizumi 1995; Tasaka et al 1996). The latter is a wedge of mesenchyme at the venous pole derived from the dorsal mesentery (mesocardium) that projects into the posterior atrial wall that accompanies the ingrowth of the atrial myocardium and endocardium (Wessels et al 1998). As shown in Fig. 7, the spina vestibuli and associated atrial myocardium follow a course or pathway toward the fused AV cushions that correlates with atrial extensions of both AV cushions. We suggest that interaction between mesenchyme populations may serve to guide the formation of the primary atrial septum. Adding to the complexity of atrial septation, Gerety and Watanabe (1997) have suggested that the endocardium at the leading edge of the atrial septum undergoes transformation to mesenchyme similar to that of the AV canal (described below). Thus, it is possible that endothelial-derived mesenchyme comingles with extracardiac mesenchyme of the spina vestibul much like what happens at the opposite pole of the heart with neural crest and the outlet cushions (see below). Unquestionably, the spina vestibuli is one of the most underappreciated structures in heart development. Its "rediscovery" (Markwald et al 1997; Webb 1997) and application to the trisomy 16 mouse are leading to a new understanding of atrial septation with the distinct possibility of engendering new molecular concepts.

Mouse chromosome 16 is syntenic to both human chromosome 21 (trisomic in Down's syndrome) and to a region of chromosome 22 that is deleted in DiGeorge syndrome (Goldmuntz and Emmanuel 1997). Deletions of the DiGeorge region (22q11) result in outflow and arterial pole defects that are thought to be caused by a lack of neural crest cells. Cardiac neural crest constitutes a population of extracardiac mesenchyme that migrates through the pharyngeal arches to enter the arterial pole of the heart. There they form the aorticopulmonary septum, which divides the arterial pole into two separate blood streams. Thus, two wedges of

---

FIGURE 16. Collagen gel culture assays for myocardialization potential of explants isolated from the midpoint of the inner curvature before (stage 18–22) or after the onset of myocardialization in vivo (stage 26–28). **a, b.** Low and high magnification (400×, 1200×, respectively) of a stage 28 explant. After 24 hours in culture, the collagen lattice had become completely cellularized with mesenchyme into which multiple, fingerlike ingrowths from the myocardial tissue had projected. **c, d.** The arrow denotes a typical invasive projection that was stained for sarcomeric myosin. Explants obtained before myocardialization (**e**, 600×), at stage 19, also mesenchymalized the lattice within 24 hours of culture but did not "muscularize" it, as few or no myosin-positive ingrowths were formed. However, if a similar explant was cocultured with the truncus region of the same embryo or the conus region of the stage 26 embryo, more numerous and longer myocardial projections were formed (**f**, 300×).

FIGURE 17. D1C4 antibody staining of a stage 24 AV canal (**a**) and conus (**b**). As shown in the superior AV cushion (center of micrograph), the antigen is expressed by most mesenchymal cells, whereas in the sinistroventral conal cushion (SVCC), the antigen is expressed in a subset of mesenchyme immediately adjacent to the myocardium and just before the onset of myocardialization. Note that expression of the antigen is usually greater along the myocardium associated with the inner curvature (arrow) 800×.

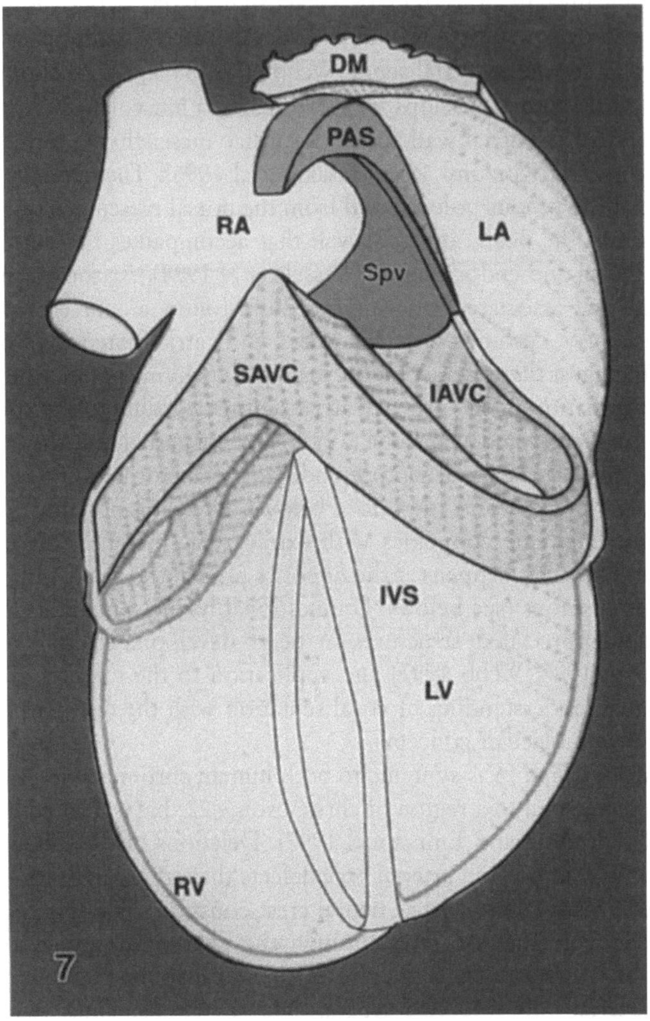

FIGURE 7. Septal primordia of the posterior limb of a stage 24 chick heart. The conus, truncus, and most of the right ventricle (RV) are above (or anterior to) the plane of this drawing (modified from one generously provided by Professor Adriana Gittenberger-de Groot, University of Leiden, Holland; see also Gittenberger-de Groot et al 1995). A figure 8-shaped primitive cardiac septum will be formed in the posterior limb by the interventricular septum (IVS), the AV septum formed by the fusion of the superior (SAVC) and inferior (IAVC) AV cushions, and the primary atrial septum (PAS). The latter forms at a point where two midline flanges from the superior and inferior AV cushions contact the dorsal-posterior atrial wall. At this point, extracardiac mesenchyme of the spina vestibuli (Spv), a derivative of the dorsal mesocardium (DM), penetrates the atrial wall accompanied by an infolding of the atrial myocardium. Note that almost all structures associated with septation of the posterior limb contact or anchor to the AV cushions, the "glue" of the figure 8-shaped septum.

extracardiac mesenchyme—spina vestibuli and neural crest—are established at each pole of the heart. We propose that one is needed for septation of the inlet, the other for the outlet limb. Interestingly, both populations appear to be influenced by genes carried on mouse chromosome 16. Therefore, one or more specific genes may exist that, if overexpressed (as may occur in Down's syndrome) or deleted (as in Di-

George syndrome), may affect atrial or outflow septation by inhibiting the formation or migration of either population of extracardiac mesenchyme. In this regard, we have found that a gene located within the 5-Mb "Down's region" of chromosome 21 (Kornenberg et al 1992)—called DS-CAM (related to neural cell adhesion molecule)—was expressed in extracardiac mesenchyme at both the inlet and outlet poles of the heart (Mjaatvedt and Kornenberg, unpublished observations). Paradoxically, genetic answers to atrial septation could lie with a well-studied cell population found at the opposite pole of the heart.

The Two Segments That Form Trabeculated Regions of Each Ventricle

Called trabeculae, ventricular invaginations, compared with atrial, are more numerous, elongated, and clustered at the junction between the two ventricular segments (Fig. 6). Each ventricular trabeculum appears to be a cone-shaped, clonal expansion of a myocardial stem cell into the lumen (Mikawa et al 1992). The traditional view is that the coalescence of trabeculae along the interventricular junction (groove) establishes the primary ventricular septum. There is no confirmation of this in living embryos. Available in vivo data (de la Cruz et al 1997) indicate that the septum develops from a single continuum of muscle that arises from a common point of origin located in the junction separating the apical region of each ventricle. Both retinoid (Sucov et al 1994) and neuregulin signaling (Meyer and Birchmeier 1995; Lee et al 1995) appear to affect formation of ventricular invaginations, including the definitive ventricular septum.

A narrow, circumferential band of myocardial cells that forms at the constriction between the two ventricular segments has been called the primary ring (Wenink 1987; Lamers et al 1992). In the human and rat heart, this ring is characterized by the expression of an antigen recognized by the antibodies G1N2 (Wessels et al 1992) and Leu7/HNK-1 (Ikeda et al 1990; Wessels et al 1996). Because cells of the ventricular septum express these markers, it was suggested that this ring is the progenitor of the interventricular septum. However, in vivo labeling studies indicate a very specific site of origin for the progenitor cells of the ventricular septum. A bead placed in the ventral fusion line of the stage 9+, linear heart at the level of the interventricular groove becomes incorporated into the ventricular septum (de la Cruz et al 1997; chapter V). The origin for the ventricular septum on the greater curvature also includes one end of the GlN2-positive ring. The opposite side of the ring passes through the inner curvature, which has not been tested by in vivo labeling for its contribution to the septum. However, as development proceeds, the right side of the AVC associated with the inner curvature and the superior AV cushion is remodeled as described in detail later. Specifically, from GlN2 expression, the right AVC expands while shifting and rotating toward the medial inferior region of this segment. As a result, GlN2 cells become positioned at the interface of the AV inlet with the muscular interventricular septum and become recognizable as the AV node, part of the atrioventricular conduction system (Wessels et al 1992).

Thus, the GlN2-positive, primary ring at the level of the inner curvature may contribute to the conduction tissue associated with the ventricular septum, although, at the point where it intersects with the left interventricular groove, it may mark a population of cells that participate in forming the muscle portion of the interventricular septum. Combining in vivo labeling with GlN2 imunostaining should resolve whether molecular regulatory mechanisms become operative within the ventral fusion line of the linear heart to direct myocardial cells into a putative septal lineage.

The Ventricular Inlet (or Atrioventricular AV) Segment

The third segment forms entirely in the posterior (caudal) limb of the heart loop. Initially it is the largest of the segments in the posterior limb. Although its lumen is directly continuous only with the left ventricle, ultimately, it will (upon remodeling) give origin to the inlet of both ventricles. Rather than forming myocardial ingrowths, the endocardium of the inlet segment transforms into mesenchymal cells that colonize an expanded cardiac jelly space to form cushion tissue (Hiltgen et al 1996) (Fig 6). Some 50 proteins have been identified within the cardiac jelly of the AVC and include collagens, fibronectin, hyaluronate, fibrillin, fibulin, proteoglycans, growth factors, growth factor binding proteins, and some glycoproteins unique to the AVC (Runyan and Markwald 1983; Rongish and Little 1995; Bouchey et al 1996; Nakajima et al 1997a).

The seeding of mesenchymal cells into this complex, expansive matrix occurs along the entire length and circumference of the AVC segment (Moreno-Rodriguez et al 1997). Over time, two conspicuously large concentrations of cellularized cushion tissue project into the lumen of the inlet, the superior and inferior AV cushions, which fuse at stage 26 to form the AV septum. The latter divides the original AV lumen into separate right (triscupid) and left (mitral) orifices (Fig. 7; chapter VI). Later, two smaller AV outgrowths, the right and left AV cushions, form on the lateral walls (in chapter VI, see fig. 6 and 11). A major unanswered question is why the lateral cushions appear later in development and whether they form by mechanisms similar to those described below for the major cushions. Perhaps there is previously unrecognized molecular heterogeneity within the AV inlet segment. Collectively, these four cushions constitute the primordia for the inlet valves (see chapter VI).

Mesenchymal cells of the superior cushion outgrow their original segmental boundaries and enter the cardiac jelly along the inner curvature where they meet up with cushion cells migrating proximally from the sinistro conal ridge (Fig. 4; also figure 9B, chapter VI). Both postmortem studies and in vivo labeling techniques indicated that this "ventricular" portion of the superior cushion also contributed significantly to the outlet for the left ventricle (chapter VII). Additionally, a less robust expansion of mesenchyme extends from the superior AV cushion (and also the inferior AV cushion) into the atrium as a midline band of cells in the plane of the future primary septum that interfaces with the mesenchyme of the spina vestibuli. From studies in mice trisomic for chromosome 16, both mesenchymal populations (extracardiac and intracardiac) contribute to atrial septation (Markwald et al 1977). Therefore, the AV segment is in many ways the "heart of the heart" for its multiple roles in septation of both the inlet and outlet limbs. Specifically, it is important to appreciate that the AV septum forms in alignment with both the future ventricular septum and primary atrial septum to form an 8-shaped septum (chapter VI) that establishes the four-chambered pattern of the mature heart (Fig. 7).

As to why cushion formation occurs in specific segments like the AV inlet, we again invoke the hypothesis that segmental genes determine the identity and fate of a specific segment. In this case, the best segmental gene candidate may be the genes encoding the bone morphogenetic proteins (*BMP-2* and *-4*). The *BMPs* are homologous to *Drosophila decapentaplegic*, another member of the TGF-β gene family, which functions in segmentation, polarity, and pattern formation (Wall and Hogan 1994). Because they are expressed uniquely in the myocardium of the AV (inlet) and outlet, but not the apical trabeculated regions of both ventricles (Jones et al 1991), *BMPs* could affect the formation of mesenchyme in a number ways, including paracrinely to directly induce target endothelial cells to transform (see below) or autocrinely to regulate myocardial secretion of signaling molecules.

THE CONCEPTUAL FRAMEWORK OF CUSHION TISSUE FORMATION

Significant progress has been made into understanding the cellular and molecular dynamics of cushion formation in the AV inlet segment and conal derivative of the first segment. Progress has largely derived from the development of a three-dimensional culture system that retains the temporal and spatial specificities (Bernanke and Markwald 1982; Runyan and Markwald 1983; Markwald et al 1984; Potts et al 1991). This model has enabled us to determine some of the mechanisms of how cushions form and differentiate, which are summarized in Fig. 8.

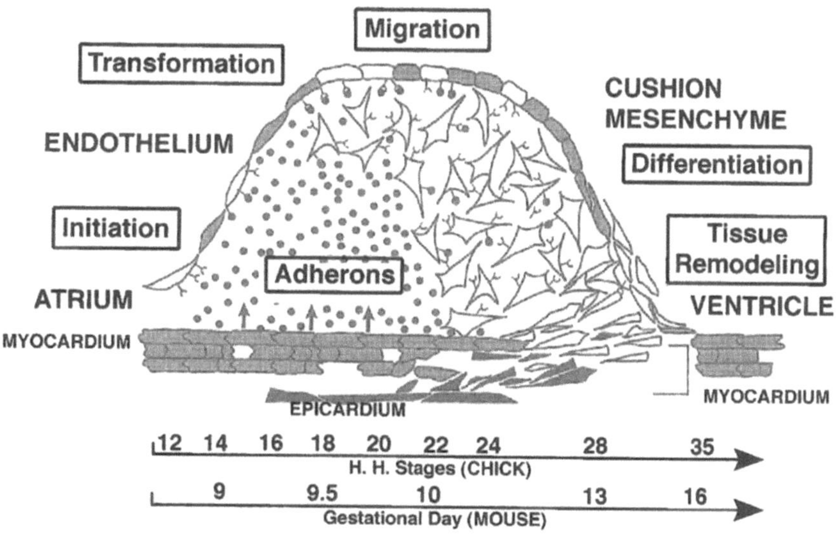

FIGURE 8. Summary of the spatial and temporal sequence of events in cushion tissue formation within the AV canal. A time-line compares chick and mouse. Myocardially derived extracellular signals (adherons) induce or initiate transformation of a subset of endothelial cells (the clear or unshaded cells) into a migratory phenotype called "cushion mesenchyme". AV cushion cells differentiate into valvular or septal fibroblasts; beginning at stage 26, a break in the continuity of the myocardium between the atrium and ventricle occurs by unknown remodeling mechanisms. (Reproduced by permission of Karger AG, Basel, from Markwald et al 1996).

Cushion Tissue Is Formed by an Inductive Interaction

The AVC myocardium induces endothelial cell transformation by a "signal" secreted into the cardiac jelly. Thus, myocardium is the stimulator and endocardium the responder in this fundamental inductive interaction (Eisenberg and Markwald 1995; Markwald et al 1996). On induction, responder cells transform or transdifferentiate into mesenchyme, which migrates to populate the cardiac jelly of the forming segment. If the AV myocardium was removed and replaced with spiczl ventricular myocardium, endothelial cells failed to form mesenchyme. Replacing spiczl ventricular with AV myocardium restored mesenchyme formation, indicating that the inductive signal is segmentally specific (Mjaatvedt et al 1987).

Target Endothelial Cell Responses to Induction

Induction engenders a cascade of dynamic changes in gene and protein expression in endothelial target cells that concludes with their transdifferentiation into mesenchyme. This cascade includes a gradual downregulation of neural cell adhesion molecule (NCAM) (Mjaatvedt and Markwald 1989) and an upregulation of serine and metalloproteinases, both of which correlate with loss of endothelial cell–cell associations (McGuire and Orkin 1992; Alexander et al 1997). Transforming endothelial cells also hypertrophy, which correlates intracellularly with their activation of the exocytic secretory pathway. Loss of cell polarity is indicated by rearrangement of the Golgi apparatus, cytoskeletal actin filaments, and cell surface markers (Krug et al 1987; DeRuiter et al 1997). Formation of migratory appendages in the chick correlates with a marked increase in expression of α-smooth muscle actin (Nakajima et al 1997b). Active, directed migration as a mesenchymal cell occurs along collagen fibrils and is causally linked with secretion of heparan and chondroitin sulfated proteoglycans (Funderburg and Markwald 1986). Cytotactin and fibulin are two de-adhesive proteins expressed by migrating cells that may function to sustain migration (Crossin and Hoffman 1991; Spence et al 1992). Migrating cushion cells also express a membrane protein (hyaluronate synthetase) that synthesizes and secretes hyaluronate (Spicer et al 1997). Hyaluronate has been shown to promote cushion cell migration (Bernanke and Markwald 1982), possibly through receptor-mediated signaling mechanisms (Hall et al 1994).

Transforming Endothelial Cells Are a Subpopulation of Endocardium

Not all endothelial cells within the AVC or conus transform to mesenchyme. The subset that does respond to inductive signals uniquely expresses JB3 antigen (Wunsch et al 1994) and a transcription factor, *Sox 4* (Ya et al 1997b). Because of their expression of JB3+ antigen (fibrillin-2, B. Rongish et al 1998), endothelial cells in a presumptive cushion lineage appear to arise from precursors within the heart-forming fields (Wunsch et al 1994, Sugi and Markwald 1996). Anterior endoderm promotes segregation of endocardial precursors from cells committed to a myocardial lineage and secretes factors (e.g., vascular endothelial growth factor) that induce expression of endothelial markers (Sugi and Markwald 1996; Y. Sugi, unpublished observations; Drake and Little 1995). Nontransforming, JB3-negative endothelial cells originate from nonprecardiac mesoderm and later migrate into the heart fields or the tubular heart (Coffin and Poole 1991; Sugi and Markwald 1996).

To summarize, the endocardium is established from two potential subsets of preendocardial cells, JB3+ and JB3−.

The Myocardial Inductive Signal

Extraction of the cardiac jelly (or myocardial basement membrane) using EDTA buffers revealed that the induction signal is a particulate complex of glycoproteins termed adherons, based on a precedent in the literature (Mjaatvedt and Markwald, 1989). Adherons are visualized as 0.1- to 0.5-μm particulates by antibody or lectin staining that are restricted to the cardiac jelly of the two mesenchyme-forming segments (Mjaatvedt et al 1987; Sinning and Markwald 1992; Sinning et al 1995). The proteins of adherons include, but are not limited to, fibronectin, ES (EDTA-soluble) proteins of Mr 28, 46, 53, 70, 93, and 130 kDa (Mjaatvedt et al 1991), and proteins recognized by antibodies made against antigens isolated by their affinity for soybean lectin, called hLAMP (heart lectin-associated myocardial proteins) (Sinning et al 1995). Directly adding adherons or hLAMP antigens to cultured AV (but not ventricular) endothelial cells induced their transformation. Development of putative receptors for adheron proteins or hLAMP antigens is envisioned as the hypothetical mechanism by which JB3+ endothelial cells become uniquely competent to respond to a transforming signal. Evidence for such a receptor is an intracellular, phosphokinase C-dependent calcium flux triggered by myocardial activation (Runyan et al 1990).

One of the ES antigens, ES130, has been cloned and sequenced and found to be a novel protein without homology to any known growth factor or candidate regulatory gene (Rezaee et al 1993; Krug et al 1995). Expression of ES130 is developmentally regulated; the protein is initially expressed in the fused heart fields at stage 6 and in the primitive heart tube within the myocardium of the AVC, conus, and truncus. At the onset of endothelial transformation (Rezeae et al 1993; Markwald et al 1995), expression of ES130 is downregulated in the myocardium but upregulated in transforming endothelial cells and their mesenchymal progeny. Expression in target cells suggests an autocrine role to sustain transformation and migration (Ramsdell et al 1997). Antisense and antibody experiments indicate ES130 is required or endothelial transformation to mesenchyme. However, although it has a membrane anchor or signal sequence and is secreted by the myocardium as part of the adheron complex, recent studies with ES130 indicate it is strongly expressed intracellularly and has homology to coiled coil proteins (e.g., kinectins or ribosome-binding proteins) that bind proteins to membranes or cytoskeleton (Krug, unpublished). Thus, we presently believe ES130 is required for inducing endothelial transformation but is not the actual ligand that initiates transformation (Ramsdell et al 1998). Because of its homology to kinectins and ribosome receptor proteins, ES130 may be required for the activation and reorganization of secretory organelles associated with the hypertrophy phase of transformation.

Another candidate for the myocardial signal responsible for transformation is the 68- to 70-kDa ES antigen. This antigen was identified as transferrin (also called conalbumin in the chick embryo) using immunopurification and microsequencing protocols (Isokawa et al 1994). Transferrin/conalbumin was isolated both from EDTA extracts of stage 14 hearts and from myocardial cell-conditioned medium, indicating its in vivo origin is from the myocardium. Preliminary findings indicated that anti–transferrin antibodies stained adheron particulates and neutralized the inductive activity of myocardial cell-conditioned medium in culture assays of endothelial transformation. As discussed by Isokawa and colleagues (1994), evidence is accumulating that, independent of iron binding, the protein itself can promote mesenchyme proliferation through receptor signaling. Antibodies directed against transferrin receptor have been shown to inhibit endothelial migration and invasion into hypertrophic cartilage. Directly adding the ligand stimulated endothelial formation and migration from a number of sources, indicating that transferrin is an angiogenic protein with chemotactic and chemokinetic properties for endothelial cells (Carlevaro et al 1997). From the above, transferrin merits further investigation as a potential myocardial morphogen.

Cushion Formation Is a Homogenetically Induced Process

Homogenetic induction as originally defined by Spemann (1938) is an inductive interaction between a stimulator (signaling) cell (or tissue) and a responder cell in which the latter on induction itself becomes a signaling tissue. As defined, it is not necessary that the stimulator and responder cells secrete the same or different inductive signals. Transforming growth factor-β-3 is a major candidate to mediate the homogenetic induction of cushion mesenchyme (Potts et al 1991). As reviewed by Runyan and coworkers (1992), TGF-β-3 is required for cushion mesenchyme formation and may operate at both stimulator and target cell levels (Brown et al 1996). On induction by the myocardium (whether by ES antigen or myocardial TGF-β is unclear), endothelial target cells upregulate expression and secretion of their own TGF-β-3 (Nakajima et al 1994; Ramsdell and Markwald 1997). Results using a growth medium harvested from cultured cushion mesenchyme indicate that TGF-β-3 secreted by cushion cells functions in an autocrine mode to sustain endothelial transformation and in a paracrine mode to amplify the original myocardial signal by inducing adjacent unactivated endothelial cells to initiate transformation (Ramsdell and Markwald 1997). Like the ripples from a stone thrown into a small pond, the secretion of TGF-β by myocardially induced target cells may be enough to insure that the myocardium does not have to directly induce each and every target endothelial cell, provided that enough endothelial cells can be stimulated to secrete TGF-β-3. This approaches a "can't miss" scenario consistent with the requirement of a threshold amount of cushion tissue for embryonic survival.

Differentiation of AVC Cushion Mesenchyme

In vivo labeling and in situ expression of marker proteins or mRNA indicate that AVC mesenchyme differentiates into valvular or septal fibroblasts (chapter VI; de la Cruz et al 1983; Wunsch et al 1994; Rongish and Little 1995; Wessels et al 1996). The differentiation of precursor mesenchyme into valve leaflets correlates with expression of transcriptional factors containing homeodomains. Few transcriptional factors have been identified in the AVC segment before endothelial transformation begins. To date, this is limited to *Sox 4* (Schilham et al 1996; Ya et al 1997b), a gene also linked to hematopoiesis. During and after cellularization of the AVC cushions, several homeobox-containing genes are expressed in the mesenchyme (Kern et al 1995). These include two paired-rule gene homologues, *Prx-1* and *Prx-2*, *Mox-1* (Candia et al 1992), and *Msx-1*. However, the knockouts of *Msx-1* (Sakota and Maas 1994), *Prx-1* or *Prx-2* (Kern et al 1995), and *Sox-4* (Shilham et al 1996; Ya et al 1997b) did not visibly affect formation or migration of AVC mesenchyme nor did they seemingly affect differentiation into mitral or tricuspid valve leaflets (although in *Sox-4* knockouts, the outlet valves were severely affected). This suggests that either redundant genetic mechanisms may exist for these genes or that the real function of these genes may not be recognized (see section of inner curvature remodeling). How cushions differentiate into valve leaflets is discussed in chapter VI and a ridge hypothesis is proposed as a molecular mechanism.

Contrasting Development Between Cushion-Forming Segments

The conus and truncus share many structural and molecular similarities to the primitive AVC inlet segment. These include formation of large cellularized cushions, which are often called "ridges", that extend along the entire length and part of the circumference of both the conus and truncus. Smaller ridges of cushion mesenchyme intercalate between the major ridges, giving the lumen of the conus and truncus the appearance of being "fluted" (Thompson et al 1979; Markwald et al 1977). The major cushion ridges fuse across the lumen to form a transitional mesenchymal septum that joins with the aorticopulmonary septum at the level of the truncus. Collectively, the conal, truncal, and aorticopulmonary septa follow a spiral course from the right ventricle through the aortic sac. A sharp bend (backward) occurs after stage 17 at the level of the truncus (Thompson et al 1979). The simplest explanation for this bending or spiraling is that the posterior (caudal) portion of the septated conus must be able to deliver blood from the left ventricle to the fourth aortic arch, and, at the same time, the anterior half of the conus must somehow get blood to the sixth, and most posterior, aortic arch. To assist in this task, neural crest cells emerge from the area between the fourth and sixth branchial arches to form the aorticopulmonary septum. The latter divides the aortic sac into the root of the aorta and the pulmonary trunk. The aorticopulmonary septum ultimately "impales" itself into the conotruncal mesenchymal septum at the level at which the future outlet valves will form (Fig. 9).

Outlet cushions express most of the same markers as the AVC cushions including one, 9G9, that is highly specific for endocardially derived mesenchymal cells (Wessels et al 1996). Adheron particulates containing ES and hLAMP proteins are present in the myocardial basement membrane of the conus and tuncus (Mjaatvedt et al 1991; Sinning et al 1995). *BMP* is expressed in the myocardium of both the AVC and conus-truncus before endothelial transformation. Newly formed cushion mesenchyme in all cushions express *Msx-1* and *Prx*. However, there are important differences. For example, *Mox-1* is expressed only in the outlet cushions and only in the mesenchyme adjacent to the myocardium (Candia et al 1992; Barton et al 1995). A proteoglycan recognized by the monoclonal antibody, d1C4, is expressed by all AVC mesenchyme, but in the conus and truncus, only by the same mesenchymal cells that express *Mox-1* (Capehart et al 1997, see also figure 17). The inhibitory-to-differentiation gene (*Id*) (Evans and O'Brien 1993) is expressed primarily in the AVC cushions. The latter is an unusual basic helix-loop-helix (HLH) protein in that it lacks a DNA-binding region. It is possible that *Id* might exert a unique effect on AVC by interacting with other HLH or Hox genes to form homodimers or heterodimers that could modify their regulatory activities in the AVC. For example, a deletion mutation of *Sox-4*, although expressed in the AVC and and truncus, inhibits valve leaflet formation only in the truncus (Schilham et al

1996; Ya et al 1997b). Thus, there is "genetic wiring" in place that could affect one cushion population more than another even though they have many, if not most genes in common. This becomes obvious as one compares the final phenotypes of the AVC, conus, and truncus.

Role of the Conal and Truncal Cushions in Valvuloseptal Morphogenesis

As in the AV inlet, the role of outlet cushions is to form septa and one-way valves. But although the process seems relatively straightforward in the AV canal, cushion-mediated septation of the conus and truncus is more complex. In part, this is because the outlet cushions of endocardial origin must fuse to form a septum that not only must align with the muscular ventricular septum proximally, but distally must integrate also with a septum of neural crest origin, the aorticopulmonary septum that divides the aortic sac. Trying to understand (and describe) septation of the outlet pathway of the tubular heart may be one of the more daunting challenges in all of embryology. It cogently underscores the advantage of studying development over time in living embryos. A single, postmortem snapshot in a fully defined, mature heart (e.g., stage 38 chick) will not easily explain (1) how the aorticopulmonary septum appears to "elongate" while the conus septum "shortens", resulting in the trunks of the great arteries seemingly taking origin directly from the ventricles; (2) how the outlet valves become positioned within the great arteries just above the level of the ventriculoarterial junction such that the valves are surrounded, not by myocardium, but by the smooth muscle of the vessel walls; and (3) why, below the level of the outlet valves and hidden by the massive walls of the ventricles, there is a small septum that is muscularized by myocardial cells that is derived not from the aorticapulmonary septum but from the original conal septum (Figs. 9 and 10).

The complexity of septating the outlet limb and arterial pole of the heart in all likelihood involves multiple genes, but the molecular concepts of regulation have been slow to emerge. Partly, this may be the result of not fully understanding the interplay between the tissues of the conus, truncus, and aortic sac, which include the cushion mesenchyme, branchial arch mesenchyme, neural crest, myocardium, and endocardium. It is possible that some of the pieces of this puzzle are there but we do not know how to integrate them for lack of any hypothetical framework to interpret their function. For example, expression of *Msx-2* uniquely occurs in the myocardial cells of the conus but not the aorticopulmonary septum nor ventricles (Chan-Thomas et al 1993); this may lead *Msx-2*-positive cells to exit the cell cycle and move toward differentiation, setting up the regional differences in proliferation (Thompson et al 1990) that shorten one septum while elongating another. *Sox-4* expression in the endocardial endothelium of the truncus may alter interactions with neural crest cells that influence formation of the outlet valves while expression of *Mox-1* or D1C4 antigens in conal cushions could promote their muscularization or becoming myocardialized. Some of these ideas are incorporated into a unifying hypothetical concept called the inner curvature hypothesis, which is presented below in *The Inner Curvature or Hub Hypothesis* section.

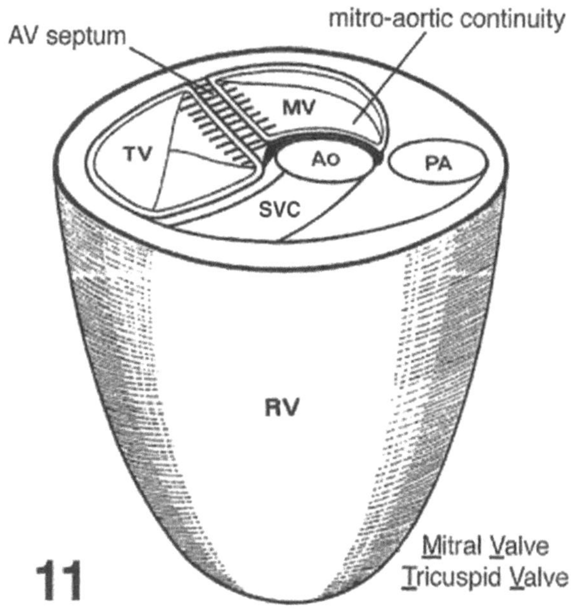

FIGURE 11. Diagram of the fibrous continuity that forms when the arterial pole of the heart wedges into the AV canal after the completion of the second phase of looping at stage 35 in a chick embryo. The figure illustrates how the backside of the mitral valve (MV) (below the plane of section) forms part of the wall of the outlet (aortic vestibule) for the left ventricle, which leads into the aorta (Ao). Note the mitroaortic continuity directly contacts both the AV septum and superventricular crest (SVC).

The Conus

To begin to understand outlet septation, it is important to recognize that the ridges of the conus do not contribute to valvular development, but rather become over time a muscularized septum. The myocardium encircling the conus extends finger-like projections similar to trabeculae into the cushion mesenchyme (Fig. 10). This process was only recently recognized (Rosenquist et al 1990) and has since been termed "myocardialization" by Lamers and colleagues (1995). Pexieder (1975) was the first to observe that the fate of many mesenchymal cells in the proximal outflow tract (i.e., the conus) was cell death or apoptosis. He did not determine its significance, perhaps because he did not recognize that the narrow developmental window in which cell death was observed closely paralleled myocardialization (Ya et al 1997a; Robert Thompson and Cheng Gang, unpublished observations). Thus, one significance of apoptosis in conal mesenchymal cells might be to provide the space or room for the invading myocardial tissue (Maurice Van Den Hoff, Academic Medical Center, University of Amsterdam, personal communication).

Myocardialization may be a mechanism for either driving fusion of the conal cushion ridges or stabilizing their union with each other or the aorticopulmonary septum. In trisomy 16 mice, myocardialization of the conal cushions does not occur and the persisting mesenchymal ridges frequently fail to form a complete septum (A. Wessels and R. Markwald, unpublished observations). We have also found in trisomy

16 mice that if the normal process of conal myocardialization does not occur, the conus remains connected to only the right ventricle, forcing the left ventricle to use the right ventricle as an outlet (viz. double-outlet right ventricle). When the fused conal ridges do not line up and contact the ventricular septum of the inlet limb as in double-outlet right ventricle, a subvalvular ventricular septal defect results that permits communication between the ventricles. Thus, from observations in trisomy 16 mice, a causal correlation may exist between myocardialization of the conal cushions and their ability to form a key septum that, if properly aligned, bridges the gap between the the ventricular septum and the aorticopulmonary septum.

The Truncus

Although never confirmed by dynamic labeling studies, the fate of the truncal cushions, like those of the AVC segment, appears on the basis of molecular makers like JB3 and 9G9 to be to form valve leaflets (Wunsch et al 1994; Bouchey et al 1996; Wessels et al. 1996). Whether the leaflets of the inlet and outlet segments form by similar mechanisms is virtually unknown but seems unlikely given the differential response to mutation of the *Sox-4* gene. Whether they ever really fuse to form a mesenchymalized septum that is impaled by the "elongating" aorticopulmonary septum also remains a controversial question. What is clear is that the truncal cushions are not myocardialized, but rather the myocardium of the truncus, like that of the AVC, disappears leaving only mesenchymal tissue (Fig. 10d). Two hypotheses have been advanced to explain the loss of truncal myocardium. The first, proposed by Thompson and colleagues (1985), is that the truncal myocardium is actively retracted back toward the right ventricle where it either participates in the myocardialization of the conus septum or it is "absorbed" into the right ventricular wall as part of the ventriculoarterial junction. It is proposed that a "septation complex" of fibromuscular tissue serves to generate a rotational, retractive force upon the truncal myocardium. A second hypothesis is that the cardiac muscle transdifferentiates into mesenchyme (Arguello et al 1978). In vivo labeling experiments in which tatoos are applied to the myocardium support the rotational retraction hypothesis. However, as shown in Fig. 10d, in those areas of the truncus where the myocardium is "disappearing", the persisting mesenchymal-like cells show evidence of faint, granular staining for myosin heavy chains. Lamers and colleagues (Ya et al 1997a) have observed a short but distinct burst of mitotic activity (from bromodeoxyuridine uptake) in these cells at the stage shown in Fig. 10. Whatever the mechanism, it is developmentally important because the persisting mesenchyme will become part of a structure called the mitroaortic continuity. The latter is established when looping of the heart is completed, i.e., when the aortic portion of the truncal mesenchyme comes into direct contact with the AV inlet segment. As a result, the backside of the developing mitral valve (derived from the superior AV cushion) literally will form part of the wall of the left ventricular outlet (Fig. 11). Thus, the existence of a mitroaortic continuity indicates that looping has been completed, and as directly demonstrated in living embryos (chapter VII), it shows how the superior AV cushion can contribute to the outlet of the left ventricle.

Another indication that the conus and truncus are under different gene regulation is the Keeshond dog (Patterson et al 1993). In this animal model, a single major gene defect affects only the conus. The mutation appears to affect myocardial development, including its ability to signal cushion tissue formation. The outcome, in this circumstance, is a defective conal septum that varies between none ("persistent truncus arteriosus") to stenosis of the right ventricular outlet ("pseudo truncus arteriosus"). The latter is similar to a serious human cardiac anomaly, tetralogy of Fallot (chapter X).

Neural Crest and the Outflow Cushions

Both the conal and truncal cushions, unlike those of the AVC segment, are invaded by neural crest cells. From studies using retroviral labeling or chimeric grafts, it has been shown that the cardiac neural crest cells gain entrance to the truncus through the aorticopulmonary septum and by migrating from the branchial arches into the lateral walls of the aortic sac and from there into the truncal cushions. Collectively, they form a column or "prong" of cells in each truncal cushion with a few isolated cells remaining beneath the myocardium (Noden et al 1995; Kirby and Waldo 1995; Bergwerff et al 1997; Waldo et al 1997). The number of cells in the prongs progressively diminishes as the crest continues to migrate into the conus ridges. A few, isolated crest cells even "turn the corner" of the inner curvature to enter the base of the superior AV cushion. The neural crest cells of the conus appear to undergo apoptosis whereas those of the truncus remain viable (Robert Poelmann and Adriana Gittenberger-deGroot, unpublished observations). Most of the viable crest cells ultimately express α-smooth muscle actin, particularly when they condense into a central aggregate that forms after the cushion ridges have fused (Ya et al 1997a; Waldo et al 1997). Although the number of mesenchymal cells in the truncal or conal ridges derived from crest cells is small compared with those derived from endothelium (Poelmann, personal communication), crest ablation experiments (Kirby 1993) or mutations in genes, e.g., *Pax-3* (the splotch mutation: Epstein et al 1991), that affect crest cell formation or migration profoundly alter the alignment of the conus and arterial pole over the ventricular septum.

Thus, a major difference between the cushion-forming segments is the immigration of neural crest. Apart from its obvious role in septation, a major question is the role of the neural crest below the level of the future outlet valves. In particular, what is the developmental significance, if any, of those condensed prongs of crest that extend through the truncus and continue as free cells even into the distal (ventricular) reaches of the superior AV cushion (Karen Waldo, personal communication; Waldo et al 1997)? Are they just aorticopulmonary septal cells that migrated too far, overshooting their intended mark (the junction of the aortic sac with the truncus)?. Or is there developmental significance that correlates with the fate of the outflow segment? For example, are they needed to seal the union of the aorticopulmonary septum with the fused truncal and conal cushions or to catalyze the fusion or stabilization of the conus ridges? If they represent, in terms of mass, only a small percentage of the total mesenchyme in the cushion ridges, is there some other function, like secretion of morphogens? Is there a connection between their presence or total cell number and the remodeling (removal) of the myocardium of the conus and truncus by myocardialization, transdifferentiation, or some other retractive mechanism? These and other questions, such as the significance of conal crest becoming apoptotic, all serve to underscore that unique genetic activities may be delivered and imparted to those cushions that host neural crest. Some of these questions may have direct bearing on the postseptal activities that serve to complete the integration of the inflow and outflow segments into the chambers of the mature, fully defined heart.

POSTSEPTAL MORPHOGENESIS: ESTABLISHING THE FOUR-CHAMBERED HEART

Transforming the primitive, U-shaped, heart tube into a four-chambered organ with all septa properly aligned is an active, ongoing process requiring (1) correct expression of segmental identity along the A-P axis; (2) correct looping and torsion of the segmented, tubular heart; (3) formation of extracardiac mesenchyme at arterial and venous poles; (4) formation of muscular and mesenchymal septa; and (5) the proper alignment of segments.

Significance of Segmental Alignment

Integration of the segments is a critical phase of septation. The reason for this is as follows. The primitive inlet (AV canal) develops initially in the posterior limb and, therefore, is in direct continuity with the left ventricle. The outlet or conus is associated with the anterior limb and is directly continuous with the right ventricle (Fig. 1, 4, and 5). Simply stated, one ventricle—the left—"owns" the inlet, the other ventricle—the right—solely possesses the outlet. For each ventricle to have its own inlet and outlet, they must share with the other. As described in more anatomical and literal terms by Lamers and coworkers (1992), "sharing" of the inlet and outlet segments between the venticles requires that the conus "shifts" to the left and the AV inlet "shifts" to the right. The morphogenetic mechanism by which these segments shift with respect to the ventricles is another relatively unexplored question. However, it is important to understand these "morphogenetic shifts" do not occur simultaneously. At stage 17 HH, the trabeculated region of each ventricle is connected through their own inlet to the atrium. In this way, the pattern of the four chambered heart is established even though the conus remains connected to the right ventricle. At later stages (26–35), the left ventricle acquires its own outlet as the conus "shifts" to the left. A visible outcome of failing to properly align the segments, i.e. and colleagues to abnormally retain the primitive condition, is considered by Anderson and colleagues (Anderson 1989; Anderson et al 1996) as one basis for double inlet of the left ventricle or double outlet of the right (namely, they do not share). Lamers and associates (1992, 1995) and Gittenberger-de Groot and coworkers (1995) suggest that the shifts (in segmental alignment) are remodeling events related to the completion of looping, particularly the second phase of looping. Recall, from above, the second phase of looping correlates with a progressive deepening of the inner curvature that ultimately brings the two limbs of the heart "face-to-face", manifested in part by the formation of a mitroaortic continuity and the wedging of the aorta between the atria.

The ventriculo-infundibular fold is that part of the inner curvature that acts as the hinge point on which the two limbs of the heart bend or fold. Is it possible that the inner curvature must physically be diminished or remodeled for the fold or crease to deepen sufficiently to bring the two limbs of the heart together and complete looping? In other words, completion of looping may require removal or redistribution of the tissues of the inner curvature.

Anatomically, the inner curvature is composed of cardiac muscle and the mesenchyme of the superior AV cushion and the sinistro-ventral conal cushion (Fig. 12). There is evidence from our studies on normal and trisomy 16 mice that the remodeling of the inner curvature and the deepening of its ventriculo-infundibular

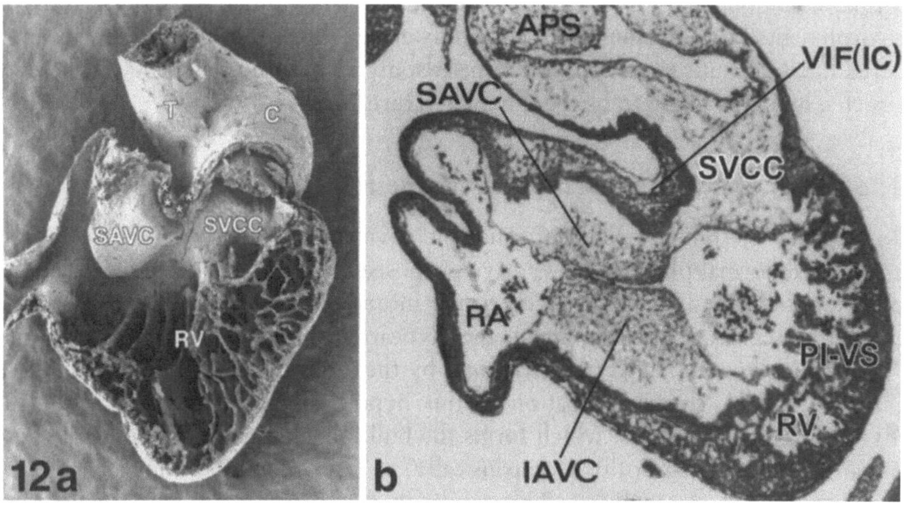

FIGURE 12. The tissues of the inner curvature of the stage 25 chick heart. **a.** A scanning electron micrograph of a heart in which the left ventricle and inferior AV cushion (IAVC of Fig. 13b) have been removed to afford a right lateral view of the heart. Notice that the inner curvature is composed of both myocardial tissue (asterisks) and the combined superior AV cushion (SAVC) and sinistroventral conal cushion (SVCC). A sharp bend occurs at the boundary between the conus (C) and truncus (T). **b.** A light microscopic, sagittal section approximating the SEM image. The tissues forming the ventricular infundibular fold or inner curvature [VIF(IC)] are clearly delineated. The union of the SVCC and SAVC will form a complete sleeve of mesenchyme. Progressive deepening of the VIF(IC) occurs during the second phase of looping, which will bring the inlet and outlet limbs into direct contact. Also observe the gradual thinning of the myocardium as one moves distally from the conus, particularly in the area where the aorticopulmonary septum (APS) has impaled the the truncal septum. (PI-VS, primary interventricular septum; RA, RV, right atrium and ventricle, respectively.)

fold occurs as a result of "myocardialization". By the latter we mean that the thickness of the wall of the inner curvature is thinned or diminished by the redistribution of the myocardium as a result of myocardial cells literally invading the underlying cushions (conal and superior SAVC cushions) (Figs. 9 and 10). As a consequence, the conus septum—initially all mesenchyme—becomes the muscular outlet septum. In trisomy 16 mice, the process of myocardialization is inhibited, and the conus septum remains mesenchymalized (Fig. 10; Wessels and Markwald, unpublished observations), looping is incomplete (Webb et al 1996), no mitroaortic continuity is established, and conotruncal defects like double-outlet right ventricle occur. A similar spectrum of cardiac abnormalities, including double-outlet right ventricle, also occurs with many other gene and environmental perturbations. These include neural crest ablation (Kirby and Waldo 1995), knockouts of endothelin-1 receptor (Kurihara et al 1995), retinoid receptors (Sucov et al 1994), the double (but not single) knockout of *msx-1* and *msx-2* (Y-P Chen, personal communication), knockout of TGF-β-2 ligand (Sanford et al 1997), trisomy 13 (Vuillemin et al 1991), treatment with retinoids (Bouman et al 1995), altering hemodynamics (Hogers et al 1997), and mechanically restricting flexure of the head and thorax (Männer et al 1995).

The question then becomes, if so many diverse genetic or environmental perturbations result in a similar phenotype, what is a spoke and what is the hub? Is there a final common pathway through which many genes function (unless affected environmentally or by mutation) to ultimately establish the mature, four-chambered heart? Results from studies on the trisomy 16 mouse suggest that if there is a such a hub, it is likely to be the inner curvature.

The "Inner Curvature or 'Hub' Hypothesis"

To explain why so many different genes and environmental perturbations result in a similar abnormal phenotype, we have proposed a working hypothesis: To complete looping (or to deepen the ventricular-infundibular fold) and bring the inlet and outlet segments into alignment, the myocardium of the inner curvature (the "hub") must be remodeled (redistributed) by the morphogenetic process of myocardialization. A conceptualization of this hypothesis is given in Fig. 13. The myocardium of the conus, which forms the bulk of the inner curvature, acquires potential (either intrinsically or extrinsically) to circumferentially invade the underlying cushion mesenchyme. This results in a concomitant thinning or loss of myocardium at the inner curvature as the cushion progenitors of the outlet septum become myocardialized.

Evidence in living embryos that the mesenchymalized cushion tissues of the inner curvature do, in fact, become muscularized (as predicted by the hypothesis) can be shown if a bead is placed into the proximal sinistro-ventral conus cushion near the sites indicated by #3 in Fig. 13 at stage 22 (before the onset of myocardialization) and examined later at stage 35 (after the second phase of looping is completed): the bead or marker is found in the supraventricular crest (see chapter VII [fig. 4]). In the mature heart, the supraventricular crest is a muscularized structure found within the

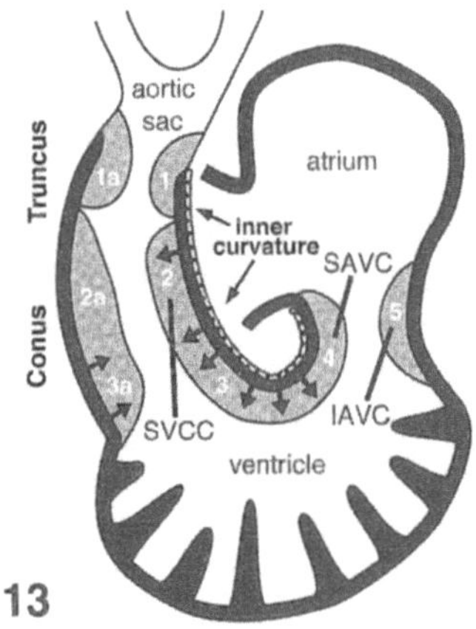

13

FIGURE 13. The concept of myocardialization is shown using the diagram described in Fig. 4. As indicated by the direction of the arrows, the myocardium of the conus region including that of the inner curvature is redistributed as a result of myocardial cells invading the underlying cushions. The outcome is a progressive thinning or removal of the myocardium along the inner curvature, except in the truncus region where the myocardium is either retracted or transdifferentiates into mesenchyme. The numbers correspond to positions that are currently being used to microinject in vivo markers to determine fate. For example, a bead inserted at position #3 at stage 19 will be found in the superventricular crest at stage 35.

right ventricle that separates the inflow and outflow blood streams of this chamber. The in vivo bead experiments indicate that the origin of the supraventricular crest is derived from the proximal dextro dorsal conal cushion after its myocardialization. It is not surprising then that in trisomy 16 mice or in mice with a targeted deletion of TGF β-2, two circumstances in which myocardioalization does not occur, there is no definitive supraventricular crest. Its mesenchymal precursor remains part of the incomplete, mesenchymalized conal septum.

A portion of the superior AV cushion also is included with the inner curvature (Fig. 13). Does this mean that an inlet cushion can also participate in remodeling of the inner curvature through the process of myocardialization, and if so, for what purpose? Again, from studies in trisomic mice, particularly by Robert Anderson and colleagues (Anderson et al 1996; Webb et al 1996; Webb 1997), it would appear that remodeling of the inner curvature at the level of the superior AV cushion might be causally related to the rightward shift of the AV canal. Depending on how much or how little a shift or remodeling occurs will determine the phenotype of the AV canal. Normally, remodeling or shifting results in an equal balance between the size of the inlet orifices. If remodeling is only partially complete, as in the trisomic 16 mouse, the right AV opening will be small compared with the left, resulting in unbalanced AV inlets and a phenotype similar to human tricuspid atresia (Fig. 14). No shift to the right at all results in retention of the primitive embryonic state or double-inlet left ventricle. Thus, the degree of shifting determines the balance in size between the two AV inlets. In the hub hypothesis, the degree of balance would be determined by the extent of remodeling of the inner curvature.

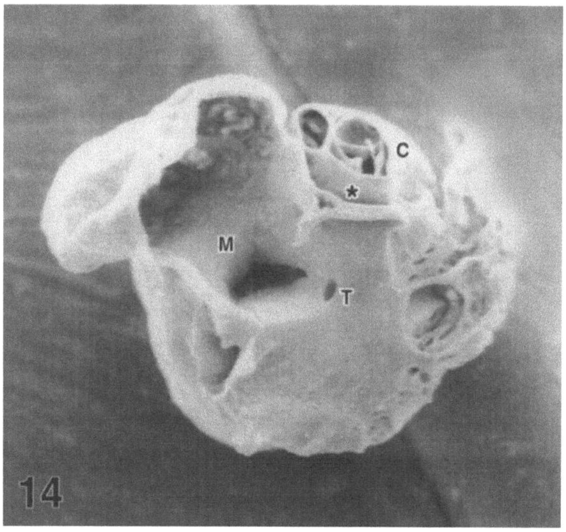

FIGURE 14. Scanning electron micrograph of a trisomy 16 mouse heart in which the atria have been removed to reveal the AV canal and conus (C). In this animal model, the second phase of looping is not completed. This correlates with the failure of the conus to contact the posterior limb as evidenced by the persistence of the ventriculo-infundibular fold (asterisk) and absence of a wedged aorta. The tricuspid (T) orifice has not been remodeled, resulting in a small right ventricular inlet and a large mitral (M) orifice (tricuspid atresia). (Micrograph kindly provided by Dr. Robert Anderson, London.)

The key to the hub or inner curvature hypothesis is remodeling, primarily through the mechanism of myocardialization (not necessarily being the only mechanism) (Fig. 13). How then is myocardialization regulated? Is it intrinsic to the myocardial cells of the inner curvature—or is it extrinsically mediated? We have proposed two corollaries to the hub hypothesis to answer these and other questions. Both envision cushion tissue as the primary causal factor (Fig. 15).

Corollary One: Cushions Induce Myocardialization

The myocardium of the inner curvature is lined by a continuous sleeve of cushion mesenchyme derived mostly from the sinistral-ventral conal ridge but includes a contribution from the superior AV cushion. There is also temporal specificity to the myocardialization of this mesenchyme. It has a specific window (Fig. 15). In the chick, it is from stage 26 to stage 34; in the mouse, day 13 to late day 15. A major

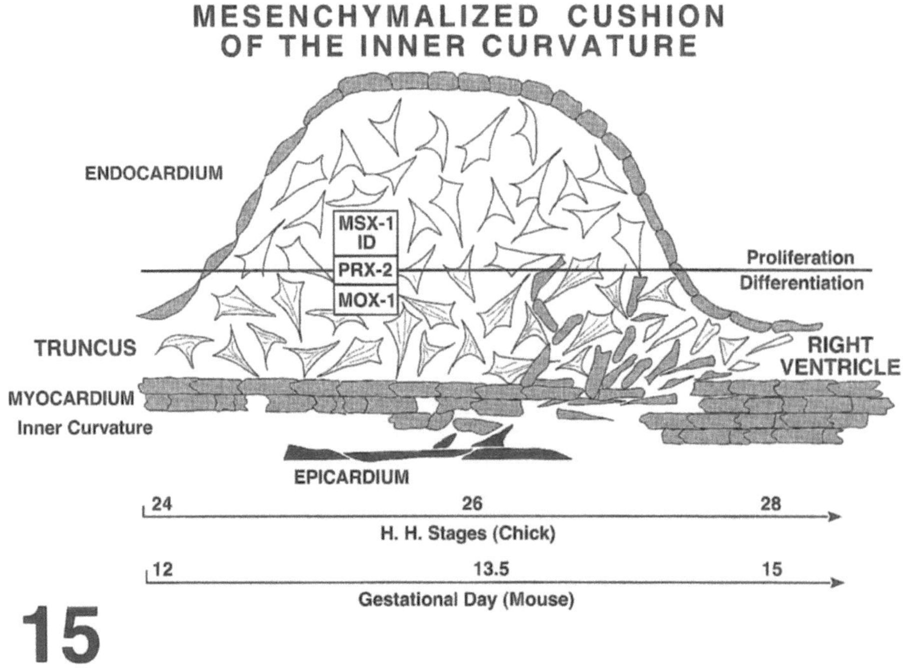

15

FIGURE 15. Conceptualization of the "inner curvature" hypothesis: mesenchymalized cushions along the inner curvature induce myocardialization at specific time points (e.g., stage 26+ in the chick), which promotes muscularization of the cushions, thinning of the myocardium, deepening of the ventriculo-infundibular fold, and the completion of looping. The potential to induce myocardialization is envisioned as a differentiative function of a subset of mesenchymal cells associated with the myocardium. These cells (indicated by shading) are under different regulatory gene control (e.g., *Mox-1*) than cells closer to the endocardium. The latter (unshaded) cells express *Msx-1* or the *Id* gene, which correlates with proliferation or antidifferentiation (as it relates to the potential to myocardialize). Other genes like the homeobox *Prx-2* are expressed throughout the cushions and may provide overlapping (redundant) regulation of proliferation or differentiation.

question is whether there are intrinsic changes that occur in the myocardium during this window that initiate invasion of the cushions or do intrinsic changes in the cushions themselves lead to their being myocardialized, e.g., by the secretion of a morphogen?

For certain, the myocardial cells of the inner curvature are different from others in that they spin off the cell cycle early, becoming the first terminally differentiated myocardial cells in the heart (Thompson et al 1990). They also are among the subpopulation of myocardial cells that express the homeobox-containing gene, *Msx-2* (Chan-Thomas et al 1993). Similarly, as described below, cushion cells immediately contiguous to the myocardium of the inner curvature also appear to be a subset of cushion mesenchyme expressing unique markers of differentiation. The presence of two, adjacent populations of potentially specialized cells suggests that a tissue interaction between them may trigger myocardialization.

To ferret out the regulatory mechanisms of myocardialization, we again turned to the collagen gel culture system (Fig. 16). Cultures of the isolated inner curvature of the conus (cushion + myocardium) were compared for potential to myocardialize, based on proximity to the developmental window for myocardialization (Fig. 15). At stages 26 and older, a robust outgrowth of cushion mesenchyme into the gel was followed by multiple, fingerlike invasive outgrowths from the myocardial portion of the explant into the mesenchyme. Myocardial outgrowths were confirmed by antibody staining for cardiac myosin heavy chains.

Conversely, an equally robust outgrowth of mesenchyme was established from conus explants taken before the normal period for myocardialization in vivo (e.g., stage 19, Fig. 16). The difference between the two explants (stage 19 versus 26+) was that no muscularized ingrowths into the mesenchyme occurred in the younger explants unless they were cocultured with the older conus tissues or their conditioned medium (Wessels and Markwald, unpublished data). Importantly, these findings were similar to those obtained by coculturing the conus of a stage 20 embryo with the truncus region of the same staged embryo. Without the truncus, there was minimal myocardialization of the young explant (Fig. 16e), but with the truncus, numerous elongated myocardial outgrowths into cushion mesenchyme were formed (Fig. 16f; A. Wessels, R. Markwald, M. Van den Hoff, and W. Lamers, unpublished findings). This was an intriguing culture finding because in vivo only the conus, not the truncus, undergoes myocardialization . So why does the truncus promote myocardialization in the conus before it normally would do so? One possible answer is the neural crest. In the conus, neural crest cells undergo apoptosis; in the truncus, they are more numerous and viable. Could apoptosis release a signal that affects the potential of cushion mesenchyme to induce myocardialization? The abundant crest population of the truncus may not have been viable under our culture conditions and, as a consequence of cell death, released a hypothetical signal that stimulated in vitro conal myocardialization. These results, although preliminary, together suggest that mesenchyme must reach a point of differentiation to induce or sustain myocardialization and that (unknown) secretory factors produced by the more differentiated cushion tissues or neural crest initiate myocardial outgrowths.

The spatiotemporal expression of two markers—d1C4 antigen and apolipoprotein J (apo-J)—support this suggestion. Two potential subpopulations of conal mesenchyme were identified by these markers at the time of myocardialization: those adjacent to the myocardium versus the lumen (myocardial versus luminal "faces"). D1C42 antigens were expressed rather uniformly in AV cushion mesenchyme, but in the conus, D1C4 was expressed immediately before the onset of myocardialization and only in mesenchyme of the myocardial face (Fig. 17).

The spatial and temporal expression of apo-J mRNA in conal mesenchyme is similar to that for D1C4 antigens (Witte et al 1996), namely, in the conus it is expressed in the mesenchyme of the myocardial face, particularly along the inner curvature. Apo-J is a protein frequently associated with remodeling events, or the processing of protein precursors.

The expression of apo-J affords one clue as to how cushions might promote or sustain myocardialization. The secreted apo-J lipoprotein can bind protease precursors known to be expressed by cushion cells, e.g., urokinase (McGuire and Alexander 1993), thrombospondin (O'Shea et al 1990), or protein precursors of activators or inhibitors of protease activity (Stefansson et al 1996). In turn, apo-J–protein complexes bind to a specific low-density lipoprotein receptor, LRP-2, which promotes endocytosis and activation of protein precursors within endosomes with the activated protease released extracellularly, much like the paradigm for antigen processing (Kounnas et al 1995). Significantly, we have found that myocardial cells of the inner curvature express the LRP-2 receptor (C. Mjaatvedt and R. Markwald, unpublished observations). Thus, the apo-J–LRP-2 system provides one, potentially site-directable, mechanism for regulating myocardialization, by secreting factors that might modify cell–cell or cell–substrate adhesions.

Corollary Two: Homeobox-Containing Genes Regulate Cushion Cell Differentiation and Potential to Induce Myocardialization (Fig. 15)

Although several homeobox-containing genes are expressed in the heart, primarily in the cushions, their role in cardiac morphogenesis remains unclear, possibly because we have not known what to look for (Kern et al 1995; Eisenberg and Markwald 1995). In Fig. 15, (Chan-Thomas et al 1993; Barton et al 1995), we propose, on the basis of in vivo pattern of expression, that two transcription factors, *Msx-1* and *Mox-1* (also called *Meox*), regulate proliferation versus differentiation of cushion mesenchyme. Specifically, *Msx-1*, perhaps in concert with two other transcription factors expressed in cushion cells, *Prx-2* and *Id* gene (inhibitory to differentiation), are envisioned as pro-proliferation or antidifferentiation.

According to this model, mesenchyme closest to the lumen (luminal face) would retain proliferative potential under *Msx-1* regulation and ultimately expand into a cushion ridge or leaflet (see also chapter VI). Conversely, as cushion mesenchymal cells migrate from the luminal face into the myocardial face, they express *Mox-1*. Under the influence of *Mox-1*, cushion cells progress in their differentiation pathway, as measured by potential to promote myocardialization and therefore to become competent to remodel the inner curvature. Thus, *Mox-1* is prodifferentiation. If true, this hypothesis would predict that a knockout of *Msx-1* would not produce a heart phenotype because only an inhibitory (antidifferentiative) function would be lost, assuming other factors (e.g., *Prx-2* or growth factors) could sustain proliferation. Indeed, consistent with this hypothesis, no cardiac phenotype was observed in mice having a targeted homozygous recombinant deletion of *Msx-1* (Sakota and Maas 1994). Conversely, a knockout for *Mox-1* would be an excellent test of the hypothesis. Because of its proposed prodifferentiation function, a knockout of *Mox-1*, if it could be developed, would be expected to inhibit looping, myocardialization, and alignment of septa with double-outlet right ventricle a likely phenotype if the hypothesis is true.

CONCLUSION

Although most current studies presently emphasize molecular genetics or gene regulation of heart development (Olson and Srivastava 1996; Fishman and Chien 1997), we must not forget that the anatomical organization of the heart is the outcome of multiple genetic events operating at different regulatory and morphological levels. Precardiac mesoderm (Lough et al 1990) and embryonic stem cells (Robbins et al 1992) growing in culture will differentiate into myocardial cells but they do not form a heart tube. As we have endeavored to show in this chapter, the potential to learn more about cardiogenesis is as dependent upon appreciating and integrating new morphological data as identifying new genes (Anderson 1989). For example, future morphological studies on the extracardiac mesenchyme of the spina vestibuli may greatly assist in understanding the function of a hypothetical "new" gene that is not expressed in the heart fields or tube but whose mutagenesis nevertheless results in atrial septal defects or abnormal pulmonary venous return. Thus, we conclude that although creating transgenic animal models obviously holds enormous potential for advancing the field, the potential is more fully realized when changes in gene function are integrated and correlated with morphological changes, particularly when viewed over time in living embryos using dynamic imaging approaches.

REFERENCES

Anderson RH. 1989. The present-day place of correlations between embryology and anatomy in the understanding of congenitally malformed hearts. In: Aranega A, Pexieder T, editors. Correlations between experimental cardiac embryology and teratology and congenital cardiac defects. University of Granada Press. p 265–95.

Anderson RH, Webb S, Brown NA. 1996. Establishing the anatomic hallmarks of congenitally malformed hearts. Trends Cardiovasc Med 6:10–5.

Alexander SM, Jackson KJ, Bushnell KM, McGuire PG. 1997. Spatial and temporal expression of the 72-kDa type IV collagenase (MMP-2) correlates with development and differentiation of valves in the embryonic avian heart. Dev Dyn 209:261–8.

Arguello C, De La Cruz MV, Sanchez C. 1978. Ultrastructural and experimental evidence of myocardial cell differentiation into connective tissue cells in embryonic chick heart. J Mol Cell Cardiol 10:307–15.

Asami I, Koizumi K. 1995. Development of the atrial septal complex in the human heart: contribution of the spina vestibuli. In: Clark EB, Markwald RR, Takao A, editors. Developmental mechanisms of heart disease. Armonk, NY: Futura Publishing Company. p 255–60.

Barton PJR, Boheler KR, Brand NJ, Thomas PJ. 1995. Molecular biology of cardiac development and growth Austin TX: Landes Co. Chapter 2; p 56.

Bergwerff M, Verberne MEM, DeRuiter MC, Poelman RE, Gittenberger-de Groot. 1997. Neural crest cell contribution to the developing circulatory system: implications for vascular morphology. Circ Res (in press).

Bernanke DH, Markwald RR. 1982. Migratory behavior of cardiac cushion tissue cells in a collagen lattice culture system. Dev Biol 91:235–45.

Bouchey D, Argraves WS, Little CD. 1996. Fibulin-1, vitronectin and fibronectin in valvuloseptal development. Anat Rec 244:540–51.

Bouman HGA, Broekhuizen MLA, Baasten MJ, Gittenberger-de Groot, AC, Wenink ACG. 1995. A spectrum of looping disturbances in stage 34 chicken hearts after retinoic acid treatment. Anat Rec 243:101–8.
Bouwmeester T, Kim T, Sasai Y, Lu B, De Robertis EM. 1996. Cerbrus is a head-inducing secreted factor expressed in the anterior endoderm of Spemann's organizer. Nature (Land) 382:595–601.
Brown CG, Boyer AS, Runyan RB, Barnett JV. 1996. Antibodies to the type II TGF beta receptor block cell activation and migration during atrioventricular cushion transformation in the heart. Dev Biol 174:248–57.
Brueckner MD, Horwich AL. 1989. Linkage mapping of a mouse gene, iv, that controls left-right asymmetry of the heart and viscera. Proc Natl Acad Sci USA 86:5035–39.
Candia A-F, Hu J, Crosby J, Lalley PA, Noden D, Nadeau JH, Wright CVE. 1992. *Mox-1* and *Mox-2* define a novel homeobox gene subfamily and are differentially expressed during early mesodermal patterning in mouse embryos. Development (Camb) 116:1123–36.
Capehart AA, Weinecke MM, Kitten GT, Solursh M, EL, Krug EL. 1997. Production of a monoclonal antibody by in vitro immunization that recognizes a native chondroitin sulfate epitope in the embryonic chick limb and heart. J Histochem Cytochem.
Carlevaro MF, Albini A, Ribatti D, Gentili C, Benelli R, Cermelli S, Cancedda R. 1997. Transferrin promotes endothelial cell migration and invasion: implication in cartilage neovascularization. J Cell Biol 136:1375–84.
Chan-Thomas P, Thompson RP, Robert B, Yacoub MH, Barton PJ. 1993. Expression of homeobox genes *Msx-1 (Hox-7)* and *Msx-2 (Hox-8)* during cardiac development in the chick. Dyn 197:203–16.
Coffin JD, Poole TJ. 1991. Endothelial cell origin and migration in embryonic heart and cranial blood vessel development. Anat Rec 231:383–95.
Crossin KL, Hoffman S. 1991. Expression of adhesion molecules during the formation and differentiation of the avian endocardial cushion tissue. Dev Biol 145:277–86.
Davis CL. 1924. The cardiac jelly of the chick embryo. Anat Rec 27:201–2.
de la Cruz MV, Sanchez-Gomez C, Arteaga MM, Arguello C. 1977. Experimental study of the development of the truncus and the conus in the chick embryo. J Anat 123: 661–86.
de la Cruz MV, Robota GM, Saravalli O, Cayre R. 1983. The contribution of the inferior cushion of the atrioventricular valves: study in the chick embryo. Am J Anat 166:63–72.
de la Cruz MV, Sanchez-Gomez C, Palomino MA. 1989. The primitive cardiac regions in the straight tube heart (stage 9^-) and their anatomical expression in the mature heart: an experimental study in the chick heart. J Anat 165:121–31.
de la Cruz MV, Castillo MM, Villavicencio L, Valencia GA, Moreno-Rodriguez RA. 1997. Primitive interventricular septum, its primordium, and its contribution in the definitive interventricular septum: in vivo labelling study in the chick embryo. Anat Rec 247: 512–20.
DeRuiter MC, Gittenberger-deGroot AC, Wenink ACG, Mentink MMT. 1995. In normal development pulmonary veins are connected to the sinus venosus segment in the left atrium. Anat Rec 243:84–92.
DeRuiter MC, Poelmann RF, VanMunsteren JC, Mironov V, Markwald R, Gittenberger-de Groot. 1997. Embryonic endothelial cells transdifferentiate into mesenchymal cells expressing smooth muscle actins in vivo and in vitro. Circ Res 80:444–51.
Drake CJ, Little CD. 1995. Exogenous VEGF induces malformed and hyperfused vessels. Proc Natl Acad Sci USA 92:7657–61.
Eisenberg LM, Markwald RR. 1995. Molecular regulation of atrioventricular valvuloseptal morphogenesis. Circ Res 77:1–6.
Epstein DJ, Vekemans M, Gros P. 1991. *Splotch* (*Sp2H*), a mutation affecting development of the mouse neural tube, shows a deletion within the paired homeodomain of *Pax-3*. Cell 67:767–74.

Evans SM, O'Brien TX. 1993. Expression of the helix-loop-helix factor *ID* during mouse embryonic development. Dev Biol 159:485–99.
Fishman MC, Chien KR. 1997. Fashioning of the vertebrate heart: earliest embryonic decisions. Development (Camb) 124:2099–117.
Franco D, Kelly R, Buckingham M, Moorman AFM. 1997. Regionalized transcriptional domains of myosin light chain 3f transgenes in the embryonic mouse heart: morphogenetic implications. Dev Biol 187:17–33.
Funderburg FM, Markwald RR. 1986. Conditioning of native substrates by chondroitin sulfate proteoglycans during cardiac mesenchymal cell migration. J Cell Biol 103:2475–87.
Garcia-Martinez V, Schoenwolf GC. 1993. Primitive steak origin of the cardiovascular system in avian embryos. Dev Biol 159:706–19.
Gerety M, Watanabe M. 1997. Polysialylated NCAM on endocardial cells of the chick primary atrial septum. Anat Rec 247:71–84.
Gittenberger-de Groot AC, Bartelings MM, Poelmann RE. 1995. Cardiac morphogenesis. In: Clark EB, Markwald RR, Takao A, editors. *Developmental mechanisms of heart disease*. Armonk, NY: Futura Publishing Company, p 157–68.
Goldmuntz E, Emmanuel BS. 1997. Genetic disorders of cardiac morphogenesis: the DiGeorge and velocardiofacial syndromes. Circ Res 80:437–43.
Hall CL, Wang C, Lange LA, Turley EV. 1994. Hyaluronan and the hyaluronan receptor RHAMM promote focal adhesion turnover and transient tyrosine kinase activity. J Cell Biol 126:575–88.
Hamburger V, Hamilton HL. 1951. A series of normal stages in the development of the chick embryo. J Morphol 88:49–92.
Hiltgen G, Litke LL, Markwald RR. 1995. Morphogenetic alterations during endocardiac cushion development in trisomy 16 (Down's) mouse. Pediatr Cardiol 17:21–30.
Hogers B, DeRuiter MC, Gittenberger-deGroot AC, Poelmann RE. 1997. Unilateral vitelline vein ligation alters intracardiac blood flow patterns and morphogenesis in the chick embryo. Circ Res 80:473–481.
Hoyle C, Brown NA, Wolpert L. 1992. Development of left/right handedness in the chick heart. Development (Camb) 115:1071–8.
Icardo JM, Sanchez MJ. 1991. Spectrum of heart malformations in mice with situs solitus, situs inversus, and associated visceral heterotaxy. Circulation 84:2547–58.
Ikeda T, Iwasaki K, et al. 1990. Leu7 immunoreactivity in human and rat embryonic hearts, with special reference to the development of the conduction tissue. Anat Embryol 182:553–62.
Isokawa K, Rezaee M, Wunsch A, Markwald R, Krug EL. 1994. Identification of transferrin as one of multiple EDTA-extractable extracellular proteins involved in early chick heart morphogenesis. J Cell Biochem 54:207–18.
Jones CM, Lyons KM, Hogan BLM. 1991. Involvement of *bone morphogenetic protein-4* (BMP-4) and *Vgr-1* in morphogenesis and neurogenesis in the mouse. Development (Camb) 111:531–42.
Kern MJ, Argao EA, Potter SS. 1995. Homeobox genes and heart development. Trends Cardiovasc Med 5:47–54.
Kirby ML. 1993. Cellular and molecular contributions of the cardiac neural crest to cardiovascular development. Trends Cardiovasc Med 3:18–23.
Kirby ML, Waldo K. 1995. Neural crest and cardiovascular patterning. Circ Res 77:211–5.
Kitten GT, Markwald RR, Bolender DL. 1987. Distribution of basement membrane antigens in cryopreserved early embryonic hearts. Anat Rec 217:379–90.
Kornenberg JR, Bradley C, Disteche CM. 1992. Down syndrome molecular mapping of the congenital heart disease and duodenal stenosis. Am J Hum Gen et 50:294–302.
Kounnas MZ, Loukinova EB, Stefansson S, Harmony JA, Brewer BH, Strickland DK, Argraves WS. 1995. Identification of glycoprotein 330 as an endocytic receptor for apolipoprotein J/clusterin. J Biol Chem 270:13070–5.

Krug EL, Mjaatvedt CH, Markwald RR. 1987. Extracellular matrix from embryonic myocardium elicits an early morphogenetic event in cardiac endothelial differentiation. Dev Biol 120:348–55.

Krug EL, Rezaee M, Isokawa K, Turner DK, Litke LL, Wunsch AM, Bain JL, Riley DA, Capehart AA, Markwald RR. 1995. Transformation of cardiac endothelium into cushion mesenchyme is dependent of ES/130: temporal, spatial, and functional studies in the early chick embryo. Cell Mol Biol Res 41:263–77.

Kurihara Y, Kurihara H, Oda H, Maemura K, Naga R, Ishikawa T. 1995. Aortic arch malformation and ventricular septal defect in mice deficient in endothelin-1. J Clin Invest 99:293–300.

Lamers WH, Wessels A, Verbeek FJ, Moorman AFM, Viragh S, Wenink ACG, Gittenberger-de Groot AC, Anderson RH. 1992. New findings concerning ventricular septation in the human heart. Circulation 86:1194–205.

Lamers WH, Viragh S, Wessels A, Moorman AFM, Anderson RH. 1995. Formation of the tricuspid valve in the human heart. Circ Res 91:111–21.

Layton WM. 1978. Heart malformations in mice homozygous for a gene causing situs inversus. In: Birth Defects: Original Article Series. 14:277–93.

Lee K, Simon H, Chen H, Bates B, Hung M, Hauser C. 1995. Requirement for neuregulin receptor erbB2 in neural and cardiac development. Nature (Lond) 378:394–8.

Levin M, Johnson RL, Stern CD, Keuhn M, Tabin C. 1995. A molecular pathway determing left-right asymmetry in chick embryogenesis. Cell 82:803–14.

Lin Q, Schwartz JA, Olsen EN. 1997. Control of cardiac morphogenesis and myogenesis by the myogenic transcription factor MEF-2C. Science (Wash DC) 276:1404–7.

Lough JW, Bolender DL, Markwald RR. 1990. A culture model for cardiac morphogenesis. In: Embryonic origins of defective heart development. Ann Acad Sci 588:421–4.

Lough J, Barron M, Brogley M, Sugi Y, Bolender DL, Zhu X. 1996. Combined BMP-2 and FGF-4 but neither factor alone, induce cardiogenesis in non-precardiac embryonic mesoderm. Dev Biol 178:198–202.

Lyons R, Parsons LM, Hartley L, Li R, Andrews JE, Robb L, Harvey RP. 1995. Myogenic and morphogenetic defects in the heart tubes of murine embryos lacking the homeo box gene *Nkx2-5*. Genes Dev 9:1654–66.

Manasek FJ. 1976. Heart development: interactions involved in cardiac morphogenesis. In: Postle R, Nicolson G, editors. The cell surface in animal embryogenesis and development. New York: Elsevier. p 545–98.

Manner J, Seidl W, Steding G. 1995. The role of extracardiac factors in normal and abnormal development of the chick embryo: cranial flexure and ventral thoracic wall. Anat Embryol 191:61–72.

Markwald RR, Fitzharris TP, Manasek FJ. 1977. Structural development of endocardial cushions. Am J Anat 148:85–120.

Markwald RR, Bernanke DH, Kitten GT, Runyan RB, Funderburg FM, Brauer PR. 1984. Use of 3-dimensional collagen gel cultures to study cell:matrix interactions in heart development. In: Trelstad R, editor. The role of extracellular matrix in development. 42nd Symposium of The Society for Developmental Biology. Alan R. Liss. New York: p 323–50.

Markwald RR, Rezaee M, Nakajima Y, Wunsch A, Isokawa K, Litke L, Krug EL. 1995. Molecular basis for the segmental pattern of cardiac cushion mesenchyme formation: role of ES/130 in the embryonic chick heart. In: Clark EB, Markwald RR, Takao A, editors. Developmental mechanisms of heart disease. Armonk, NY: Futura Publishing Company. p 185–94.

Markwald RR, Eisenberg L, et al. 1996. Epithelial mesenchymal transformations in early avian heart development. Acta Anat 156:173–86.

Markwald RR, Trusk T, Gittenberger-de Groot AC, Poelman R. 1997. Cardiac morphogenesis: formation and septation of the primary heart tube. In: Kavlock R, Datson G, editor. Handbook of experimental pharmacology. 124/I. Berlin: Springer-Verlag. p 11–40.

McGuire PG, Orkin RW. 1992. Urokinase activity in the developing avian heart: a spatial and temporal analysis. Dev Dyn 193:24–33.

McGuire PG, Alexander SM. 1993. Inhibition of urokinase synthesis and cell surface binding alters the motile behavior of embryonic endocardial derived mesenchymal cells in vitro. Development (Camb) 118:931–9.

Meyer D, Birchmeier C. 1995. Multiple essential functions of neuregulin in development. Nature (Land) 378:386–90.

Mikawa T, Borisov A, Brown AMC, Fischman DA. 1992. Clonal analysis of cardiac morphogenesis in the chicken embryo using a replication-defective retrovirus: I. Formation of the ventricular myocardium. Dev Dyn 195:133–141.

Mjaatvedt CH, Lepera RC, Markwald RR. 1987. Myocardial specificity for initiating endothelial-mesenchymal cell transition in embryonic chick heart correlates with a particulate distribution of fibronectin. Dev Biol 119:59–67.

Mjaatvedt CH, Markwald RR. 1989. Induction of epithelial-mesenchymal transition by an *in vivo* adheron-like complex. Dev Biol 136:118–128.

Mjaatvedt CH, Krug EL, Markwald RR. 1991. An antiserum (ES1) against a particulate form of extracellular matrix blocks the transformation of cardiac endothelium into mesenchyme in culture. Dev Biol 145:219–230.

Moreno-Rodriguez RA, de la Cruz MV, Krug EL. 1997. Temporal and spatial asymmetries in the initial distribution of mesenchyme cells in the atrioventricular canal cushions of the developing chick heart. Anat Rec 248:84–92.

Nakajima Y, Krug EL, Markwald RR. 1994. Myocardial regulation of transforming growth factor-beta expression by outflow tract endothelium in the early embryonic chick heart. Dev Biol 165:615–626.

Nakajima Y, Miyazono K, Kato M, Takase M, Yamagishi T, Nakamura H. 1997a. Extracellular fibrillar structure of latent TGF beta binding protein-1: role in TGF beta-dependent endothelial-mesenchymal transformation during endocardial cushion formation in mouse embryonic hearts. J Cell Biol 136:193–204.

Nakajima Y, Mironov V, Yamagishi T, Nakamura H, Markwald RR. 1997b. Expression of smooth muscle alpha-actin in mesenchymal cells lduring formation of avian endocardial cushion tissue: a role for transforming growth factor beta 3. Dev Dyn 209: 296–309.

Noden DM. 1991. Origins and patterning of avian outflow tract endocardium, Development (Camb) 111:857–861.

Noden DM, Poelmann RE, Gittenberger-de Groot AC. 1995. Cell origins and tissue boundaries during outflow tract development. Trends Cardiovasc Med 5:69–75.

Olsen EN, Srivastava D. 1996. Molecular pathways controlling heart development. Science (Wash DC) 272:671–676.

O'Shea KS, Liu LH, Kinnunen LH, Dixit VM. 1990. Role of extracellular matrix protein thrombospondin in the early development of the mouse embryo. J, Cell Biol 111:2713–23.

Patterson DF, Pexieder T, Schnarr WR, Navratil T, Alaili R. 1993. A single major-gene defect underlying cardiac conotruncal malformations interferes with myocardial growth during embryonic development: studies in the CTD line of Keeshond dogs. Am J Hum Genet 52:388–97.

Pexieder T. 1975. Cell death in the morphogenesis and teratogenesis of the heart. Adv Anat Embryol Cell Biol 51 Fasc. 3:1–100.

Pexieder T, Wenink ACG, Anderson RH. 1989. A suggested nomenclature for the developing heart. Int. J. Cardiol 25:255–64.

Pexieder T. 1995. Conotruncus and its septation in the advent of the molecular biology era. In: Clark EB, Markwald RR, Takao A, editors. Developmental mechanisms of heart disease. Armonk, NY: Futura Publishing Co. Inc. p 227–47.

Potts JD, Dagle JM, Walder JA, Weeks DL, Runyan RB. 1991. Epithelial-mesenchymal transformation of embryonic cardiac endothelial cells is inhibited by a modified antisense oligodeoxynucleotide to transforming growth factor b3. Proc Natl Acad Sci USA 88:1516–20.

Ramsdell AF, Moreno-Rodriguez RA, Weinecke MM, Sugi Y, Turner DK, Mjaatvedt CH, Markwald R. 1997. Patterning of ES/130 expression in the avian heart suggests induction of endocardial cushion tissue is mediated, in part, by an autoregulatory pathway. Acta Anat (submitted)

Ramsdell A, Markwald R. 1997. Induction of endocardial cushion tissue in the avian heart is regulated, in part, by TGF beta-3-mediated autocrine signalling. Dev Biol 187:64–74.

Rawles ME. 1943. The heart-forming areas of the early chick blastoderm. Physiol Zool 16:22–42.

Rezaee M, Isokawa K, Krug EL, Markwald RR. 1993. Identification of a 130kDa protein potentially involved in cardiac morphogenesis. J Biol Chem 268:14404–11.

Robbins J, Doetschman T, Jones WK, Sanchez A. 1992. Embryonic stem cells as a model for cardiogenesis. Trends Cardiovasc Med 2:44–50.

Rongish BJ, Little CD. 1995. Extracellular matrix in heart development. Experentia 51:873–82.

Rongish BJ, Drake CJ, Argraves WS and Little CD. 1998. Identification of the developmental marker, JB3, antigen as fibrillin-2 and its de novo organization into embryonic microfibrillous arrays. Dev Dyn (in press).

Rosenquist TH, Fray-Gavalas C, Waldo K, Beall AC. 1990. Development of the musculoelastic septation complex in the avian truncus arteriosus. Am J Anat 189:339–56.

Ross RS, Navankasattusas S, Harvey RP, Chien KR. 1996. An HF-1a/HF-1b/MEF-2 combinatorial element confers cardiac ventricular specificity and establishes an anterior posterior gradient of expression. Development (Camb) 122:1799–809.

Runyan RB, Markwald RR. 1983. Invasion of mesenchyme into three-dimensional gels: a regional and temporal analysis of interaction in embryonic heart tissue. Dev Biol 95:108–14.

Runyan RB, Potts JD, Sharma RV, Loeber CP, Chiang JJ, Bhalla RC. 1990. Signal transduction of a tissue interaction during embryonic heart development. Cell Regul 1:301–13.

Runyan RB, Potts JD, Weeks DL. 1992. TGF beta-3 mediated tissue interaction during embryonic heart development. Mol Reprod Dev 32:152–9.

Ruzicka DL, Schwartz RJ. 1988. Sequential activation of alpha-actin genes during avian cardiogenesis: vascular smooth muscle alpha-actin gene transcripts mark the onset of cardiomyocyte differentiation. J Cell Biol 107:2755–2588.

Sakota I, Maas R. 1994. Msx-1 deficient mice exhibit cleft palate and abnormalities of craniofacial and tooth development. Nat Genet 6:34–356.

Sanford LP, Ormsby I, Gittenberger-de Groot AC, Sariola H, Friedman R, Boivin GP, Cardell EL, Doetschman T. 1997. TGF beta-2 knockout mice have multple developmental defects that are non-overlapping with other TGF beta knockout phenotypes. Development (Camb) 124:2645–57.

Satin J, Fuji S, DeHaan RL. 1988. Development of cardiac beat rate in early chick embryos is regulated by regional cues. Dev Biol 129:103–13.

Schilham MW, Oosterwegel MA, et al. 1996. *Sox-4* gene is required for cardiac outflow tract formation and pro-B lymphocyte expansion. Nature (Lond) 380:711–4.

Schultheiss TM, Burch JBE, Lassar AB. 1997. A role for bone morphogenetic proteins in the induction of cardiac myogenesis. Genes Dev 11:451–62.

Sinning AR, Markwald RR. 1992. Multiple glycoproteins localize to a particulate form of extracellular matrix in regions of the embryonic where endothelial cells transform into mesenchyme. Anat Rec 232:285–92.

Sinning AR, Hewitt CC, Markwald RR. 1995. A subset of SBA lectin-binding proteins isolated from myocardial-conditioned media transforms cardiac endothelium into mesenchyme. Acta Anat 154:111–9.

Spemann H. 1938. Embryonic Development and Induction. New Haven, CT: Yale University Press.

Spence SG, Argraves WS, Walters L, Hungerford JE, Little CD. 1992. Fibulin is localized at sites of epithelial-mesenchymal transitions in the early embryo. Dev Biol 151:73–484.

Spicer AP, Augustine M, McDonald JA. 1997. Molecular cloning and characterization of a putative mouse hyaluronan synthase. J Biol Chem 272:8957–8691.

Srivastava D, Thomas T, Lin Q, Kirby ML, Brown D, Olson EN. 1997. Regulation of cardiac mesodermal and neural crest development by the bHLH transcription factor dHAND. Nat Genet 16:154–60.

Stefansson S, Lawrence DA, Argraves WS. 1996. Plasminogen activator inhibitor-1 and vitronectin promote the cellular clearance of thrombin by low density lipoprotein receptor-related proteins 1 and 2. J Biol Chem 271:8215–8200.

Sucov HM, Dyson E, Gumeringer CL, Price J, Chien C, Evans RM. 1994. RXR alpha-mutant mice establish a genetic basis for vitamin A signalling in heart morphogenesis. Genes Dev 8:1007–18.

Sugi Y, Markwald RR. 1996. Formation and early morphogenesis of endocardial precursor cells and the role of endoderm. Dev Biol 175:66–83.

Tasaka H, Krug EL, Markwald RR. 1996. Origin of the pulmonary venous orifice in the mouse and its relationship to the morphogenesis of the sinus venosus, extracardiac mesenchyme (spina vestibuli) and atrium. Anat Rec 246:107–13.

Thompson RP, Fitzharris TP. 1979. Morphogenesis of the truncus arteriosus of the chick embryo heart: tissue reorganization during septation. Am J Anat 156:251–64.

Thompson RP, Lindroth JR, Wong YM. 1990. Regional differences in DNA-synthetic activity in the preseptation myocardium of the chick. In: Clark EB, Takao A, editors. Developmental cardiology: morphogenesis and function. Mt. Kisco, NY: Futura Publishing Co. p 219–34.

Thompson RP, Fitzharris TP. 1985. Division of the cardiac outflow. In: Ferrans V, Rosenquist G, Weinstein C, editors. Cardiac morphogenesis. Elsevier Science. p 169–80.

Tsuda T, Philp N, Zile JH, Linask KK. 1996. Left-right asymmetric localization of *flectin* in the extracellular matrix during heart looping. Dev Biol 173:39–50.

Vuillemin M, Pexieder T, Winking H. 1991. Pathogenesis of various forms of double outlet right ventricle in mouse fetal trisomy 13. Int J Cardiol 33:281–304.

Waldo K, Miyagawa-Tomita S, Kumiski D, Kirby ML. 1997. Cardiac neural crest cells provide new insight into septation of the cardiac outflow tract: aortic sac to ventricular septal closure. Dev Biol (in press).

Wall NA, Hogan B. 1994. TGF-beta related genes in development. Curr Opin Genet Dev 4:517–22.

Webb S, Anderson RH, Brown N. 1996. Endocardial cushion development and heart loop architecture inthe trisomy 16 mouse. Dev Dyn 206:301–9.

Webb S, Brown NA, Wessels A, Anderson RH. 1997a. The development of the murine pulmonary vein and its relationship to the embryonic venous sinus. Anat Rec (in press).

Webb S, Brown NA, Anderson RH. 1997b. Formation of the atrioventricular septal structures in the normal mouse. Circ Res (in press).

Webb S. 1997. Development of the atrioventricular septum in trisomy 16 and normal mice. Doctoral Dissertation, Faculty of Science of the University of London, Imperial College School of Medicine at the National Heart and Lung Institute, London. p 142–79.

Wenink ACG. 1987. Embryology of the heart. In: Anderson RH, Macartney FJ, Shinebourne EA, Tynan M, editors. Paediatric Cardiology. Edinburgh: Churchill Livingston. p 83–107.

Wessels A, Vermeulen JLM, Viragh Sz, Lamers WH, Moorman AFM. 1991. Spatial distribution of "tissue-specific" antigens in the developing human heart and skeletal muscle: II) an immunohistochemical analysis of myosin heavy chain isoform expression patterns in the embryonic heart. Anat Rec 229:355–68.

Wessels A, Vermeulen JLM, Verbeek FJ, Viragh Sz, Kalman F, Lamers WH, Moorman AFM. 1992. Spatial distribution of "tissue-specific" antigens in the developing human heart and skeletal muscle: III) an immunohistochemical analysis of the distribution of the neural tissue antigen G1N2 in the embryonic heart; implications for the development of the atrioventricular conduction system. Anat Rec 231:97–111.

Wessels A, Markman MWM, Vermeulen JLM, RH Anderson, Sz Viragh, AFM Moorman, WH Lamers. 1996. The development of the atrioventricular junction in the human heart: an immunohistochemical study. Circ Res 78:110–7.

Wessels A, Markwald R, Webb S, Brown NA, Anderson RH, Moorman AFM, Lamers WH. 1998. Atrial development in the human heart: the role of the dorsal mesocardium in the development of the pulmonary veins and primary atrial septum. (submitted)

Winnier G, Blessing M, Labosky PA, Hogan BLM. 1995. Bone morphogenetic protein-4 is required for mesoderm formation and patterning in the mouse. Genes Dev 9:2105–16.

Witte DP, Aronow BJ, Dry JK, Harmony J. 1996. Temporally and spatially restricted expression of apolipoprotein J in the developing heart defines discrete stages of valve morphogenesis. Dev Dyn 201:290–6.

Wunsch A, Markwald RR, Little CD. 1994. Cardiac endothelial heterogeneity defines valvular development as demonstrated by the diverse expression of JB3 antigen, a fibrillin-like protein of the endocardial cushion tissue. Dev Biol 165:585–601.

Ya J, Van den Hoff MJB, de Boer PAJ, Tesink-Taekema S, Franco D, Moorman AFM, Lamers WH. 1997a. The normal development of the outflow tract in the rat. Circ Res (in press)

Ya J, Schilham MW, de Boer PAJ, Moorman AFM, Clevers H, Lamers WH. 1997b. *Sox4*-deficient mice provide an animal model for the development of common trunk. (submitted)

Yamamura H, Zhang M, Markwald RR, Mjaatvedt CH. 1997. A heart segmental defect in the anterior/posterior axis of a transgenic mutant mouse. Dev Biol 186:58–72.

Yost H. 1992. Regulation of vertebrate left-right asymmetries by extracellular matrix. Nature (Lond) 357:158–61.

Yutzey KE, Rhee JT, Bader DM. 1994. Expression of the atrial-specific myosin heavy chain AMHC1 and the establishment of anteroposterior polarity in the developing chicken heart. Development (Camb) 120:871–83.

Zhang H, Bradley A. 1996. Mice deficient for BMP-2 are nonviable and have defects in amnion/chorion and cardiac development. Development (Camb) 122:2977–86.

Zou Y, Evans S, Chen J, Kuo H-C, Harvey RP, Chien KR. 1997. CARP, a cardiac ankyrin repeat protein, is downstream in the Nkx2-5 homeobox gene pathway. Development (Camb) 124:793–809.

CHAPTER 3

Straight Tube Heart. Primitive Cardiac Cavities vs. Primitive Cardiac Segments

María V. de la Cruz and Concepción Sanchez-Gomez

In integrating the postmortem study of morphological structures with their prospective fate in the straight tube heart in man and in chick, interpretations were made that are not consistent with results ascertained by in vivo labeling, because the prospective fate of developing structure can be only investigated by in vivo studies. For that reason, traditional discriptions of the straight tube heart in both species may need further clarification including our own early studies (De la Cruz et al 1972) as well as those of others (Davis 1927; Streeter 1942; Patten 1948; Romanoff 1960; DeVries and Saunders 1962; Grant 1962; Rosenquist and DaHaan 1966; Netter and Van Mierop 1969; Dor and Corone 1973; Steding and Seidl 1980; Pexieder et al 1989; Viragh et al 1989). For example, the embryological constitution of the definitive ventricles appears to be much different based on in vivo labeling than originally thought when only fixed and embedded materials were studied.

Our purpose in this chapter is to clarify information obtained from postmortem studies in ligtht of new knowledge obtained from in vivo studies of the chick embryonic heart (DeHaan 1963; Stalsberg and DeHaan 1969; Castro-Quezada et al 1972; de la Cruz et al 1977, 1987, 1989, 1991; Linask and Lash 1993; Eisenberg and Bader 1995; Markwald 1995).

By means of in vivo labeling studies of the precardiac mesoderm in the chick embryo at stage 6HH, DeHaan (1963) demonstrated that the cardiogenic areas fuse in the cephalic midline to form an inverted U-shaped crescent that circumscribes the anterior end of notochord. He designated this crescent the "cardiogenic plate". As shown in Fig. 1A, the cardiogenic plate is associated dorsally with the ectoderm and with the endoderm ventrally (Fig. 1B). According to the recent investigations of Peng and colleagues (1990) between stages 4HH and 5HH, the precardiac mesoderm forms a true epithelium. Subsequently, Linask and Lash (1993) and Eisenberg and Bader (1995) showed that the precardiac mesodermal epithelium has the capability of forming myocardium and endocardium. From preliminary studies of primary cultures, Markwald (1995) proposed that the endoderm may induce segregation of the precardiac mesodermal epithelium into myocardial and endocardial lineages. It is obvious we do not know whether there are cardiogenic cells within a crescent in the human embryo because this information was obtained by

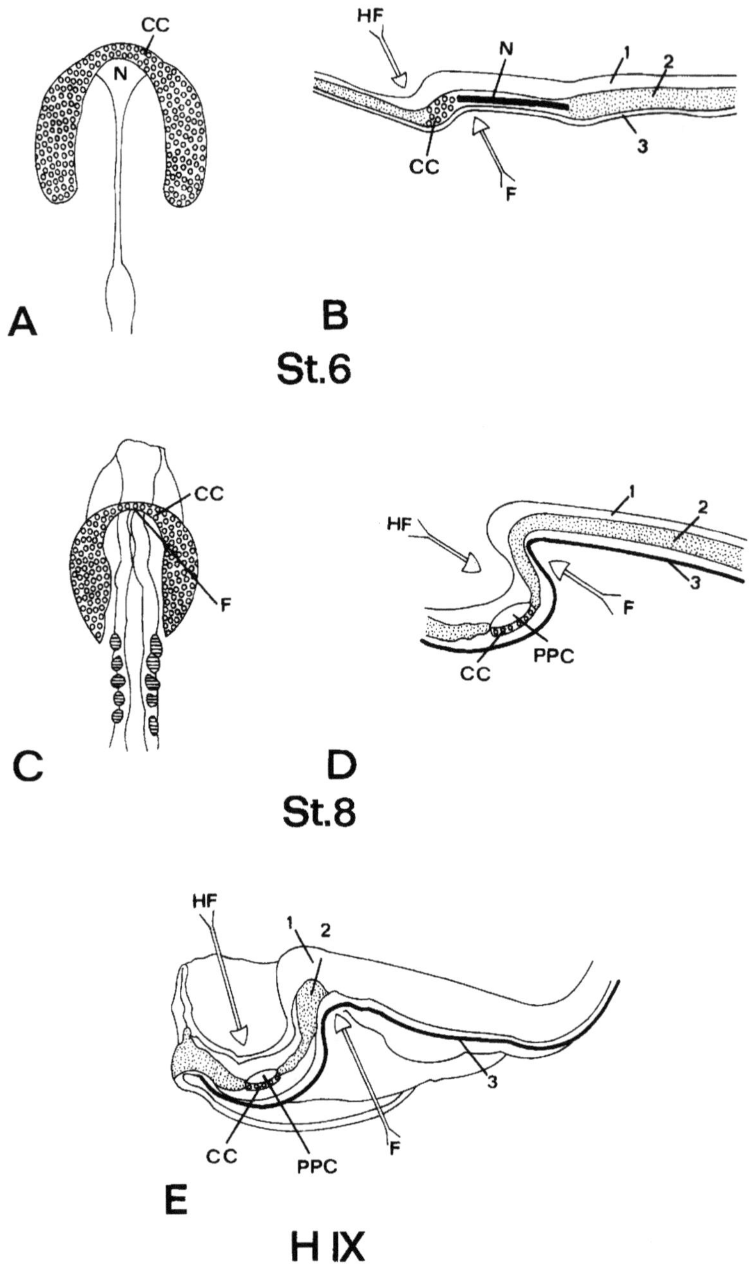

FIGURE 1. The appearance of the cardiogenic plate or crescent (CC) formed by the fusion of the paired heart fields in the chick, its location, its changes in position, and the appearance of the primitive pericardial cavity (PPC) both in chick and in man. **A, B.** Chick embryo at stage 6HH. **A.** Ventral view showing the cardiogenic crescent rostral to the notochord (N). **B.** Median longitudinal section of the same embryo. Notice the beginning of the development of the head fold (HF) and of the foregut (F) and the position of the cardiogenic crescent rostral to the notochord. **C, D.** Chick embryo at stage 8HH. **C.** Ventral view showing the cardiogenic crescent in a ventral position with respect to the foregut. **D.** Median longitudinal section of the same embryo. Notice the appearance of the primitive pericardial cavity and of the cardiogenic crescent in a ventral position with respect to the foregut. **E.** Median longitudinal section of the human embryo at Horizon IX showing the cardiogenic crescent, which is the first morphological manifestation of the heart, and the primitive pericardial cavity. The cardiogenic crescent or plate is in a ventral position with respect to the foregut. 1 = ectoderm; 2 = mesoderm; 3 = endoderm.

means of in vivo labeling in the chick embryo. However, using the expression of cardiac-specific genes, e.g., GATA-4 or CSX, to visualize the heart fields in mice indicates that the heart fields of mammals similarly fuse to form a U-shaped crescent (chapters I and II).

The cardiogenic plate undergoes a morphological change in the chick embryo between stages 7HH and 8HH (Stalsberg and DeHaan 1969) (Fig. 1, C and D). The mesoderm becomes divided with formation of the coelom in two layers, one adjacent to the ectoderm (somatopleure) and the other to the endoderm (splanchnopleure). The splanchnopleure contains the paired heart-forming fields (Fig. 1, C and D). The space between the somatopleure and the cardiogenic region of the splanchnopleure is the primitive pericardial cavity (Fig. 1D). Moreno-Rodriquez (personal communication, 1996), by means of scanning electron microscopy, did a careful study of the morphological changes that take place in this region during the formation process of the primitive pericardial cavity in the chick. He found results similar to those of Davis (1927) in the human embryo and Linask (1992), who used confocal laser scanning microscope to study coelomic formation in avian embryo.

The first morphological manifestation of the human heart was found by Davis (1927) in embryo 5080, in which the first pair of somites was being formed at horizon IX of Streeter (1942). He described a U-shaped plate that he called the cardiogenic plate, which was found within the splanchnopleure. It circumscribed the cephalic end of the neural plate. Between the cardiogenic plate and the somatopleure he observed numerous vesicles that he suggested were in the process of coalescing to form the primitive pericardial cavity (Fig. 1E). This description by Davis (1927) of the human embryo heart at horizon IX corresponds to that of the chick embryo heart at stage 7HH to 8HH as initially described by Stalsberg and DeHaan (1969) (Fig. 1, D and E).

The morphological changes that occur in the cephalic end of the chick embryo between stages 7HH and 8HH are initiated by the folding of the ectoderm and the endoderm to form, respectively, the early head fold and the foregut. In this manner the foregut acquires its ventral wall (Stalsberg and DeHaan 1969) (Fig. 1D). At the same time, the cardiogenic plate that originally had a cephalic position with respect to the notochord (Fig. 1, A and B) becomes ventrally positioned beneath the foregut (Fig. 1, C and D). The same morphogenetic folding takes place in human embryo 5080 of horizon IX (Davis 1927) (Fig. 1E).

The straight tube heart appears in the chick embryo at stage 9+HH (Fig. 2A) and at horizon X in man (embryo 3709 of 4 somites, De Vries and Saunders 1962). In both species the cardiogenic plate acquires a canal-shape, which is myocardial in the chick (Manasek 1969; Männer 1993) and myoepicardial in man (Davis 1927), that forms the ventral and lateral walls of the heart tube. The dorsal wall of the tube is the ventral wall of the foregut, which exhibits a marked cellular thickening at this level (Fig. 2B). In the cavity of this cardiac tube or "trough" there is an endothelial plexus in man (Davis 1927) but two endocardial tubes in the chick (Patten 1922; de la Cruz et al 1972) (Fig. 2B). Separating the myocardial and endocardial tubes is the cardiac jelly (Davis 1927) or extracellular matrix, which according to the findings of Kitten and associates (1987) in the chick embryo is secreted by the myocardium. Hurlé and Ojeda's studies (1977) in the chick embryo have shown that the extracellular matrix between the myocardiac mantle and the endocardial tubes is sparse and scant in fibrillar structures compared with that present between the endocardial tubes and the ventral wall of the foregut.

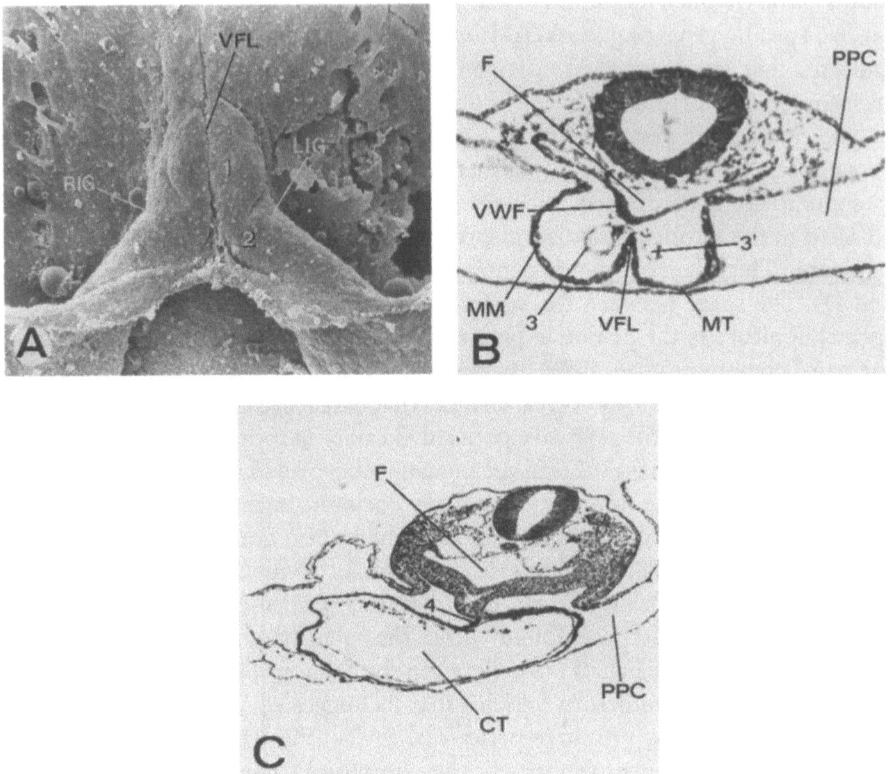

FIGURE 2. Scanning electron micrograph (**A**) of the straight tube heart and histological sections (**B, C**) of the chick embryo heart at stages 9+HH and 12HH. **A.** Ventral view of the straight tube heart (stage 9+HH). **B.** Transverse section of the straight tube heart showing the myocardial trough (MT), the ventral wall of the foregut (VWF), the myocardial mantle (MM), and the developing endocardial tubes (3, 3′). **C.** Transverse section through the cardiac loop (stage 12HH). RIG = right interventricular groove; LIG = left interventricular groove; VFL = ventral fusion line of both cardiac primordia (Ventral mesocardium is a temporary structure located in the fusion line in chick); F = foregut; CT = looped cardiac tube; PPC = primitive pericardial cavity; 1 = primordium of the apical trabeculated region of the right ventricle; 2 = primordium of the apical trabeculated region of the left ventricle; 4 = dorsal mesocardium. Fig. 2A and C reprinted with permission of from de la Cruz et al. (1989) J Anat 165:121.

Davis (1927) established, on the basis of postmortem studies of the straight tube heart in man, that this heart is constituted by different segments and that each segment gave origin to a definitive cardiac cavity, which he designated this segment primitive cardiac cavities. In a cephalocaudal order, the primitive cardiac cavities were designated by Davis (1927) as follows: aortic bulb, bulbus cordis, left ventricle, and atria (right and left), which gave origin respectively to the great arteries, the right ventricle, the left ventricle, and the right and left atria (Davis 1927) (Fig. 3A). These cavities were separated by incomplete dorsoventral grooves with their corresponding internal ridges. He termed these grooves the right and left interbulbar sulcus between the aortic bulb and the bulbus cordis; the right and left bulboventricular sulcus between the bulbus cordis and the left ventricle; and the right and left atrioventricular sulcus between the left ventricle and the atria (Davis 1927) (Fig.

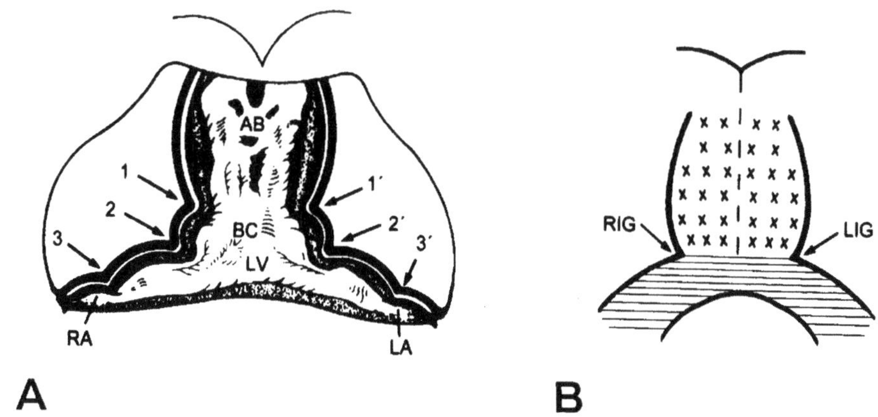

FIGURE 3. Schematic representation of the different segments that constitute the straight tube heart from postmortem studies and in vivo labeling experiments. **A.** Diagram of the straight tube heart from postmortem studies. **B.** Diagram of the straight tube heart from in vivo labeling experiments. AB = aortic bulb; BC = bulbus cordis; LV = left ventricle; RA = right atrium; LA = left atrium; RIG = right interventricular groove; LIG = left interventricular groove; 1, 1′ = right and left interbulbar sulcus; 2, 2′ ± right and left bulboventricular sulcus (interventricular groove); 3, 3′ = right and left atrioventricular sulcus. Crossed area (**x**'s) represents the primordium of the apical trabeculated region of the right ventricle. Striped area denotes the primordium of the apical trabeculated region of the left ventricle. Reprinted with permission of from de la Cruz et al. (1989) J Anat 165:121.

3A). The deeper and most clearly defined grooves were the right and left bulboventricular sulcus. Davis's (1927) concept, based on postmorten studies that showed that the human straight tube heart was formed by different segments (primitive cardiac cavities) and that each one of them gave origin to a complete definitive cardiac cavity, was generally accepted in the study of the chick embryo heart, obviously using the same nomenclature (Patten 1948; Romanoff 1960; Rosenquist and DeHaan 1966; de la Cruz et al 1972; Dor and Corone 1973; Virágh et al 1989).

Postmortem studies, however, do not permit any given embryological structure to be dynamically studied from its initial appearance up to its anatomical expression in the mature heart in a continuous and uninterrupted sequence; in other words, postmortem studies do not allow direct determination of the prospective fate of an embryological structure. Consequently, the only way to investigate whether there is a primordium (primitive cardiac cavities) in the straight tube heart for each of the definitive cardiac cavities as suggested by Davis (1927) is to label this primordium in vivo and trace the label up to the mature heart to determine its anatomical expression (de la Cruz et al 1977, 1987, 1989, 1991). Such labeling studies must be done in an adequate biological model like the chick embryo heart since for obvious reasons they cannot be done in man.

Using in vivo labeling studies, de la Cruz and associates (1977, 1987, 1989, 1991) mapped the fate of the straight tube heart in the chick embryo (stage 9+HH). These studies demonstrated that this tube is constituted entirely of just two regions, the primordium of the apical trabeculated region of the right ventricle, cephalically (Fig. 4) and the primordium of the apical trabeculated region of the left ventricle, caudally (Fig. 5). Thus, it was demonstrated that there are no primitive cardiac cavities that correspond to the definitive cardiac cavities. This information was

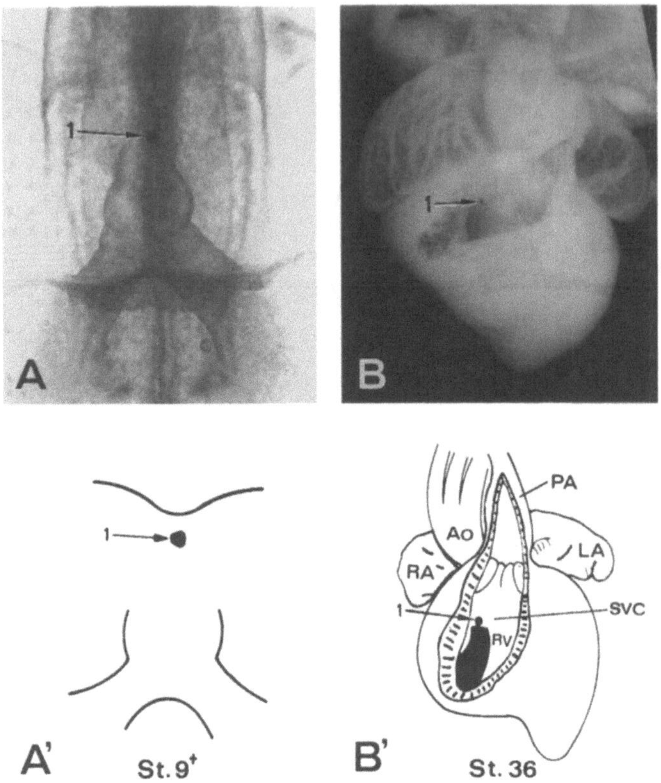

FIGURE 4. Photographs and diagrams of an in vivo labeling experiment in the chick embryo heart that show that the cephalic region of the straight tube heart is the primordium of the apical trabeculated region of the anatomical right ventricle. **A, A′**. Notice the label (1) that was placed at the cephalic end of the straight tube heart (stage 9+HH). **B, B′**. Notice the same label (1) in the proximal border of the supraventricular crest (SVC), which corresponds to the anatomical limit between the apical trabeculated region and the outlet of the anatomical right ventricle in the mature heart. This experiment shows that the most cephalic (anterior) end of the straight tube heart corresponds to the limit between the outlet and the apical trabeculated region of the right ventricle; consequently, the cephalic region of the straight tube heart is the primordium of the apical trabeculated region of the anatomical right ventricle. PA = pulmonary artery; Ao = aorta; RA = right atrium; LA = left atrium; RV = right ventricle.

obtained by placing a label in the cephalic end (de la Cruz et al 1987, 1989, 1991) (Fig. 4, A and A′) and another one in the caudal end (de la Cruz et al 1987, 1989, 1991) (Fig. 5, A and A′) of the straight tube heart at stage 9+HH. The cephalic label was traced to the mature heart where it was found in the proximal border of the supraventricular crest, which is the anatomical boundary between the ventricular outlet (infundibulum) and the apical trabeculated region of the right ventricle (de la Cruz et al 1977, 1987, 1989, 1991) (Fig. 4). The caudal label was found in the mature heart between the smooth and the apical trabeculated regions of the left ventricle, a site that corresponds to the anatomical limit between the inlet of the left ventricle and its apical trabeculated region (de la Cruz et al 1987, 1989, 1991) (Fig. 5). As described in chapters IV, VI, VII, and VIII, the remaining segments, i.e., primitive ventricular outlet (conus), the primitive ventricular inlets, and the sino-

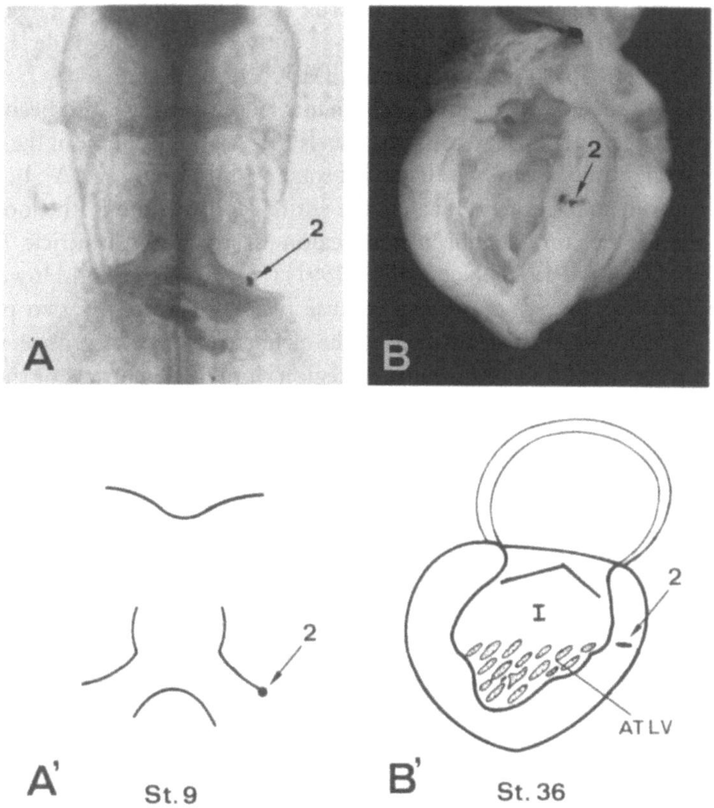

FIGURE 5. Photographs and diagrams of in vivo labeling experiments in the chick embryo heart that show that the most caudal (posterior) region of the straight tube heart is the primordium of the apical trabeculated region of the anatomical left ventricle. **A, A′**. Notice the label (2) that was placed at the caudal end of the straight tube heart (stage 9^+ HH). **B, B′**. Notice the same label (2) in the mature heart at the limit between the apical trabeculated region of the left ventricle and its smooth portion (inlet). This experiment shows that the caudal end of the straight tube heart corresponds to the limit between the inlet (I) and the apical trabeculated region of the left ventricle (ATLV); consequently, the caudal region of the straight tube heart is the primosdium of the apical trabeculated region of the anatomical left ventricle. Fig 5 A and B reprinted with permission of from de la Cruz et al. (1989): J. Anat 165:121.

atrial segment, are not present at the stage 9+HH tubular heart but appear during looping and torsion (stage 12HH to 14HH).

The important points are that (1) the primitive cardiac cavities do not give origin to future definitive ones, and (2) during the development of the heart from the straight tube heart to the early looping period, new segments appear in the heart. Each segment gives origin to only a specific region of a definitive cardiac cavity in the mature heart (de la Cruz et al 1977, 1987, 1989, 1991). These segments are designated as primitive cardiac segments (de la Cruz et al 1989, 1991). By example, the definitive ventricles are anatomical units, but not embryological units, because the apical trabeculated region of the anatomical right ventricle has its own primordium and the same is true of the apical trabeculated region of the anatomical left ventricle (de la Cruz et al 1989, 1991). The inlet of each ventricle originates from a single primordium (primitive inlet) (de la Cruz et al 1987, 1989, 1991); likewise the outlet of each ventricle is derived from the primitive outlet (conus) (de la Cruz et al 1977, 1987, 1989, 1991) (Fig. 6) (chapters IV, V, VI, and VII).

The results of the in vivo labeling experiments mentioned have also been verified with deletion experiments (Castro-Quezada et al 1972). For example, if the cephalic half of the straight tube heart was deleted at stage 9+HH (Fig. 7, A, A′, B, and B′), the same embryo at stage 12HH lacked the entire cephalic limb of the loop or the primordium of the apical trabeculated region of the right ventricle (Castro-Quezada et al 1972; de la Cruz et al 1989, 1991) (Fig. 7, C, and C′). However, the caudal limb of the loop was present because it is constituted by two primitive cardiac segments, one of them adjacent to the left interventricular groove, which is the primordium of the apical trabeculated region of the left ventricle or the caudal

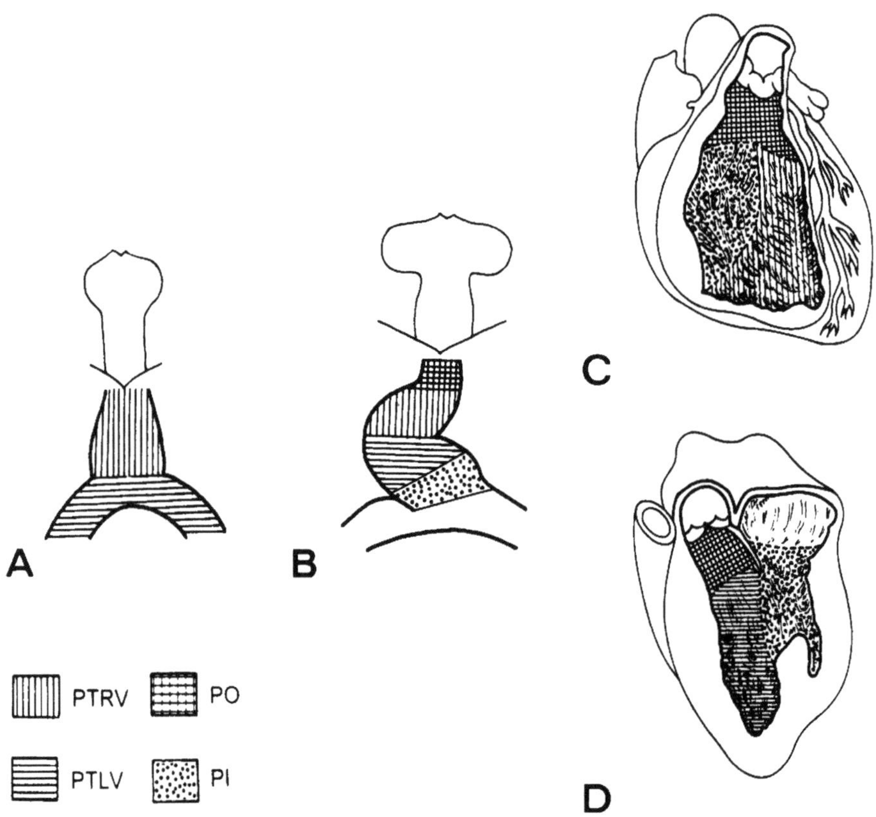

FIGURE 6. Diagrams summarizing the origins of the ventricles. Each ventricle is constituted by three primordia that give origin to a specific anatomical region of the mature ventricle. **A.** The cephalic region of the straight tube heart is the primordium of the apical trabeculated region of the right ventricle, and its caudal region, the primordium of the apical trabeculated region of the left ventricle. **B.** In the C-shaped looped heart a new cephalic segment, the primitive outlet (conus), develops, which forms the primordium of the outlet of both ventricles. Also a new caudal segment, the primitive inlet, develops, which becomes the primordium of the inlet of both ventricles. **C, D.** Internal aspect of the anatomical right and left ventricle, respectively, showing the contribution's of the 3 primordia. PTRV = primordium of the apical trabeculated region of the right ventricle; PTLV = primordium of the apical trabeculated region of the left ventricle; PO = primordium of the primitive outlet (conus); PI = primordium of the primitive inlet.

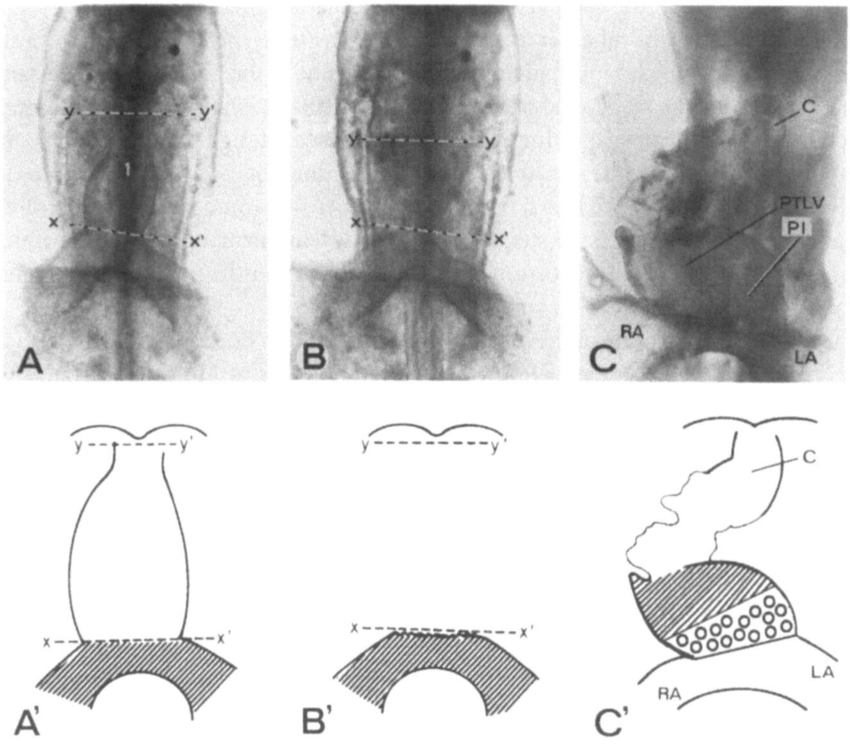

FIGURE 7. Photographs and diagrams of a typical deletion experiment in the straight tube heart of the chick embryo to show that the cephalic region of the straight tube heart (primordium of the apical trabeculated region of the right ventricle) gives origin to the cephalic limb of the loop, as had been shown with the in vivo labeling experiments. **A, A′**. Straight tube heart before removing its cephalic segment, corresponding to the primordium of the apical trabeculated region of the right ventricle (1). **B, B′**. The same embryo after removing that region. **C, C′**. The same embryo at the C-shaped loop stage. Notice that the cephalic limb of the loop is absent, demonstrating that the cephalic region of the straight tube heart (primordium of the apical trabeculated region of the right ventricle) gives origin to the cephalic limb of the loop. 1 = primordium of the apical trabeculated region of the right ventricle; C = primordium of the outlet of both ventricles or conus; RA = right atrium; LA = left atrium; y, y′ = iniscion in the cephalic end of the straight tube heart; x, x′ = iniscion at the level of the interventricular grooves; striped area = primordium of the apical trabeculated region of the left ventricle; circles area = primitive inlet; PI = primitive inlet; PTLV = primordium of the apical trabeculated region of the anatomical left ventricle.

region of the straight tube heart; the other one is adjacent to the right atrioventricular groove and is the primitive inlet that appears in this stage of development (stage 12HH) and gives origin to the inlet of both ventricles (de la Cruz et al 1987, 1989, 1991) (Fig. 7, C and C′) (chapters IV, V, and VI).

The term bulbus cordis was used by Davis (1927) to designate a region of the human straight tube heart that would give origin to the entire right ventricle, and the term left ventricle, to designate another region of this heart, which would form the left ventricle also in its entirety. Because of the fact that in the straight tube heart there is no region that gives origin either to the right or to the left ventricle in their entirety, this nomenclature is both obsolete and erroneous. With respect to the aortic bulb, which would give origin to the great arteries (Davis 1927), it is important to point out that the great arteries are not cardiac cavities, nor is the aortic bulb present in the straight tube heart. Furthermore this term means a structure in the shape of a bulb, which would give origin exclusively to the aorta, and at the same time it excludes the stage of development in which the primordium of the great arteries has a tubular shape, for which reason it was designated as truncus. We propose that the correct designation for the primordium of each of the great arteries is the "arterial pole" of the heart, because it includes the primordium of each of the great arteries and changes in shape during its development up to its anatomical expression as the ascending portion of the aortic arch and the trunk of the pulmonary artery.

The straight tube heart in the chick and in man has two borders, a right one and a left one (Davis 1927; Patten 1948). Each of these borders exhibits a lateral groove, which de la Cruz and coworkers (1989, 1991) and DeVries and Saunders (1962) termed the interventricular grooves and which was called by Davis (1927) the bulboventricular sulcus (Figs. 2A and 3). These grooves divide the straight tube heart into two regions, one cephalic and the other caudal (Fig. 2A), each corresponding respectively to the primordium of the apical trabeculated regions of the right and left ventricles, as shown by in vivo labeling and deletion experiments (Castro-Quezada et al 1972; de la Cruz et al 1977, 1987, 1989, 1991) in the chick (Figs. 4, 5, and 7). Furthermore, in both species the straight tube heart exhibits a ventral groove, which extends in a cephalocaudal direction from the middle region of the subcephalic fold, to the medial area of the anterior intestinal portal (Fig. 2, A and B). This groove corresponds to the ventral fusion line of both cardiac primordia (the heart-forming fields) and forms part of the ventral mesocardium in the chick.

Davis (1927), using postmortem material, studied the straight tube heart in the human embryo and concluded that its right and left borders gave origin respectively to the right border or convex surface of the loop (greater curvature) and to the left border or concave surface of the loop (inner curvature). He also pointed out that the right interventricular groove disappears, whereas the left interventricular groove becomes deeper. These conclusions by Davis with respect to the prospective fate of the borders and the grooves of the straight tube heart and their morphological expression in the loop have been evaluated by in vivo labeling experiments in the chick embryo heart (Castro-Quezada et al 1972; de la Cruz et al 1977, 1987, 1989).

Castro-Quezada and colleagues (1972), in the chick embryo, placed a label at the right interventricular groove in the straight tube heart (Fig. 8, A and A′), and de la Cruz and associates (1989) did the same in the left interventricular groove (Fig. 8, C and C′). In each case the labels were traced up to the loop stage 12HH. The right-positioned label was found in the dorsal wall of the loop, in the proximity of the left interventricular groove (inner curvature) (Castro-Quezada et al 1972) (Fig. 8, B and B′); the second left-sided label was found in the ventral wall of the loop, also in the proximity of the left interventricular groove (inner curvature) (de la Cruz et al 1989) (Fig. 8, D and D′). These findings indicate that (1) the right and left borders of the straight tube heart form the left or concave border of the loop (inner curvature) (Castro-Quezada et al 1972; de la Cruz et al 1989) (Fig. 8, A–D′); and (2) both the right and left interventricular grooves of the straight tube heart contribute to the development of the left interventricular groove of the loop (de la Cruz et al 1989). Consequently, the right interventricular groove of the straight tube heart does not disappear (de la Cruz et al 1989) as had been originally proposed by Davis (1927)

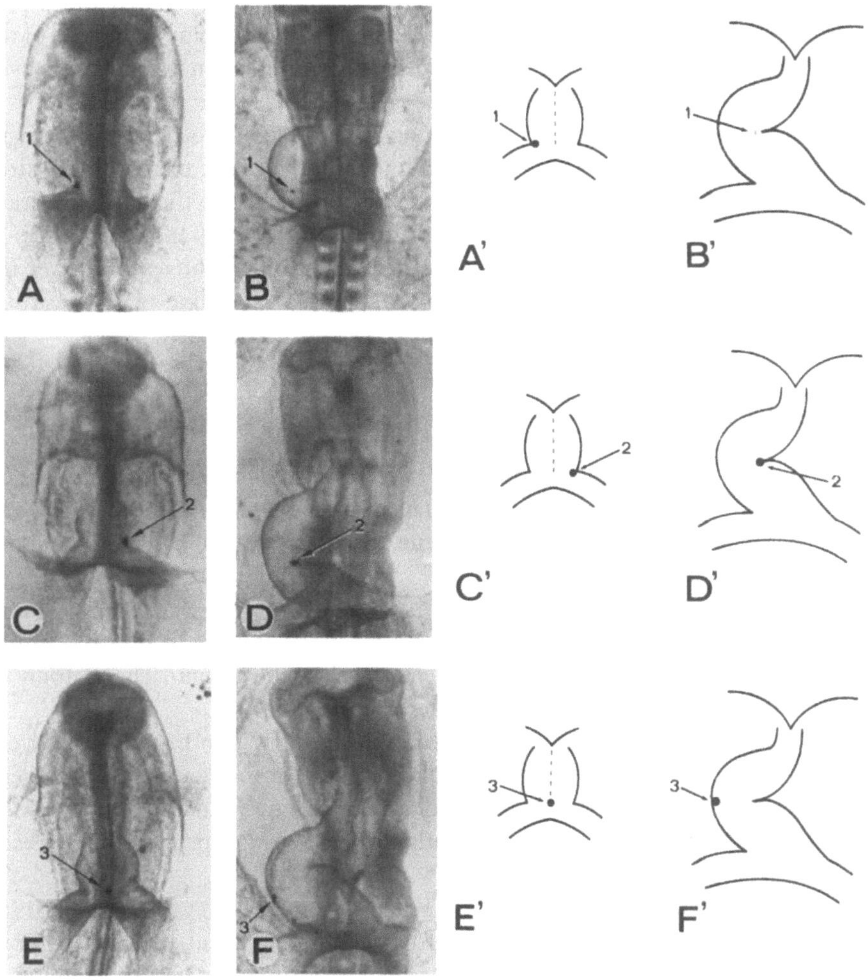

FIGURE 8. Photographs and diagrams of in vivo labeling experiments in the chick embryo heart that show that both the right and left borders of the straight tube heart give origin to the left border or inner curvature of the heart loop, whereas the ventral fusion line of both cardiac primordia of the straight tube heart becomes the right border or great curvature of the loop. **A, A′**. Straight tube heart (stage 9+HH) showing the label (1) that was placed into the right interventricular groove. **B, B′**. The same embryo but now at stage 12HH. The label (1) is now in the dorsal wall of the loop, in the proximity of the left interventricular groove (inner curvature). **C, C′**. The second label (2), which was initially placed in the left interventricular groove of the straight tube heart. **D, D′**. The same embryo at stage 12HH showing the label (2) is now in the ventral wall of the loop, also in the proximity of the left interventricular groove (inner curvature). E, E′. A label (3) was placed at stage 9+HH into the ventral fusion line of both cardiac primordia at the level of the interventricular grooves. F, F′. The same embryo at stage 12HH, showing the label (3) is now present in the right border of the loop (great curvature). Fig. 8 C–F reprinted with permission of from de la Cruz et al. (1989) J Anat 165:121.

(Fig. 8, A–D′). Likewise, the transverse histological sections of the straight tube heart and of the loop show that the right and left borders of the straight tube heart are the ones that fuse and constitute the concave or left border of the loop (inner curvature) (de la Cruz et al 1989) (Fig. 2, B and C). Furthermore, de la Cruz and colleagues (1989) showed that the right or convex border of the loop (greater curvature) originates from the ventral fusion line of both cardiac primordia in the straight tube heart; as shown (Fig. 8, E, E′, F, and F′), when a label is placed on this line at the level of the interventricular grooves in a straight tube heart, they found it on the right or convex border of the loop (greater curvature) at the stage 12HH.

In summary, the results of in vivo labeling in the straight tube heart on the right and left borders and on the ventral fusion line of both cardiac primordia (Castro-Quezada et al 1972; de la Cruz et al 1991) demonstrate that the left or concave border of the loop (inner curvature) originates from the right and left borders of the straight tube heart (Fig. 8, A–D′), whereas the right or convex border of the loop (greater curvature) originates from the ventral fusion line of both cardiac primordia (Fig. 8, E, E′, F, and F′).

CONCLUSIONS

Because of the morphological similarity between the straight tube heart in man and in the chick, we suggest that the data obtained by in vivo labeling experiments in chick can be extrapolated also to man. If true, then the following can be said of both man and chick:

1. The ventral and lateral walls of the straight tube heart are formed by cardiac muscle, while the dorsal wall is the ventral wall of the foregut. The anatomy of this heart corresponds to a “myoendocardial trough”.
2. The straight tube heart is constituted exclusively by two primordia, one cephalic, i.e., that of the apical trabeculated region of the anatomical right ventricle, and the other caudal, that of the apical trabeculated region of the anatomical left ventricle. Consequently there is no single primordium for each of the definitive cardiac cavities.
3. The primordium of the apical trabeculated regions of each ventricle appears in the straight tube heart. The primordia of the outlet and the inlet of both ventricles, the primitive atria, and the sinus venosus appear during looping to complete the formation of the primitive cardiac segments. During cardiogenesis these segments or regions become integrated to give origin to the definitive cardiac cavities.
4. The right and left borders of the straight tube heart both form the left or concave border of the loop (inner curvature).
5. The ventral fusion line of both cardiac primordia forms the right or convex border of the loop (greater curvature).
6. Both the right and left interventricular grooves of the straight tube heart contribute to the development of the left interventricular groove of the looped heart that forms on the inner curvature.

REFERENCES

Castro-Quezada A, Nadal-Ginard B, de la Cruz MV. 1972. Experimental study of the formation of the bulboventricular loop in the chick. J Embryol Exp Morphol 27:623–37.

Davis CL. 1927. Development of the human heart from its first appearance to the stage found in embryos of twenty paired somites. Carnegie Contrib Embryol 19:245–84.

DeHaan RL. 1963. Organization of the cardiogenic plate in the early chick embryo. Acta Embryol Morphol Exp 6:26–38.

de la Cruz MV, Muñoz-Armas S, Muñoz Castellanos L. 1972. Development of the Chick Heart. Baltimore, MD: Johns Hopkins University Press.

de la Cruz MV, Sánchez-Gómez C, Arteaga M, Argüello C. 1977. Experimental study of the development of the truncus and the conus in the chick embryo. J Anat 123:651–86.

de la Cruz MV, Sánchez-Gómez C, Robledo Tovi JL. 1987. Experimental study of the development of the ventricular inlets in the chick embryo. Embryologische Hefte. 1:25–37.

de la Cruz MV, Sánchez-Gómez C, Palomino MA. 1989. The primitive cardiac regions in the straight tube heart (Stage 9^-) and their anatomical expression in the mature heart: an experimental study in the chick embryo. J Anat 165:121–31.

de la Cruz MV, Sánchez-Gómez C, Cayré R. 1991. The developmental components of the ventricles: their significance in congenital cardiac malformations. Cardiol Young 1:123–8.

DeVries PA, Saunders JB. 1962. Development of the ventricles and spiral outflow tract in the human heart. A contribution of the development of the human heart from age group IX to age group XV. Carnegie Contrib Embryol 256:89–114.

Dor X, Corone P. 1973. Role du conus dans la morphogenese cardiaque. Essau d' etude sur l'embryon de poulet. Coeur 4:207–307.

Eisenberg C, Bader D. 1995. QCE-6: a clonal cell line with cardiomyogenic and endothelial cell potentials. Dev Biol 177:469–81.

Grant RP. 1962. The embryology of ventricular flow pathways in man. Circulation 25:756–779.

Hurlé JM, Ojeda JL. 1977. Cardiac jelly arrangement during the formation of the tubular heart of the chick embryo. Acta Anat 98:444–55.

Kitten GT Markwald RR, Bolender DL. 1987. Distribution of basement membrane antigens in cryopreserved early embryonic hearts. Anat Rec 217:379–390.

Linask KK. 1992. N-cadherin localization in early heart development and polar expression of Na^+,K^+-ATPase, and integrin during pericardial coelom formation and epithelialization of the differentiating myocardium. Dev Biol 151:213–224.

Linask KK, Lash JW. 1993. Early heart development: dynamics of endocardial cell sorting suggests a common origin with cardiomyocytes. Dev Dyn 195:62–69.

Manasek FJ. 1969. Embryonic development of the heart. II. Formation of the epicardium. J Embryol Exp Morphol 22:333–48.

Männer J. 1993. Experimental study on the formation of the epicardium in chick embryos. Anat Embryol 187:281–89.

Markwald RR. 1995. Overview: formation and early morphogenesis of the primary heart tube. In: Clark EB, Markwald RR, Takao A, editors. Developmental mechanisms of heart disease. Armonk, NY:. Futura Publishing Co. 149–55.

Netter FH, Van Mierop LHS. 1969. Embryology. In: Netter FH, editor. CIBA collection of medical illustrations. Ardsley, New Jersey. CIBA Pharmaceutical Co: Vol. 5, p. 119–25.

Patten BM. 1922. The formation of the cardiac loop in the chick. Am J Anat 30:373–97.

Patten BM. 1948. The Early Embryology of the Chick. 3rd ed. Philadelphia: The Blakiston Co. 184–92.

Peng I, Dennis JE, Rodriguez-Boulan E, Fischman DA. 1990. Polarized release of enveloped viruses in the embryonic chicken heart: demonstration of epithelial polarity in the presumptive myocardium. Dev Biol 141:164–72.

Pexieder T, Wenink AC, Anderson RH. 1989. A suggested nomenclature for the developing heart. Int J Cardiol 25:255–64.

Romanoff AL. 1960. The Avian Embryo. New York: Macmillan. p 680–780.

Rosenquist GC, DeHaan RL. 1966. Migration of precardiac cells in the chick embryo: a radioautographic study. Carnegie Contrib Embryol 263:111–21.

Stalsberg H, DeHaan RL. 1969. The precardiac areas and formation of the tubular heart in the chick embryo. Dev Biol 19:128–59.

Steding G, Seidl W. 1980. Contribution to the development of the heart. Part I: Normal development. Thorac Cardiovasc Surgeon 28:386–409.

Streeter GL. 1942. Development horizon in human embryos. Description of age group XI, 13 to 20 somites and age group XII, 21 to 29 somites. Carnegie Contrib Embryol 30:211–30.
Virágh S, Szabo E, Challice CE. 1989. Formation of the primitive myo and endocardial tubes in the chick embryo. J Mol Cell Cardiol 21:123–37.

CHAPTER 4

Torsion and Looping of the Cardiac Tube and Primitive Cardiac Segments. Anatomical Manifestations

María V. de la Cruz

Torsion of the cardiac tube takes place during the looping period of embryological development, i.e., between stage 9+HH of the straight tube heart (de la Cruz et al 1989, 1991) and stage 17HH, when septation begins (de la Cruz et al 1997). Septation will culminate with the formation of a four-chambered heart.

During the torsion period, highly interesting events occur in the development of the heart: (1) The heart acquires the shape of a tube whose walls are constituted by cardiac muscle, which in later stages will give origin to the free walls of the definitive cardiac cavities; it is important to remember that the straight tube heart (stage 9+HH) is not a myocardial tube but rather a myocardial trough, because its dorsal wall is the ventral wall of the foregut (Manasek 1969; Stalsberg and DeHaan 1969; de la Cruz et al 1989). (2) The primordium of the outlet of both ventricles (de la Cruz et al 1977, 1991) (primitive outlet), the primordium of the inlet of both ventricles (de la Cruz et al 1987, 1991) (primitive inlet), and the primitive right and left atria (Stalsberg and DeHaan 1969; Castro-Quezada et al 1972; de la Cruz et al 1991) appear, which together with the primordium of the apical trabeculated regions of each of the ventricles appearing in the straight tube heart (de la Cruz et al 1989, 1991), constitute a tubular heart in which the primitive cardiac segments (de la Cruz et al 1989, 1991) are present for the first time. Each of these primitive cardiac segments corresponds to a segment of the primary tubular heart and each one of these segments gives origin to a specific anatomical region of a definitive cardiac cavity (de la Cruz et al 1989, 1991). Therefore, a definitive cardiac cavity in the adult is constituted by the integration of multiple primitive cardiac segments (de la Cruz et al 1989, 1991). (3) By means of the process of torsion and looping of the cardiac tube, the different primitive cardiac segments change their spatial position and establish new relations with each other, leading to the normal septation of the heart (Männer et al 1993; de la Cruz et al 1997). Septation of the heart tube begins when the torsion is completed (de la Cruz et al 1997) (stage 17HH).

The period of torsion and looping includes several stages of development. We will select those with a greater relevance to the study: (1) morphological aspects of the complex torsion process in the cardiac tube and its anatomical expression, and (2) the causal factors of the torsion.

MORPHOLOGICAL ASPECTS OF THE TORSION IN THE CARDIAC TUBE AND ITS ANATOMICAL EXPRESSION

The torsion process is characterized by a spectrum of sequential morphological changes. We will focus on the developmental stages with special importance to the prospective fate of the primitive cardiac segments during which their spatial position and the relation with each other play a very important role. In addition, we will integrate the postmortem information in the chick (Patten 1948; Romanoff 1960; de la Cruz et al 1972) and in man (Von Haller 1758; Davis 1927; Kramer 1942; Streeter 1942; De Vries and Saunders 1962; Grant 1962; Netter and Van Mierop 1969; Steding and Seidl 1980) with that acquired from in vivo studies in the chick embryo (Stalsberg 1969a, 1969b; Stalsberg and De Haan 1969; Castro-Quezada et al 1972; de la Cruz et al 1977, 1983, 1989, 1991; Männer et al 1993).

We selected the following stages: (1) C-shaped loop (Fig. 1), i.e., stage 12HH in the chick and embryo 3707 of 12 somites, horizon X in man (De Vries and Saunders 1962); (2) S-shaped loop (Fig. 2), i.e., stage 14HH in the chick and embryo 6344 of 14 somites, horizon XI in man (De Vries and Saunders 1962); and (3) terminal stage (Fig. 3), i.e., stage 16HH in the chick and embryo 2053 of 20 somites, horizon XI in man (De Vries and Saunders 1962).

C-Shaped Loop

The chick embryo heart at stage 12HH and that of human embryo 3707 of 12 somites, horizon X, are representative examples of the C-shaped loop, i.e., the convex surface (greater curvature) is to the right and concave border (inner curvature) to the left when viewed in the frontal plane. The loop is more clearly seen in the ventral view of the heart (Fig. 1A). The dorsal wall of the loop is parallel and adjacent to the ventral wall of the foregut (Fig. 1B).

In this stage, for the first time the heart is constituted by all of the primitive cardiac segments, each one of which gives origin to a specific anatomical region of a definitive cardiac cavity (de la Cruz et al 1977, 1987, 1989, 1991) (Fig. 4 B, F, and G). This information was obtained by means of in vivo labeling experiments in the chick embryo heart (de la Cruz et al 1989, 1991), which show that at this stage of development the following primitive cardiac segments appear: (1) the primordium of the outlet of the right ventricle (de la Cruz et al 1977, 1989, 1991) (primitive outlet), also designated as conus (Figs. 5 and 6); (2) the primitive ventricular inlet, i.e., the primordium of the inlet of both ventricles (de la Cruz et al 1987, 1989, 1991), also designated as atrioventricular (AV) canal (Fig. 7); and (3) the primordium of each of the atria (Stalsberg and DeHaan 1969; Castro-Quezada et al 1972) or primitive right and left atria (Figs. 1C and 4B). Also present are the primordium of the apical trabeculated region of the right and left ventricles, which formed the straight tube heart (de la Cruz et al 1989, 1991) (chapter III, Figs. 4 and 5) (Fig. 4 A and B).

We use the term primitive outlet because it gives origin to the outlet of both ventricles (de la Cruz et al 1977, 1991), i.e., it comprises the outlet of the right

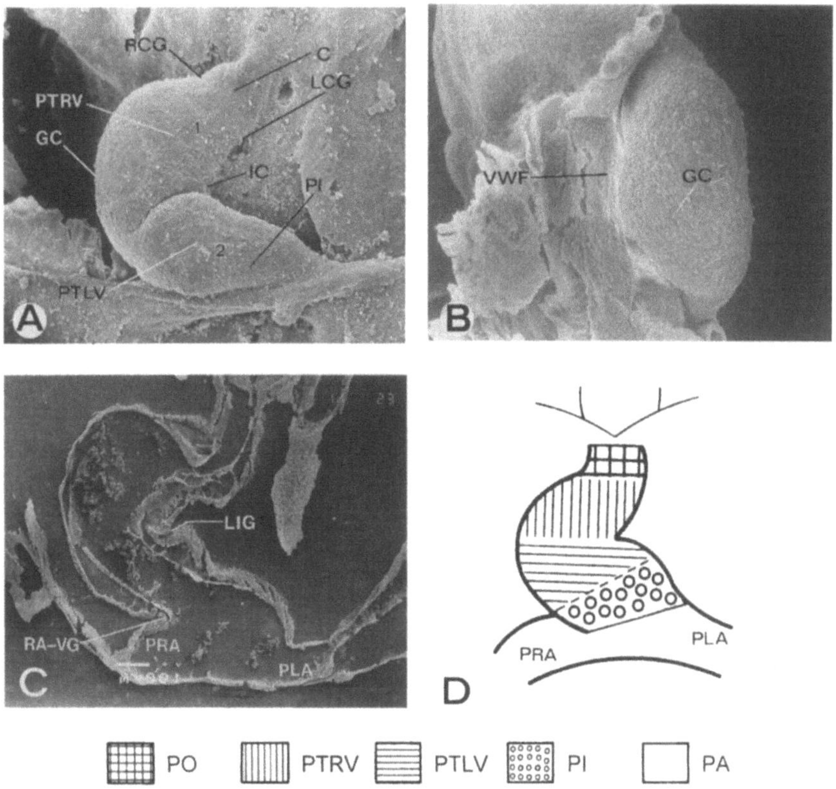

FIGURE 1. Photographs obtained with the scanning electron microscope, histological section, and diagram of the C-shaped loop heart of the chick embryo at stage 12HH. **A.** Ventral view of the heart. Notice the convex surface of the loop or greater curvature (GC) to the right and the concave surface or inner curvature (IC) to the left **B.** Right laterial view of the heart. Notice the convex surface of the loop or greater curvature (GC) and the dorsal wall of the heart adjacent to the ventral wall of the foregut (VWF). **C.** Frontal section of the heart photographed with the scanning electron microscope. **D.** Diagram representing the primitive cardiac segments. Notice in C and D, the greater curvature to the right and the inner curvature to the left. C = conus or primitive outlet; RCG = right conus groove; LCG = left conus groove; PO = primitive outlet or conus; LIG = left interventricular groove; RA-VG = right atrioventricular groove; PRA = primitive right atrium; PLA = primitive left atrium; PTRV = primordium of the apical trabeculated region of the right ventricle; PTLV = primordium of the apical trabeculated region of the left ventricle; PI = primitive inlet; PA = primitive atria; 1 = cephalic limb of the loop (primordium of the apical trabeculated region of the right ventricle); 2 = caudal limb of the loop (primordium of the apical trabeculated region of the left ventricle plus the primitive inlet).

ventricle or infundibulum and contributes to the development of the outlet of the left ventricle or aortic vestibule (de la Cruz et al 1982). We prefer not to use the term "conus" because this term refers only to the geometric form of the segment, and has no meaning with respect to its prospective fate. We use the term "primitive inlet" because it gives origin to the inlet of both ventricles (de la Cruz et al 1983, 1991, 1997). We do not use the term AV canal because it does not constitute the entire inlet.

For study purposes, we will divide the C-shaped loop into three regions: (1) the

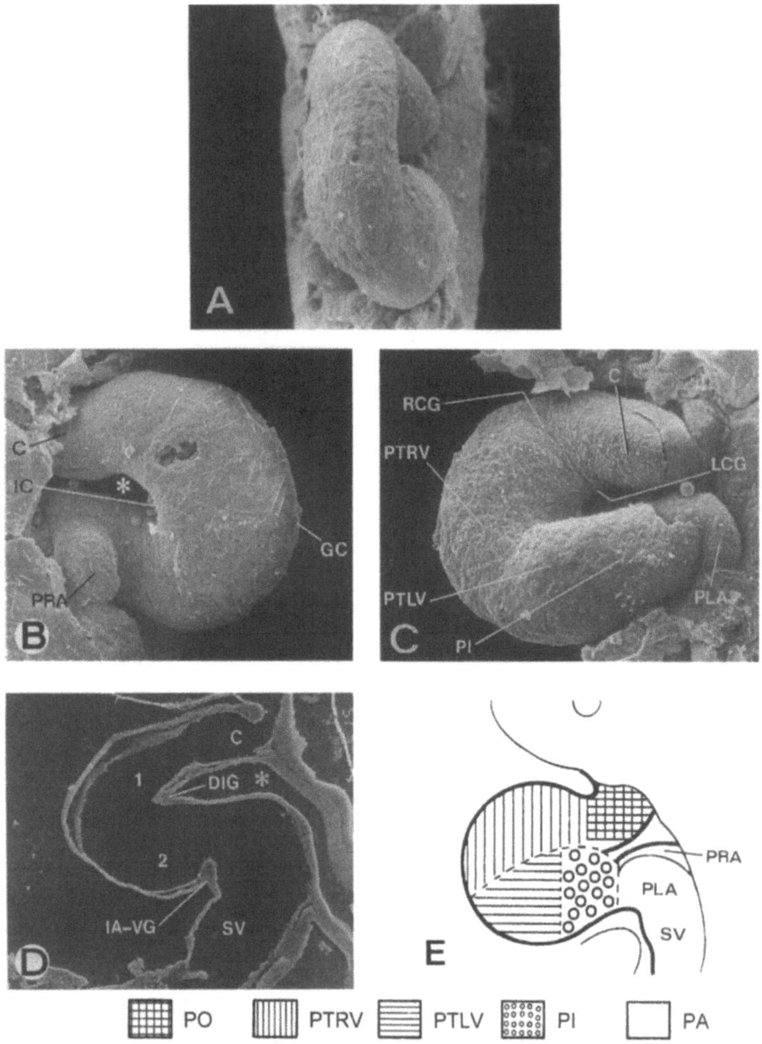

FIGURE 2. Photographs obtained with the scanning electron microscope, histological section, and diagram of the S-shaped loop heart of the chick embryo at stage 14HH. **A.** Ventral view of the heart. Notice the greater curvature (convex surface of the loop) perpendicular to the frontal plane. **B.** Right lateral view of the heart, showing the convex surface of the loop (greater curvature) in a ventral position, the concave surface of the loop (inner curvature) in a dorsal position, both limbs of the loop in a dorsoventral and caudocephalic direction, and the presence of the free retrocardiac space (*). **C.** Left lateral view of the heart. **D.** Sagittal section of the heart photographed with the scanning electron microscope. Notice the dorsal interventricular groove (DIG) and the inferior atrioventricular groove (IA-VG), which at stage 12HH are the left interventricular groove (LIG) and the right atrioventricular groove (RA-VG), respectively; compare with Fig. 1C. **E.** Diagram representing the primitive cardiac segments. C = conus or primitive outlet; RCG = right conus groove; LCG = left conus groove; PO = primitive outlet or conus; PRA = primitive right atrium; PLA = primitive left atrium; PTRV = primordium of the apical trabeculated region of the right ventricle; PTLV = primordium of the apical trabeculated region of the left ventricle; PI = primitive inlet; PA = primitive atria; GC = greater curvature; IC = inner curvature; SV = sinus venosus; 1 = cephalic limb of the loop (primordium of the apical trabeculated region of the right ventricle); 2 = caudal limb of the loop constituted by the primordium of the apical trabeculated region of the left ventricle plus the primitive inlet.

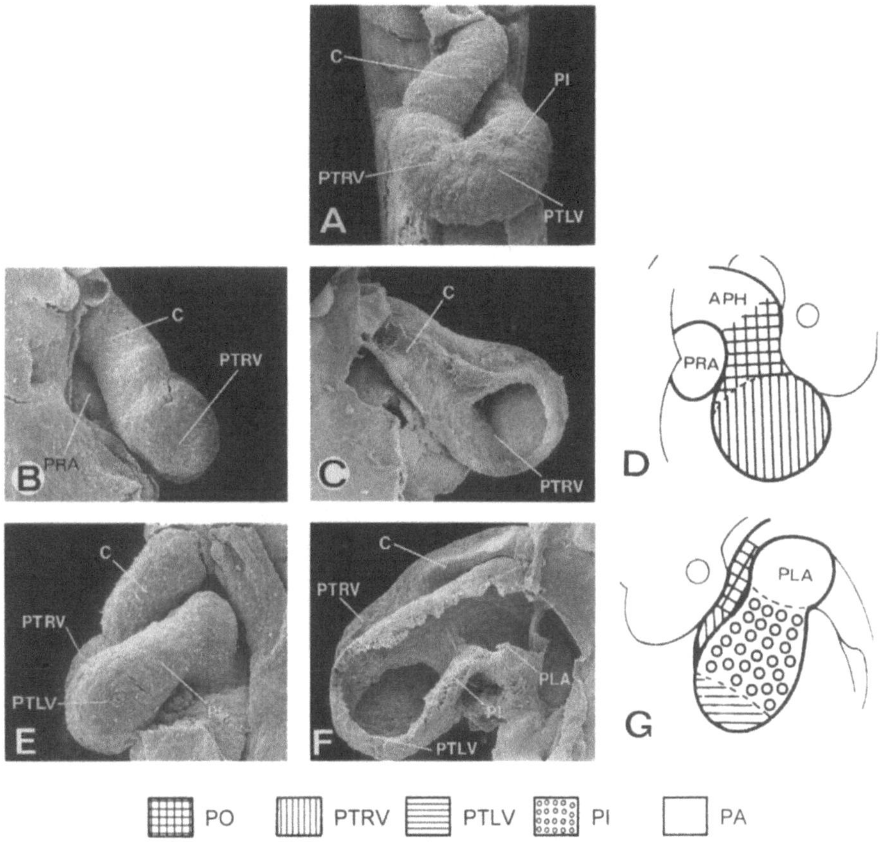

FIGURE 3. Photographs obtained with the scanning electron microscope and diagrams showing the primitive cardiac segments of the chick embryo heart in the terminal stage or stage 16HH. The primitive cardiac segments show the relations that they have in the mature heart. Notice the relation of proximity between the primitive right atrium (PRA), the primitive inlet (PI), and the primordium of the apical trabeculated region of the right ventricle (PTRV), also between the conus (C) or primitive outlet (PO) and the primordium of the apical trabeculated region of the left ventricle (PTLV). The primordium of the apical trabeculated region of the right ventricle (PTRV) is not yet connected with the primitive right atrium (PRA), nor the primordium of the apical trabeculated region of the left ventricle (PTLV) with the conus (C). **A.** Ventral view of the heart. Notice the primordium of the apical trabeculated region of the right ventricle to the right and that of the left ventricle to the left and adjacent to each other. **B.** Right lateral view of the heart. Notice the primitive right atrium in a dorso-cephalic position and in a proximity relation with the primordium of the apical trabeculated region of the right ventricle. **C.** Right lateral view of a dissection of the conus and the primordium of the apical trabeculated region of the right ventricle. Notice the conus is connected with the primordium of the apical trabeculated region of the right ventricle. **D.** Diagram of the right lateral view of the heart showing the primitive cardiac segment. **E.** Left lateral view of the heart showing the primordium of the apical trabeculated region of the right ventricle to the right and adjacent to the primordium of the apical trabeculated region of the left ventricle to the left. Observe that the conus is cephalic and in a proximity relationship with the primordium of the apical trabeculated region of the left ventricle. **F.** Left lateral view of a dissection of the primitive left atrium the primitive inlet, and the primordium of the apical trabeculated region of the left ventricle. Notice the primitive inlet adjacent to the primordium of the apical trabeculated region of the right ventricle and connecting the primitive left atrium with the primordium of the apical trabeculated region of the left ventricle. **G.** Diagram of the left lateral view of the heart showing the primitive cardiac segments. PA = primitive atria.

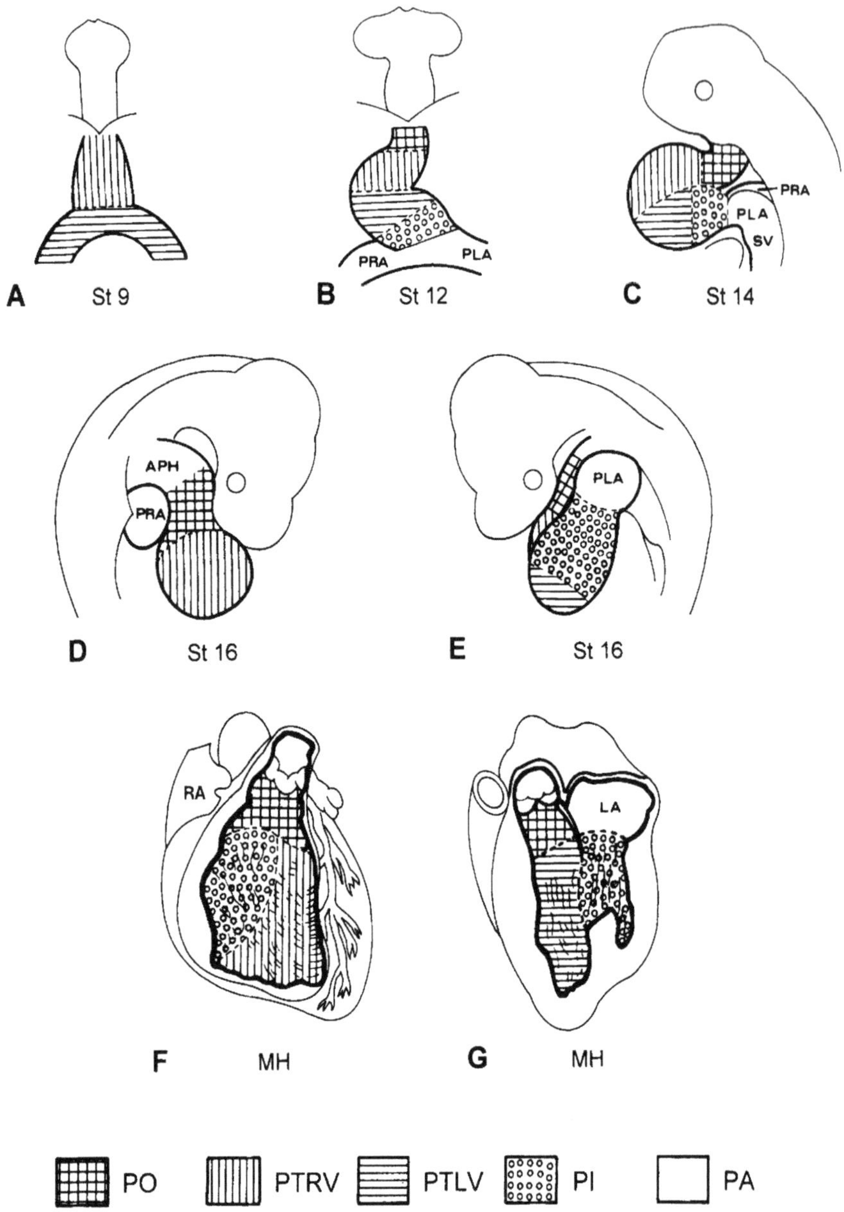

FIGURE 4. Diagrams representing the primitive cardiac segments, the stages of development at which they appear, and their anatomical manifestation in the mature heart. Besides the changes of shape, spatial position and the relationships among each other also change. **A.** Straight tube heart. **B.** Frontal view of the C-shaped loop heart. **C.** Left lateral view of the S-shaped loop heart. **D.** Right lateral view of the heart in the terminal stage. **E.** Left lateral view of the heart in the terminal stage. **F.** Internal view of the anatomical right ventricle of the mature heart (MH). **G.** Internal view of the anatomical left ventricle of the mature heart. PTRV = primordium of the apical trabeculated region of the anatomical right ventricle; PTLV = primordium of the apical trabeculated region of the anatomical left ventricle; PO = primitive outlet; PI = primitive inlet; PRA = primitive right atrium; PLA = primitive left atrium; APH = arterial pole of the heart; SV = sinus venosus; RA = right atrium; LA = left atrium; PA = primitive atrium.

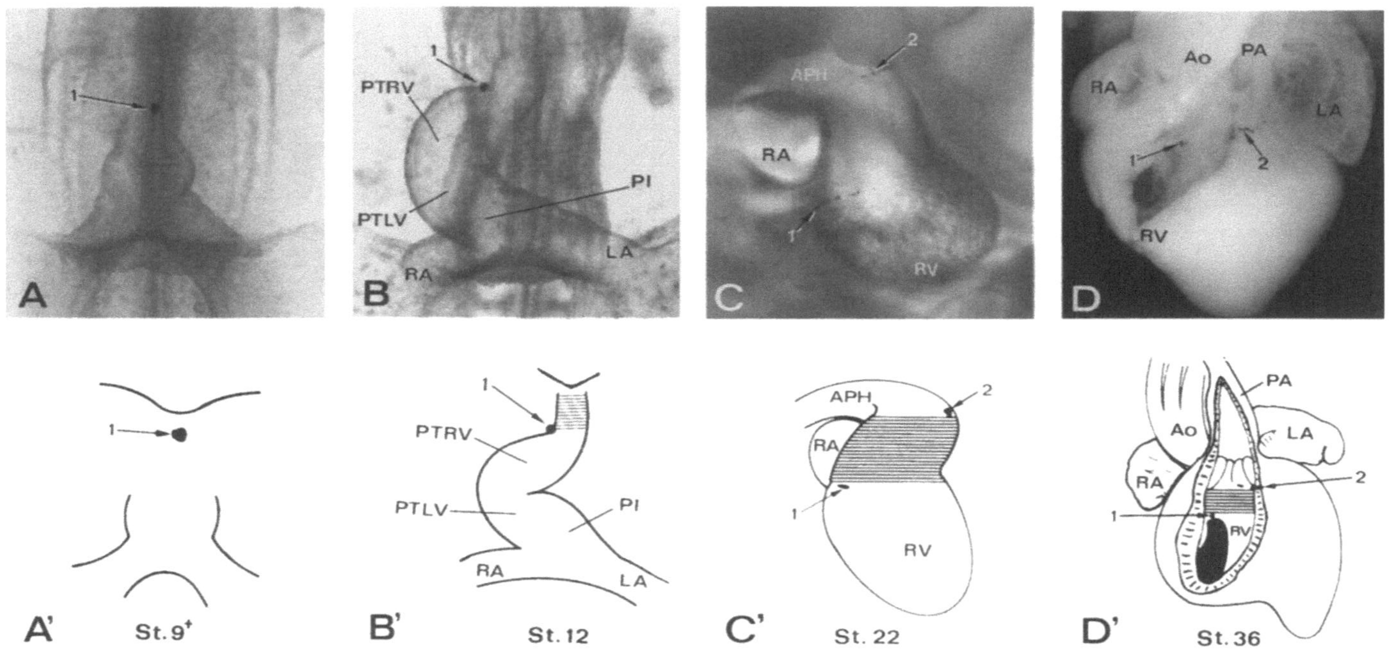

FIGURE 5. Photographs and diagrams of in vivo labeling experiments in the chick embryo heart, which show that the primordium of the ventricular outlet (primitive outlet or conus) appears at stage 12HH and that it become the most cephalic segment of the heart tube. **A, A′**. Notice the label (1) in the cephalic end of the straight tube heart at stage 9+HH. **B, B′**. The same label (1) in the same embryo now at stage 12HH. Note the label is located in the caudal end of a new segment (primitive outlet or conus), which constitutes the most cephalic region of this heart. **C, C′**. The same label (1) in the caudal end of the conal ridges at stage 22HH. **D, D′**. The same label (1) in the mature heart is found in the proximal border of the supraventricular crest, which is the anatomical limit between the apical trabeculated region of the anatomical right ventricle and its outlet or infundibulum. Thus, this experiment shows that the new segment is the primitive outlet or conus. A second label (2) was placed at the cephalic limit of the conal ridges at stage 22HH (C, C′). The same label (2) appears in the mature heart beneath the pulmonary cusps (D, D′). This experiment shows that the cephalic end of the conal ridges corresponds to the boundary between the outlet of the right ventricle and the pulmonary artery. PA = pulmonary artery; Ao = aorta; RA = right atrium; LA = left atrium; RV = right ventricle; PTRV = primordium of the apical trabeculated region of the right ventricle; PTLV = primordium of the apical trabeculated region of the left ventricle; PI = primitive inlet; APH = arterial pole of the heart; Striped area = ventricular outlet. Reprinted with permission of from de la Cruz et al. (1991) Cardiol Young 1:123.

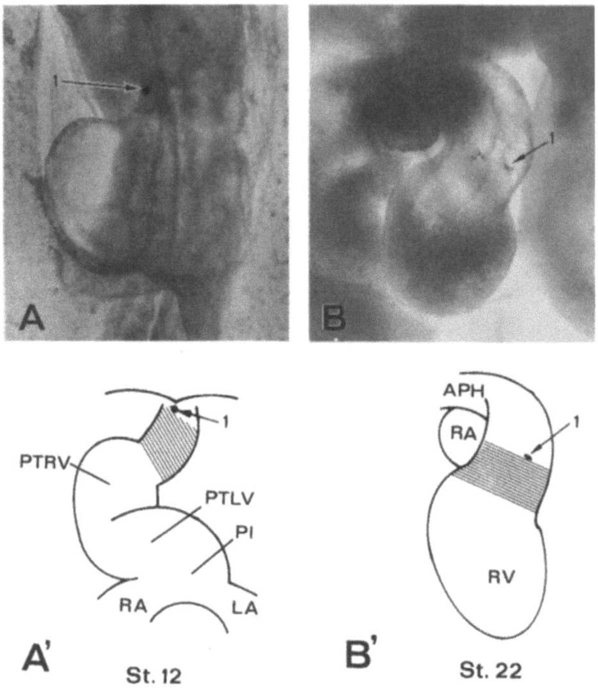

FIGURE 6. Photographs and diagrams of in vivo labeling experiments in the chick embryo heart, which show that the new segment that appears at stage 12HH, cephalic to the conal grooves, is the primordium of the outlet of the right ventricle (conus) and that the primordium of the great arteries or arterial pole of the heart is not present. **A, A′**. Notice label (1) in the cephalic end of the heart at stage 12HH. **B, B′**. The same embryo at stage 22HH showing the same label (1) in the middle zone of the conus. In addition, these experiments show that the new cephalic segment or conus at stage 12HH corresponds, at stage 22HH, to the region of the primitive outlet or conus adjacent to the primordium of the apical trabeculated region of the right ventricle. PTRV = primordium of the apical trabeculated region of the right ventricle; PTLV = primordium of the apical trabeculated region of the left ventricle; PI = primitive inlet; RA = right atrium; LA = left atrium; RV = right ventricle; APH = arterial pole of the heart; Striped area = the conus region adjacent to the primordium of the apical trabeculated region of right ventricle. Fig. 6A and B reprinted with permission of from de la Cruz et al. (1977) J Anat 123:661.

cephalic region, or the primitive outlet (de la Cruz et al 1977, 1991) (Figs. 1, A and D; 4, B and F; and 5, B, B′, D and D′); (2) the middle region, or the loop region constituted in a cephalocaudal order by the primordium of the apical trabeculated region of the right ventricle, the primordium of the apical trabeculated region of the left ventricle, and the primitive inlet (de la Cruz et al 1987, 1989, 1991) (Figs. 1, A and D; 4, B, F and G; and 7, B–H); and the (3) caudal region, or the primitive atria (Stalsberg and De Haan 1969; Castro-Quezada et al 1972) (Figs. 1, C and D and 4, B, F and G).

Cephalic Region or Primitive Outlet

By means of in vivo labeling experiments in the chick embryo heart, de la Cruz and colleagues (1977, 1991) showed that the conus is the primordium of the outlet of

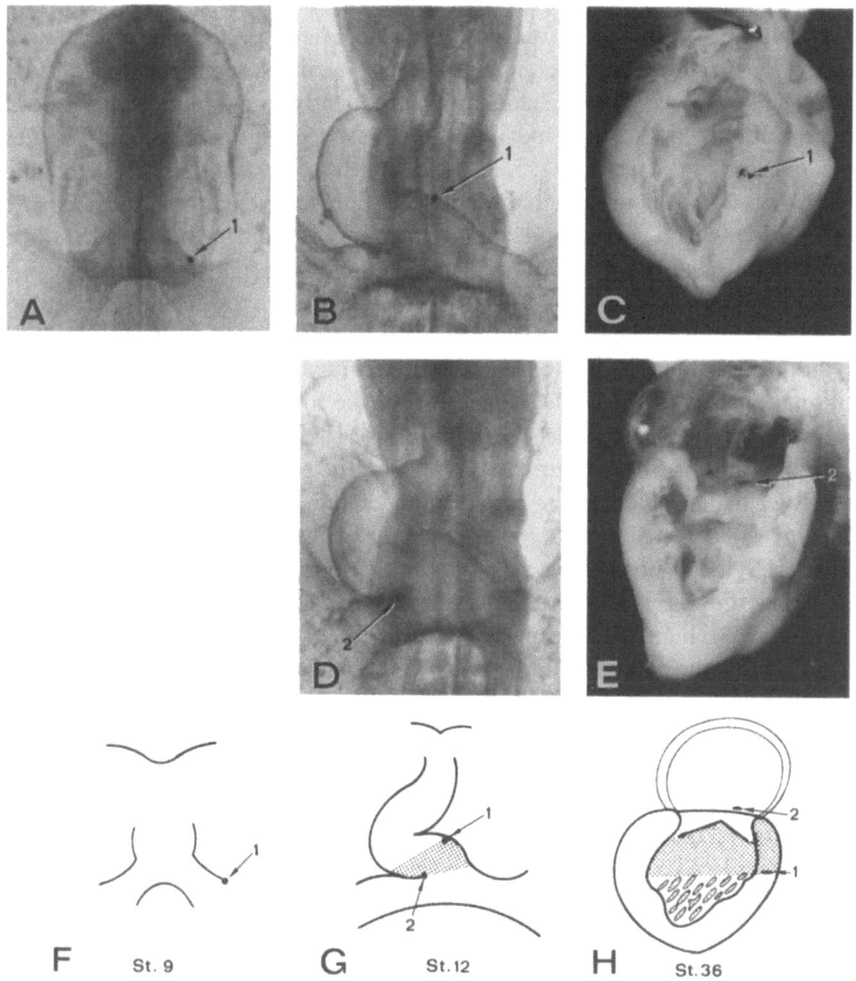

FIGURE 7. Photographs and diagrams of in vivo labeling experiments in the chick embryo heart, which show that the primordium of the ventricular inlet (primitive inlet) appears at stage 12HH, and that it is the segment adjacent to the right atrioventricular groove in the caudal limb of the loop and connects both primitive atria with the primordium of the apical trabeculated region of the left ventricle. **A, F.** Notice the label (1) in the caudal end of the straight tube heart at stage 9+HH. **B, G.** The same label (1) in the same embryo but now at stage 12HH is seen in the caudal limb of the loop in the cephalic limit of a new segment. **C, H.** The same label (1) was found in the mature heart at the limit between the smooth region (inlet) and the apical trabeculated region of the left ventricle. This experiment shows that the site at which label (1) was found at stage 12HH, has become the boundary between the smooth region (inlet) and the apical trabeculated region of the left ventricle in the mature heart. **D, G.** Notice a second label (2) was placed in the right atrioventricular groove at stage 12HH. **E, H.** This same label (2) was found in the mature heart in the insertion of the anteroseptal leaflet of the mitral valve, which is the limit between the atrium and the inlet of the left ventricle (primitive inlet). Collectively those experiments show that the new segment comprised between labels (1) and (2) is the primordium of the inlet of the left ventricle or primitive inlet. It is important to note that this segment is located in the caudal limb of the loop adjacent to the right AV groove and connects both primitive atria with the primordium of the apical trabeculated region of the left ventricle. **F, G, H.** Schematic synthesis of the in vivo labeling experiments described above. In addition these experments show that the primitive right and left atria first appear at stage 12HH as the caudal segment of the heart. PRA = primitive right atrium; PLA = primitive left atrium; LV = left ventricle; Dotted area = ventricular inlet. Reprinted with permission of from de la Cruz et al. (1991) Cardiol Young 1:123.

the right ventricle; it appears at this stage of development (stage 12HH) and forms the cephalic region of thè heart (Figs. 4, B and F and 5). This information was obtained by placing a label at the cephalic end of the straight tube heart (stage 9+HH) and observing that the label was subsequently found in the conal grooves at stage 12HH, which is the caudal limit of a new segment that becomes the new cephalic region of the heart (Fig. 5, A, A′, B, and B′). This same label was found in the mature heart at the proximal border of the supraventricular crest (de la Cruz et al 1977, 1991), which correspond's to the anatomical boundary between the outlet (infundibulum) and the apical trabeculated region of the right ventricle (Fig. 5, D and D′) (chapters III and VII). Therefore, the conal grooves in the heart at stage 12HH correspond to the boundary between the primordium of the outlet (conus) and the primordium of the apical trabeculated region of the right ventricle; in addition, that part of the conus, which is cephalic to these grooves, becomes the primordium of the outlet of the right ventricle (de la Cruz et al 1977, 1991) (Fig. 5).

The same authors (de la Cruz et al 1977), with the purpose of clarifying whether this new cephalic region is the primordium of the outlet of the right ventricle (conus) or whether in addition, the arterial pole of the heart (primordium of both great arteries) is also present, placed a label at the cephalic end of this region at stage 12HH; they found this label at the middle zone of the conus at stage 22HH (de la Cruz et al 1977) (Fig. 6). This experiment shows that the new segment that appears at stage 12HH (the conus), and that is cephalic to the conal grooves, is exclusively the primordium of the outlet of the right ventricle and that at this stage the primordium of the great arteries (arterial pole of the heart) is still not present (de la Cruz et al 1977) (Figs. 5 and 6). Furthermore, with the purpose of investigating the limit between the primordium of the outlet of the right ventricle (conus) and of the great arteries (arterial pole of the heart) at stage 22HH, de la Cruz and associates (1977, 1991) placed a label at the cephalic end of the conal ridges at this stage and found it in the mature heart beneath the leaflet of the pulmonary valve. This experiment shows that the cephalic end of the conal ridges at stage 22HH corresponds to the limit between the great arteries (arterial pole) and the outlet of the right ventricle (Fig. 5, C, C′, D, and D′) (chapter VII).

The in vivo labeling experiments show that the new cephalic segment, which appears at stage 12HH, gives origin to the outlet of the right ventricle (de la Cruz et al 1977, 1991), but it also contributes to the development of the outlet of the left ventricle. For that reason, the conus is correctly designated as the primitive outlet (chapter VII).

The results of the in vivo labeling experiments (de la Cruz et al 1977, 1991) show that the findings concerning the cephalic region of the chick embryo heart at stage 12HH are valid also for the human embryo 3707 of similar cardiac morphology. Consequently, this new information argues against the assumptions made by Davis (1927) and DeVries and Saunders (1962), which maintained that the cephalic region of the human embryo heart 3707 is the primordium of the great arteries.

Middle Region or Loop Region

The limit of the loop are cephalically the conal grooves and caudally the right atrioventricular groove, since at this stage there is a shallow left atrioventricular groove (Fig. 1, A and C).

The loop has two borders, a right convex (greater curvature) and a left concave (inner curvature) (Fig. 1, A and C). de la Cruz and coworkers (1989, 1997) have shown by means of in vivo labeling experiments in the chick embryo heart that the right border or greater curvature of the loop originates from the ventral fusion line of both cardiac primordia of the straight tube heart (chapter III, Fig. 8, E, F, E′, and F′). Postmortem studies with the scanning electron microscope of the loop of the chick embryo at stage 12HH show a groove in its convex surface, which corresponds to the ventral fusion line of the straight tube heart. The left border of the loop originates from the right and left borders of the straight tube heart, as de la Cruz and associates (1989, 1991) have shown by means of in vivo labeling experiments (chapter III, Fig. 8, A–D′).

The loop has two limbs, a cephalic or ascending limb situated to the right and a caudal or descending limb situated to the left (Fig. 1A).

Cephalic Limb of the Loop In the chick embryo it is exclusively constituted by the primordium of the apical trabeculated region of the right ventricle, which appears in the straight tube heart (de la Cruz et al 1977, 1989, 1991) (chapter III, Figs. 4 and 6) (Figs. 1D; and 4, B and F). The cephalic limits of the loop are the conal grooves, which separate it from the primitive outlet or conus (de la Cruz et al 1977, 1991) (Fig. 5), and its caudal limit is the left interventricular groove, which separates it from the primordium of the apical trabeculated region of the left ventricle (de la Cruz et al 1989, 1991) (Fig. 7, A–C). This information was obtained by means of in vivo labeling experiments in the chick embryo (de la Cruz et al 1977, 1989, 1991) (chapter III). The removal experiments in the chick embryo, by Castro-Quezada and associates (1972) also show that the cephalic limb of the loop is constituted by the primordium of the apical trabeculated region of the right ventricle (chapter III, Fig. 7).

The cephalic limb of the loop of human embryo 3707 and of the chick at stage 12HH (C-shaped loop) are similar morphologically. Davis (1927) points out that in the human embryo this limb is constituted by the bulbus cordis or primordium of the entire right ventricle. Our experimental results using in vivo labeling (de la Cruz et al 1977, 1989, 1991) and removal techniques (Castro-Quezada et al 1972) do not support Davis's (1927) view in man.

Caudal Limb of the Loop The in vivo labeling experiments in the chick embryo (de la Cruz et al 1987, 1989, 1991) have shown that this limb is constituted by two primordia, one adjacent to the left interventricular groove, i.e., the primordium of the apical trabeculated region of the left ventricle, and the other adjacent to the right atrioventricular groove, which is the primitive inlet (de la Cruz et al 1987, 1991) (Figs. 1D; 4, B, and G; and 7). It is important to point out that there is no groove or morphological structure to identify the limit between these two primordia in either species (Figs. 1 A and C; and 7B).

The in vivo labeling experiments (de la Cruz et al 1987, 1991), which show that the caudal limb of the loop is constituted by two primordia, were carried out by placing a label at the caudal end of the straight tube heart (stage 9+HH), which was found in the caudal limb of the loop (stage 12HH) at 110 μm from the left interventricular groove, and in the nature heart, at the limit between the smooth region (inlet) and the apical trabeculated region of the left ventricle (Fig. 7A–C and F–H). The results of this experiment show that the zone where the label was found in the caudal limb of the loop (stage 12HH) corresponds to the limit between the primordium of the apical trabeculated region of the left ventricle (adjacent to the left interventricular groove) (chapter III) and the primitive ventricular inlet (adjacent to the right atrioventricular groove) (de la Cruz et al 1987, 1991) (Figs. 1D and 7). The segment adjacent to the right atrioventricular groove is a new segment because it appears in the loop at stage 12HH immediately caudal to the label that was initially placed at the caudal end of the straight tube heart at stage 9+HH (de la Cruz et al 1987, 1991) (chapter III) (Fig. 7, A, B, F, and G). With the purpose of investigating the prospective fate of the right atrioventricular groove, de la Cruz and associates (1987, 1991) placed a label in this groove (stage 12HH) and traced it up to the mature heart; they found it in the region of the anteroseptal leaflet of the mitral valve, which inserts into the septum, thus showing that the limit between the primitive inlet and the primitive atria is the right atrioventricular groove (Fig. 7 D, E, G, and H). Furthermore, when the inferior cushion of the AV canal was labeled, the same zone of the anteroseptal leaflet of the mitral valve appeared labeled (de la Cruz et al 1983); therefore, the right atrioventricular groove is the primordium of this cushion (chapter VI, Fig. 4D) (Fig. 7, D, E, G, and H).

The information regarding the appearance of the primitive inlet at stage 12HH has also been supported by in vivo labeling of the extracardiac cell populations adjacent to the caudal end of the straight tube heart (stage 9+HH). When these cells were traced up to stage 12HH, they were found in the caudal limb of the loop, at the segment adjacent to the right atrioventricular groove or primitive inlet (George 1993).

Thus it is important to understand that at this stage of development there is only one inlet connecting both primitive atria with the primordium of the apical trabeculated region of the left ventricle. This single inlet should be designated as the primitive inlet, because at stage 17HH when the septation of the heart takes place, it gives origin to the right ventricular inlet and to the left ventricular inlet (Van Mierop et al 1962; Netter and Van Mierop 1969; de la Cruz et al 1983, 1997; Wenink and Gittenberger-de Groot 1985) (chapter VI, Fig. 2).

The results of the in vivo labeling experiments in the chick embryo heart (de la Cruz et al 1987, 1991) show that the caudal limb of the loop at stage 12HH is constituted by two primordia, i.e., that of the trabeculated region of the left ventricle and that of the inlet of both ventricles (de la Cruz et al 1987, 1991), or the primitive inlet. This new information negates that the caudal limb of the loop of the human embryo 3707 of similar cardiac morphology to that of the chick is constituted by the primordium of the left ventricle entirely, as proposed by Davis (1927) and by DeVries and Saunders (1962), which they designated as primitive ventricle and left ventricle, respectively.

Caudal Region or Primitive Atria

The atrial region in the chick embryo has a crescent shape that circumscribes the anterior portal gut, and its boundary with the caudal limb of the loop is the right atrioventricular groove (Fig. 1C). According to the in vivo labeling experiments by Stalsberg and DeHaan (1969) and Castro-Quezada and coworkers (1972), this region appears at stage 12HH. Experimental results by de la Cruz and colleagues (1987, 1991) (Fig. 7) also confirmed these earlier findings.

The atrial region of human embryo 3707 and of the chick embryo heart at stage 12HH are morphologically similar in both species. It is separated from the caudal limb of the loop by the right atrioventricular groove, which is very deep. Likewise the primordium of the right atrium is larger than that of the left atrium in both species.

S-Shaped Loop

The chick embryo heart at stage 14HH and that of the human embryo 6344 of 13 to 14 somites, horizon XI, are typical examples of a ventricular loop, convex ventrally and concave dorsally, or an S-shaped loop (Fig. 2A). This loop is in the sagittal plane and it is more clearly seen in the right or the left lateral views of the heart (Fig. 2, B–E).

The most relevant occurrence in the heart at this stage of development in both species is the fact that the loop is convex ventrally and concave dorsally (S-shaped loop) in the sagittal plane. Consequently, the dorsal wall of the loop has ceased to be parallel and adjacent to the ventral wall of the foregut as was the case at stage 12HH (Fig. 1B); then a retrocardiac space appears (Fig. 2, B–D) and the dorsal wall of the loop is now right and its ventral wall is left. We will divide this heart also into three regions for its study.

Cephalic Region or Primitive Outlet

This primitive cardiac region maintains its cephalic position but it acquires a dorsoventral direction, is situated more to left, and remains connected with the cephalic limb of the loop (primordium of the apical trabeculated region of the right ventricle) (de la Cruz et al 1977, 1991) (Figs. 2, B, C, and E; and 4C).

Middle Region or Loop Region

Owing to the fact that the loop is convex ventrally and concave dorsally, both limbs are in the sagittal plane in a dorsoventral direction (Fig. 2, B–E). The two segments that constitute the caudal limb of the loop have a different direction; the long axis of the segment adjacent to the left interventricular groove (primordium of the apical trabeculated region of the left ventricle) (de la Cruz et al 1987, 1989, 1991) is oblique, dorsoventral, and caudocephalic (Figs. 2, B–E; and 4C), whereas the long axis of the segment adjacent to the right atrioventricular groove or primitive inlet (de la Cruz al 1987, 1989, 1991) is perpendicular to the frontal plane (Fig. 2, D, and E). Therefore this latter segment cannot be seen in the frontal or anterior view of the heart (Fig. 2A). It is important to point out that the left interventricular groove and the right atrioventricular groove at stage 12HH (C-shaped loop) (Fig. 1C), are dorsal and inferior respectively at stage 14HH (S-shaped loop) (Figs. 1C and 2D).

Caudal Region or Primitive Atria

The atria have acquired a dorsal position because they have become displaced cephalically within the retrocardiac space; however, they remain connected by way of the primitive inlet with the primordium of the apical trabeculated region of the left ventricle (de la Cruz et al 1987, 1989, 1991) (Figs. 2, B–E; and 4C). The dorsal mesocardium has disappeared.

Terminal Stage

The chick embryo heart at stage 16HH and that of human embryo 2053 of 20 somites, horizon XI, are the most representative of the last phase of the torsion process of the cardiac tube.

The most outstanding feature of this phase is the fact that the primitive cardiac segments occupy the spatial position and their relationship of proximity that they have in the mature heart. This fact plays a very important role in the normal septation of this organ, which begins at the next developmental stage (Steding and Seidl 1980; de la Cruz et al 1983, 1997; Männer et al 1993) (stage 17HH).

The primordium of the apical trabeculated region of the right ventricle, which is cephalic in the S-shaped loop, and the primordium of the apical trabeculated region of the left ventricle, which is caudal (Figs. 2, C and E; and 4C), become situated right and left, respectively, and adjacent to each other at the concluding phase of the torsion process or terminal stage (stage 16HH) (Figs. 3 and 4, D and E). The atria maintain the dorsal position that they had in the S-shaped loop stage. The new relationship of proximity between the primordia of the apical trabeculated region of the right ventricle, the primitive inlet (Figs. 3, E and G; and 4E), and the primitive right atrium (Figs. 3B and 4D) determine that when the 8-shaped septum appears at stage 17HH to divide the primitive inlet into a right and a left inlet, the primordium of the apical trabeculated region of the right ventricle becomes connected with the right atrium by way of its own inlet (de la Cruz et al 1983, 1997) (chapter VI, Fig. 2). Furthermore, the primitive outlet or conus has established a close relationship with the primordium of the apical trabeculated region of the left ventricle (Figs. 3, E and F; and 4E), which will facilitate the connection between them at later developmental stages (chapter VII).

The histological features of the walls of the cardiac tube during the torsion period are similar in man and in chick: both have a myocardial mantle, endocardium, and extracellular matrix (cardiac jelly). There is little or no extracellular matrix at the atrial level.

CAUSAL FACTORS OF THE TORSION

The search for causal factors of the cardiac tube torsion, particularly the development of a ventricular loop convex to the right (C-shaped loop), has been the subject of numerous studies. These searches have been done, for obvious reasons, in the preloop stages, targeting the cardiogenic areas and the straight tube heart. The following subjects have been studied: extrinsic factor (Patten 1922; Butler 1952; Orts-Llorca and Jiménez-Collado 1967; Castro-Quezada et al 1972); the differential growth (Sissman 1966; Stalsberg 1969a, 1969b); the cell population movement (Lepori 1967); the heart contraction (Manasek and Monroe 1972); hemodynamics (Roux 1895; Spitzer 1951); the morphological and molecular aspects of the myocardium (Manasek and Monroe 1972; Manasek et al 1972; Itasaki et al 1991; Shiraishi et al 1992); the cadiac jelly (Nakamura and Manasek 1978; Nakamura and Manasek 1981; Manasek et al 1984; Baldwin and Solursh 1989); the endocardium; morphogens (Orts-Llorca and Ruano-Gil 1967; Brown and Wolpert 1990; Easton et al 1992; Hoyle et al 1992); and the genetic factors (Osmond et al 1991; Van Keuren et al 1991; Yost 1992; Yokoyama et al 1993).

We will refer briefly to some of the published work on the causal factors of development of the C-shaped loop and finally we will deal with the S-shaped loop.

Extrinsic Factors

The most commonly quoted publication related to extrinsic factors is Patten's (1922). This author maintained that the ventricular loop is formed because the cardiac tube grows longitudinally at a greater speed than the pericardial cavity in which it is contained. However, Butler (1952), Orts-Llorca and Jiménez-Collado (1967), Orts-Llorca and Ruano-Gil (1967), and Castro-Quezada and associates (1972) showed that the cardiac tube bends outside the pericardial cavity.

Differential Growth

Differential growth in its cell proliferation aspect has been proposed by different investigators. Sissman (1966), through the study of radioactive index using tritiated thymidine in the chick embryo heart at stages 11HH to 17HH, concluded that his results were not sufficient to support the view that differential growth is a causal factor for looping. Stalsberg (1969a) studied the radioactive index with tritiated thymidine in the right and left cardiogenic areas of the chick embryo. His results, according to Manasek (1981), did not show a significant quantitative difference between the right and the left cardiogenic areas. Stalsberg (1969b) also used colchicine to study the mitotic activity in the cardiogenic areas, in the straight tube heart, and in the loop and found no differences in rates of cell proliferation.

Cell Population Movements

The difference in rate of movement of cells in the cardiogenic areas (heart-forming fields), together with the cardia bifida of the chick embryo in which both cardiac primordia have a "C" shape with their concave aspects facing each other, were considered by Lepori (1967) as causal factors of the D-loop or L-loop. However, Nadal-Ginard and García (1972) showed that in the cardia bifida of the chick embryo both cardiac primordia have a "C" shape, but with their convex aspects facing each other. Therefore, it is impossible that the caudal part of either of the two primordia enters inside the concavity of the other.

The Heart Contraction

Contraction of the cardiac muscle as a causal factor of the torsion of the cardiac tube was studied by Manasek and Monroe (1972) in the chick embryo at stage 9HH. They used potassium chloride in the culture media instead of sodium chloride to inhibit contraction. They obtained a normal loop and they concluded that the myocardial contraction was not a causal factor of the torsion.

Hemodynamics

Roux (1895) and Spitzer (1951) suggested the hemodynamic factor as a causal agent of the torsion of the cardiac tube. The fact that there is no blood flow at the stage preceding the torsion of the cardiac tube negates the views of these authors.

Morphological and Molecular Aspects of the Myocardium

Concerning the morphological and molecular characteristics of the myocardium and their participation as causal factors in the development of the ventricular loop, Manasek and coworkers (1972) proposed that the looping is a consequence of regional differences in size and orientation of the myocardial cells. They found that at the preloop stage, the size and orientation of the long axes of the myocardial cells were different from those at the loop stage, and they concluded that these changes in form and orientation of the myocardial cells may be the cause or the result of looping of the cardiac tube. Manasek (1972) pointed out that the development of the loop occurred simultaneously with myocardial differentiation, i.e., formation of myofibrils and the onset of contraction. Manasek (1972), using cytochalasin-B in the chick embryo at the preloop stage, blocked the looping; after the removal of cytochalasin-B, the same embryos developed a normal loop. Also, in older embryos (stage 10HH to 11HH) after the myocardium had differentiated, he added cytochalasin-B and observed that the myofibrils disappeared and the heart lost its characteristic shape. After the removal of cytochalasin-B, the myofibrils reappeared and the heart loop recovered (Manasek 1972).

Itasaky and associates (1991) found actin bundles distributed in a circumferential arrangement at the caudal part of the straight tube heart in the chick embryo. These were more apparent in the right side. By placing cytochalasin-B crystals into the right caudal part of the heart, the bundles disintegrated and an inverted loop ensued. On the contrary, when the crystals were placed onto the left caudal part of the heart, a normal loop was obtained. These authors suggested that the normal loop is caused by the tension exerted by the actin bundles at the right caudal part of the straight tube heart. These data suggest that the looping process has two mechanisms, one to produce the loop and the other to produce the type i.e., D- or L-loop.

Shiraishi and colleagues (1992, 1993) studied the orientation of the myofibrils and the shape of the cells in the different layers of the myocardium from the preloop period up to the loop stage in the chick embryo with the use of phalloidin and the confocal microscope. These authors concluded that the circumferentially arranged myofibrils at the bottom of the inner layer may play a most important role in the looping process. These same authors (Shiraishi et al 1993) studied the development of myocyte cell junctions during the looping process and proposed that the adhession molecule, N-cadherin, played an important role; however they did not reach any conclusion concerning their contribution in the torsion process.

Cardiac Jelly

The participation of the cardiac jelly (extracellular matrix) in the looping process has frequently been suggested as a causal mechanism. We will refer to some of the studies. Nakamura and Manasek (1978, 1981) and Manasek (1981) proposed that the accumulation of hyaluronic acid in the extracellular matrix (cardiac jelly) in the cardiac tube and its hydration were the cause of normal heart looping in vertebrates. On the other hand, Baldwin and Solursh (1989) cultivated rat embryos in the presence of hyaluronidase and showed that the loop formed despite the absence of hyaluronic acid.

Endocardium

This structure has not been considered as a causal factor of the torsion of the cardiac tube. Nevertheless the endocardial tube bends even in the absence of the myocardium, as seen in the experiment of Castro-Quezada and colleagues (1972), who removed the cephalic region of the straight tube heart (stage 9+HH) and obtained a loop whose cephalic limb was exclusively constituted by an endocardial tube that showed the normal orientation of this limb.

Morphogens

The importance of morphogens in the development of the loop has been studied by different investigators. We will refer to the studies of some of them. Easton and associates (1992) grafted the caudal region of the quail precardiac area into the cephalic precardiac mesoderm of the chick; they obtained a large percentage of hearts without a curvature (compact heart) and also inverted loops. These authors (Easton et al 1992) thought their results were caused by the fact that the cephalic region of the precardiac areas or heart fields produced a looping promoter morphogen, while the caudal region produces a looping inhibitor morphogen. With the purpose of investigating whether any intrinsic differences existed in the right and left precardiac areas that might participate in the development of the loop, Orts-Llorca and Ruano-Gil (1967), Brown and Wolpert (1990), and Hoyle and coworkers (1992) performed right-left switching experiments of these areas in the chick embryo at stages 5HH to 6HH and found differences in their morphogenetic capability to form a loop. Brown and Wolpert (1990) and Hoyle and coworkers (1992) also suggested retinoic acid as a morphogen that influenced looping by affecting direction of looping but not the motor.

Genetic Factors

Van Keuren and associates (1991), Yost (1992), and Yokoyama and colleagues (1993) have pointed out that there are at least two genes implicated in the development of the loop. Osmond and associates (1991) proposed that the action of these genes is possibly triggered by retinoic acid.

Most of the investigative search for the causal factors of the cardiac tube looping and torsion have been directed to the stages in which the loop was convex to the right and concave to the left (12HH or C-shaped loop). However, experimental study of causal factors that direct or influence the movement of the convex surface ventrally and the concave surface dorsally, i.e., formation of an S-shaped loop, are scant. His (1881) pointed out that the S-shaped might be caused by cervical flexure of the embryo, whereas Patten (1922) ascribed it to the cranial flexure. The most relevant study concerning the causes for S-shaped loop formation is that of Männer et al (1993); these authors did experimental work in the chick embryo at stage 12HH, the end of the C-loop period. They prevented the cervical and cranial flexures of the embryo and obtained abnormal "S" loops, which ultimately resulted in cardiac septal defects (Männer et al 1993).

Despite the numerous experimental studies undertaken with the purpose of ascertaining the causes for looping and torsion of the cardiac tube, we still do not know the genetic factors that determine, at the beginning of this process, why the loop is convex to the right and concave to the left; nor why it becomes convex ventrally and concave dorsally (S-shaped); nor at the end of the process, ultimately how the primitive cardiac regions or segment come to occupy the spatial position and have their relationship of proximity that they have in the mature heart. These sequential changes are of great importance because they determine the normal cardiac septation and they lead to the constitution of each of the definitive cardiac cavities that form the mature heart.

CONCLUSIONS

The torsion and looping of the cardiac tube are processes that take place during the period of development comprising the time between the straight tube heart at stage 9+HH in the chick embryo and stage 17HH when cardiac septation begins. During this period, the different primitive cardiac segments acquire relationships among themselves leading to the process of septation, which will give origin ultimately to the four-chambered heart. The information acquired by means of in vivo studies in the chick embryo is applicable in the evaluation of postmortem studies of human embryos of similar cardiac morphology.

In the process of torsion and looping, the most significant stages are C-shaped loop, S-shaped loop, and terminal stage.

1. C-shaped loop. The heart acquires the shape of a tube and its walls are cardiac muscle. The loop is convex to the right and concave to the left and its dorsal wall is adjacent to the ventral wall of the foregut. The heart is constituted by all of the primitive cardiac segments, which are in a cephalocaudal order: the primitive outlet, the primordium of the apical trabeculated region of the right ventricle, the primordium of the apical trabeculated region of the left ventricle, the primitive inlet, and the right and left primitive atria. All of them appear at this stage of development, with the exception of the primordia of the apical trabeculated regions of the right and left ventricle, which appear in the straight tube heart.
2. S-shaped loop. The loop is convex ventrally and concave dorsally; consequently the dorsal wall of the C-shaped loop, which was adjacent to the foregut, becomes right, the ventral becomes left, and the retrocardiac space appears. The primitive atria begin to displace within this space and acquire a dorsal position.
3. Terminal stage. The primordium of the apical trabeculated region of both ventricles become side-by-side, the right one to the right and the left one to the left; furthermore, a proximity relationship is established between the primitive right atrium, the primitive inlet, and the primordium of the apical trabeculated region of the right ventricle. In addition, a proximity relationship is established between the primitive outlet and the primordium of the apical trabeculated region of the left ventricle. In conclusion, the primitive cardiac segments acquire the positions and interrelationships which eventually will determine the normal septation of the heart in the ensuring periods.
4. As yet, we do not know the causal factors of the torsion and looping of the cardiac tube, but the information we have permits us to propose that several factors participate in this process and that, according to the developmental

stage at which they act, the anatomical manifestations in the mature heart will be different.

REFERENCES

Baldwin HS, Solursh M. 1989. Degradation of hyaluronic acids does not prevent looping of the mammalian heart "in situ". Dev Biol 136:555–9.

Brown NA, Wolpert L. 1990. The development of handedness in left/right asymmetry. Development (Camb) 109:1–9.

Butler JK. 1952. An experimental analysis of cardiac loop formation in the chick. M.A. Thesis. Austin: University of Texas.

Castro-Quezada A, Nadal-Ginard B, de la Cruz MV. 1972. Experimental study of the formation of the bulboventricular loop in the chick. J Embryol Exp Morphol 27:623–37.

Davis CL. 1927. Development of the human heart from its first appearance to the stage found in embryos of twenty paired somites. Carnegie Contrib Embryol 19:245–84.

de la Cruz MV, Castillo MM, Villavicencio L, Valencia A, Moreno-Rodriguez RA. 1997. Primitive interventricular septum, its primordium, and its contribution in the definitive interventricular septum: in vivo labelling study in the chick embryo heart. Anat Rec 247:512–20.

de la Cruz MV, Giménez-Ribotta M, Saravalli O, Cayré R. 1983. The contribution of the inferior endocardial cushion of the atrioventricular canal to cardiac septation and to the development of the atrioventricular valves: study in the chick embryo. Am J Anat 166:63–72.

de la Cruz MV, Muñoz-Armas S, Muñnoz-Castellanos L. 1972. Development of the Chick Heart. Baltimore, MD: Johns Hopkins University Press.

de la Cruz MV, Quero-Jiménez M, Arteaga M, Cayré R. 1982. Morphogénèse du septum interventriculaire. Coeur 13:443–8.

de la Cruz MV, Sánchez-Gómez C, Arteaga M, Argüello C. 1977. Experimental study of the development of the truncus and the conus in the chick embryo. J Anat 123:661–86.

de la Cruz MV, Sánchez-Gómez C, Cayré R. 1991. The developmental components of the ventricles: their significance in congenital cardiac malformations. Cardiol Young 1:123–8.

de la Cruz MV, Sánchez-Gómez C, Palomino MA. 1989. The primitive cardiac regions in the straight tube heart (Stage 9−) and their anatomical expression in the mature heart: an experimental study in the chick embryo. J Anat 165:121–31.

de la Cruz MV, Sánchez-Gómez C, Robledo Tovi JL. 1987. Experimental study of the development of the ventricular inlets in the chick embryo. Embryologische Hefte 1:25–37.

DeVries PA, Saunders JB. 1962. Development of the ventricles and spiral outflow tract in the human heart. A contribution to the development of the human heart from age group IX to age group XV. Carnegie Contrib Embryol 256:89–114.

Easton H, Veini M, Bellairs R. 1992. Cardiac looping in the chick embryo: the role of the posterior precardiac mesoderm. Anat Embryol 185:249–58.

George TR. 1993. Contribución de las poblaciones celulares adyacentes al extremo caudal del corazón en el tubo recto (ST9-HH) en el desarrollo del asa bulboventricular (ST12HH). Estudio experimental en el embrión del pollo. Thesis, México Universidad Nacional Autónoma de México.

Grant RP. 1962. The embryology of ventricular flow pathways in man. Circulation 25:756–79.

His W. 1881. Mittheilungen zur Embryologie der Säugethiere und des Menschen. Arch Anat Entwickl Gesch JG 1881:303–29.

Hoyle C, Brown NA, Wolpert L. 1992. Development of left/right handedness in the chick heart. Development (Camb) 115:1071–8.

Itasaki N, Nakamura H, Sumida H, Yasuda M. 1991. Actin bundles on the right side in the

caudal part of the heart tube play a role in dextro-looping in the embryonic chick heart. Anat Embryol 183:29–39.
Kramer TC. 1942. The partitioning of the truncus and conus and the formation of the membranous portion of the inverventricular septum in the human heart. Am J Anat 71:343–70.
Lepori NG. 1967. Research on heart development in chick embryo under normal and experimental conditions. Monit Zool Ital 1:159–83.
Manasek FJ. 1969. Embryonic development of the heart II. Formation of the epicardium. J Embryol Exp Morphol 22:333–48.
Manasek FJ. 1972. A descriptive and experimental analysis of cardiac looping. Anat Rec 172:362A.
Manasek FJ. 1981. Determinants of heart shape in early embryos. Fed Proc 40:2011–6.
Manasek FJ, Burnside MB, Waterman RE. 1972. Myocardial cell shape change as a mechanism of embryonic heart looping. Dev Biol 29:349–71.
Manasek FJ, Isobe Y, Shimada Y, Hopkins W. 1984. The embryonic myocardial cytoskeleton, interstitial pressure, and the control of morphogenesis. In: Nora JJ, Takao A, editors. Congenital heart disease: cause and processes. New York: Futura Publishing Co. p 359–76.
Manasek FJ, Monroe RG. 1972. Early cardiac morphogenesis is independent of function. Dev Biol 27:584–8.
Männer J, Seidl W, Steding G. 1993. Correlation between the embryonic head flexures and cardiac development. An experimental study in chick embryos. Anat Embryol 188:269–85.
Nadal-Ginard B, García MP. 1972. The morphologic expression of each cardiac primordium in the chick embryo. J Embryol Exp Morphol 28:141–152.
Nakamura A, Manasek FJ. 1978. Cardiac jelly fibrils: their distribution and organization. In: Resenquist GC, Bergsma D, editors. Morphogenesis and malformation of the cardiovascular system. Birth Defects: Original Article Series. Vol. 14, Number 7. New York: AR Liss Inc. p 229–50.
Nakamura A, Manasek FJ. 1981. An experimental study of the relation of cardiac jelly to the shape of the early chick embryonic heart. J Embryol Exp Morphol 65:235–56.
Netter FH, Van Mierop LHS. 1969. Embryology. In Netter FH, editor. CIBA collection of medical illustrations. Ardsley, New Jersey. CIBA Pharmaceutical Co: Vol. 5, p 119–25.
Orts-Llorca F, Jiménez-Collado J. 1967. Determination of heart polarity (arterio venous axis) in the chicken embryo. Wilhelm Roux' Archiv Entwicklungsmech. Org 158:147–63.
Orts-Llorca F, Ruano-Gil D. 1967. A causal analysis of the heart curvatures in the chicken embryo. Wilhelm Roux' Archiv Entwicklungsmech Org 158:52–63.
Osmond MK, Butler AJ, Voon FCT, Bellairs R. 1991. The effects of retinoic acid on heart formation in the early chick embryo. Development (Camb) 113:1405–17.
Patten BM. 1922. The formation of the cardiac loop in the chick. Am J Anat 30:373–97.
Patten BM. 1948. The Early Embryology of the Chick. 3rd ed. Philadelphia: The Blakiston Co. p 184–92.
Romanoff AL. 1960. The Avian Embryo. New York: Macmillan. p 680–780.
Roux W. 1895. Gesammelte Abhandlungen über Entwickelungsmechanik der Organismen. 2 vol. Leipzig, Engelmann.
Shiraishi I, Takamatsu T, Fujita S. 1993. 3-D observation of N-cadherin expression during cardiac myofibrillogenesis of the chick embryo using a confocal laser scanning microscope. Anat Embryol 102:115–20.
Shiraishi I, Takamatsu T, Minamikawa T, Fujita S. 1992. 3-D observation of actin filaments during cardiac myofibrinogenesis in chick embryo using a confocal laser scanning microscope. Anat Embryol 185:401–8.
Sissman NJ. 1966. Cell multiplication rates during development of the primitive cardiac tube in the chick embryo. Nature (Lond) 210:504–7.

Spitzer A. 1951. The Architecture of Normal and Malform Hearts. Springfield, IL: Charles C. Thomas.
Stalsberg H. 1969a. The origin of heart asymmetry: right and left contributions to the early chick embryo heart. Dev Biol 19:109–27.
Stalsberg H. 1969b. Regional mitotic activity in the precardiac mesoderm and differentiating heart tube in the chick embryo. Dev Biol 20:18–45.
Stalsberg H, DeHaan RL. 1969. The precardiac areas and formation of the tubular heart in the chick embryo. Dev Biol 19:128–59.
Steding G, Seidl W. 1980. Contribution to the development of the heart. Part I: Normal development. Thorac Cardiovasc Surgeon 28:386–409.
Streeter GL. 1942. Development horizon in human embryos. Description of age group XI, 13 to 20 somites and age group XII, 21 to 29 somites. Carnegie Contrib Embryol 30:211–45.
Van Keuren M, Layton WM, Iacob RA, Kurnit DM. 1991. Situs inversus in the developing mouse: proteins affected by the iv mutation (genecopy) and the teratogen retinoic acid (phenocopy). Mol Reprod Dev 29:136–44.
Van Mierop LHS, Alley RD, Kausel HW, Stranahan A. 1962. The anatomy and embryology of endocardial cushion defects. J Thorac Cardiovasc Surg 43:71–83.
Von Haller A. 1758. Sur la Formation du Coeur. Lausanne, Switzerland, M.M. Bousquet Publishing Co..
Wenink ACG, Gittenberger-de Groot AC. 1985. The role of atrioventricular endocardial cushions in the septation of the heart. Int J Cardiol 8: 25–44.
Yokoyama T, Copeland NG, Jenkins NA, Montgomery CA, Elder FFB, Overbeek PA. 1993. Reversal of left-right asymmetry: a situs inversus mutation. Science (Wash DC) 260:679–82.
Yost HJ. 1992. Regulation of vertebrate left-right asymmetries by extracellular matrix. Nature (Lond) 357:158–61.

CHAPTER 5

Embryological Development of the Apical Trabeculated Region of Both Ventricles. The Contribution of the Primitive Interventricular Septum in the Ventricular Septation

María V. de la Cruz and Ricardo Moreno-Rodriguez

The apical trabeculated region of the anatomical right ventricle has two boundaries, one with its inlet and the other with its outlet, which correspond to the base of the papillary muscles and to the proximal or free border of the supraventricular crest, respectively. The apical trabeculated region of the anatomical left ventricle also has two limits, one with its inlet and the other with its outlet, which are the base of the papillary muscles and a tangential plane at the free border of the free portion of the anteroseptal leaflet of the mitral valve (mitroaortic continuity), respectively (chapter X).

Owing to the fact that the apical trabeculated region of each ventricle has its own primordium and specific anatomical expression and also the important contribution of the primitive interventricular septum to the ventricular septation, we will divide their study into two sections: (1) the primitive apical trabeculated segments of each ventricle, and (2) the primitive interventricular septum.

THE PRIMITIVE APICAL TRABECULAR SEGMENT OF EACH VENTRICLE

By means of in vivo labeling experiments in the chick embryo heart, de la Cruz and associates (1989, 1991) showed that the primordium of the apical trabeculated region of each ventricle appeared in the straight tube heart (stage 9+HH). The primordium of the apical trabeculated region of the anatomical right ventricle is the cephalic segment of this heart and the primordium of the apical trabeculated region of the anatomical left ventricle is its caudal segment (chapters III, Figs. 4 and 5). These two segments are separated by the right and left interventricular grooves, and the cephalic segment is larger than the caudal segment (chapter III, Fig 2A). In addition, its dorsal wall is the ventral wall of the foregut (chapter III, Fig 2B). The heart of this embryo is morphologically similar to that of human embryo 3709 horizon X (chapter III).

The primordium of the apical trabeculated region of each ventricle is morphologically expressed only after the torsion and looping period, during which they establish new relationships with each other and they acquire connections with new primitive cardiac segments (chapter IV, Figs. 1, 2, 3, and 4, A–E). Because of these facts, we give a brief account of their most significant changes in morphology and position during this process of torsion and looping.

At stage 12HH (C-shaped loop), these segments become tubular even as they remain adjacent to the ventral wall of the foregut; furthermore, they retain their cephalic and caudal position, respectively. However, the first (cephalic) one connects with the primitive outlet and the second (caudal) segment with the primitive inlet, which appear at this stage of development (chapter IV, Fig. 1). The heart of human embryo 3707 of 12 somites, horizon X (DeVries and Saunders 1962) is similar morphologically to that of the chick embryo at stage 12HH (chapter IV). At stage 14HH (S-shaped loop) the primordium of the apical trabeculated region of the right ventricle continues to be cephalic and the primordium of the apical trabeculated region of the left ventricle caudal. At this stage, both primordia no longer remain adjacent to the ventral wall of the foregut, because the retrocardiac space has developed and the atria are now located in a position dorsal to the primordia of the apical trabecular region of both ventricles (chapter IV, Fig. 2). The same is true in human embryo 6344 of 13 to 14 somites, horizon XI (DeVries and Saunders 1962), of a similar cardiac morphology (chapter IV). At stage 16HH (terminal stage of torsion and looping), the primordia of the apical trabeculated regions of both ventricles become situated with the cephalic segment to the right and the caudal segment to the left and adjacent to each other. Therefore, the primitive right atrium and the primitive inlet have established direct relationship with the apical trabeculated region of the right ventricle, as exhibited in the mature heart (chapter IV, Fig. 3). The same is observed in human embryo 2053 of 20 somites, horizon XI (DeVries and Saunders 1962) of similar cardiac morphology (chapter IV). It is of interest to point out that during the torsion and looping period no trabeculated cardiac muscle is seen in either primordium nor is there any indication of the primitive interventricular septum (de la Cruz et al 1997) (Fig. 1B).

After torsion and looping, at stage 17HH, trabeculated cardiac muscle appears for the first time on either side of the interventricular groove at the apical region of the heart, in the zones corresponding to the primordium of the apical trabeculated region of each ventricule (de la Cruz et al 1997) (Fig. 1, A–C). These facts permit us to propose that for the primordium of the apical trabeculated region of each ventricle, which appeared initially in the straight tube heart (stage 9+HH) (de la Cruz et al 1989, 1991), to have a morphological expression, it is necessary that the torsion and looping process take place.

THE PRIMITIVE INTERVENTRICULAR SEPTUM

By means of in vivo labeling experiments in the chick embryo heart, de la Cruz and colleagues (1997) found that the primordium of the primitive interventricular septum appears in the straight tube heart (stage 9+HH) in the ventral fusion line of both cardiac primordia at the level of the interventricular grooves, which give

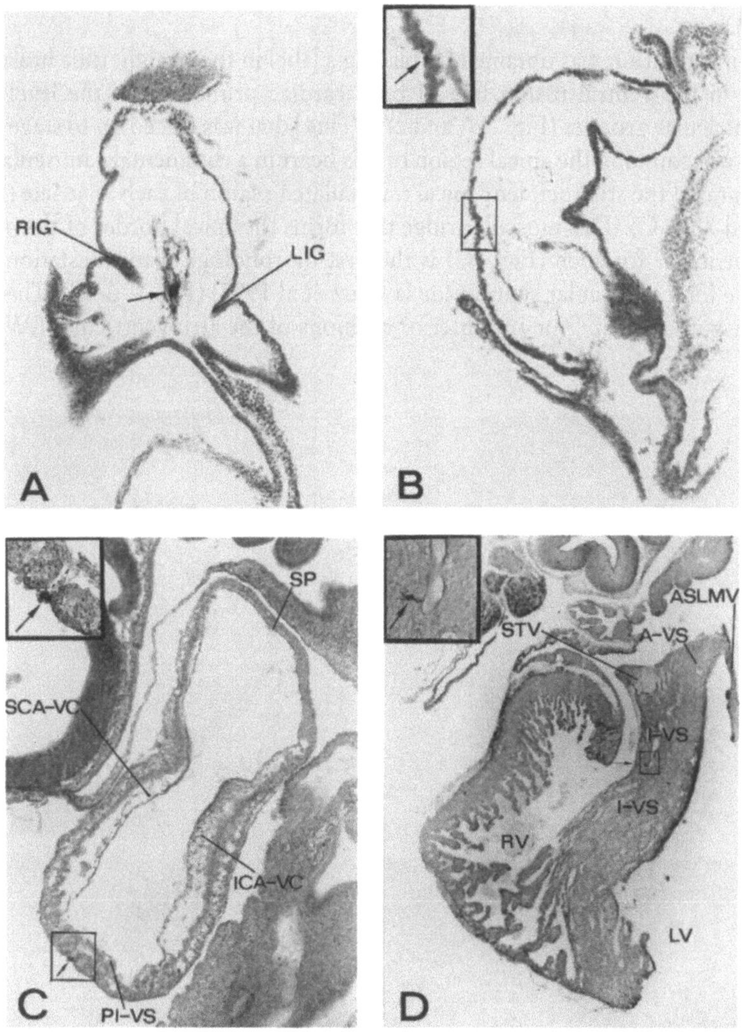

FIGURE 1. Photographs of the histological study of in vivo labeling experiment on the chick embryo heart, showing the site of the primordium of the primitive interventricular septum at stage 9+HH, its first morphological manifestation at stage 17HH, and its contribution to the definitive interventricular septum in the mature heart (stage 36HH). **A.** Frontal section of the straight tube heart (stage 9+HH), showing the label at the ventral fusion line of both cardiac primordia at the level of the interventricular grooves (arrow). **B.** Sagittal section of the heart at stage 14HH (S-shaped loop) showing that there is no morphological manifestation of septation where the label (arrow) was found, nor in any other part of the heart. **C.** Sagittal section of the heart at stage 17HH. Observe in the apex of the heart a label (arrow) in the incipient primitive interventricular septum, which is part of the first cardiac septum (8-shaped septum) that is constituted in addition by the superior and inferior cushions of the the AV canal and by the incipient septum primum. **D.** Four-chamber section of the mature heart (stage 36HH). Notice the label (arrow) in the definitive interventricular septum at the limit between the basal and the middle third. The insets in B, C, and D are amplifications of the cardiac zones in which the labels were found (arrows). SCA-VC = superior endocardial cushion of the atrioventricular canal; ICA-VC = inferior endocardial cushion of the atriventricular canal; SP = septum primum; PI-VS = primitive interventricular septum; I-VS = interventricular septum; A-VS = atrioventricular septum; STV = septal tricuspid valve; ASLMV = anteroseptal leaflet of the mitral valve; RV = right ventricle; LV = left ventricle; RIG = right interventricular groove; LIG = left interventricular groove. Reprinted with permission of from de la Cruz et al (1997) Anat Rec 247:512.

origin to the apical and middle third of the definitive interventricular septum (Figs. 1 and 2).

This information was obtained by placing a label in the straight tube heart (stage 9+HH) in the ventral fusion line of both cardiac primordia, at the level of the interventricular grooves (Figs. 1A and 2A). This label was traced up to stage 17HH when it was found in the apical region of this heart in a rudimentary muscular ridge that separated the still incipient apical trabeculated region of each ventricle (Figs. 1, A–C and 2, A–C). This muscular ridge that forms the apical border of the primary interventricular foramen (Fig. 1C) is the first morphological manifestation of the primitive interventricular septum (de la Cruz et al 1997) (Fig. 1, A–C). This ridge, together with the superior and inferior cushions of the atrioventricular (AV) canal

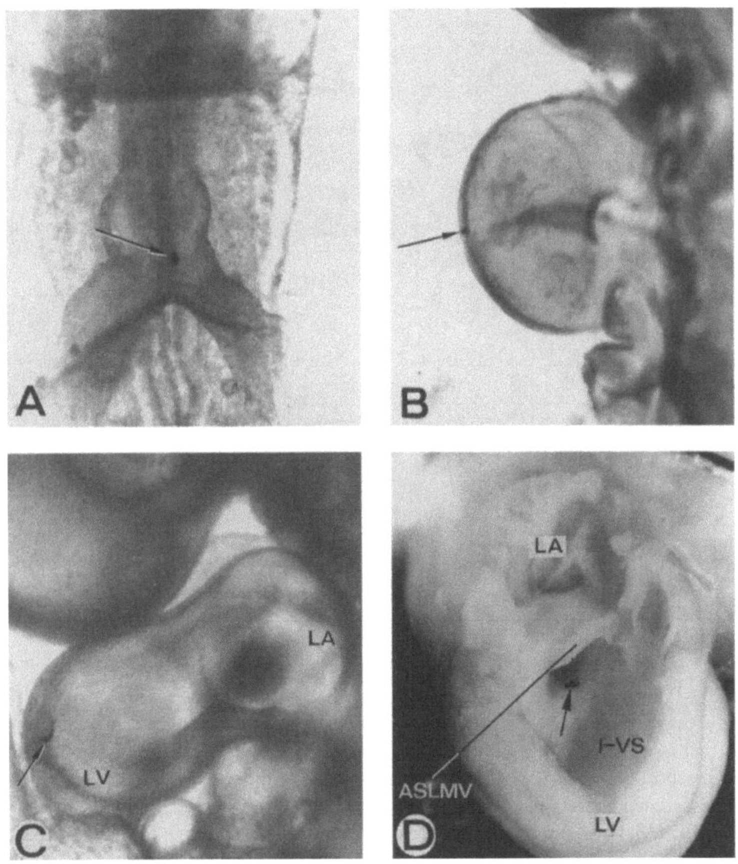

FIGURE 2. In vivo labeling showing the stage in which the primordium of the primitive interventricular septum appears, and its tracing up to stage 36HH (mature heart). **A.** Embryo at stage 9+HH after placing the label (arrow) in the ventral fusion line of both cardiac primordia at the level of the interventricular grooves. **B.** The same embryo at stage 14HH showing the label (arrow) in the greater curvature of the loop, opposite the left interventricular groove. **C.** Notice the same label (arrow) at stage 17HH in the apical region of the interventricular groove. **D.** Mature heart (stage 36HH) showing the same label (arrow) in the limit between the basal and the middle third of the definitive interventricular septum. I-VS = interventricular septum; LA = left atrium; LV = left ventricle; ASLMV = anteroseptal leaflet of the mitral valve. Reprinted with permission of from de la Cruz et al (1997) Anat Rec 247:512.

and with developing atrial septum primum, constitutes an 8-shaped septum or primitive cardiac septum, the first septum to appear in the heart (de la Cruz et al 1983, 1997) (chapter VI, Fig. 2). In addition, the histological studies of the 8-shaped septum (stage 17HH) show that the primitive interventricular septum is constituted from its first appearance by trabeculated cardiac muscle, the endocardial cushions of the AV canal by mesenchymal tissue, and the septum primum by compact cardiac muscle (Fig. 1C).

The heart of the chick embryo at stage 17HH corresponds morphologically to that of human embryo at horizon XIV, in which DeVries and Saunders (1962) and Wenink and Gittenberger-de Groot (1985) describe that the superior and inferior cushions of the AV canal are continuous with the incipient primitive interventricular septum and that both embryological structures appear simultaneously at this stage of development.

de la Cruz and colleagues (1997), with the purpose of investigating the contribution of the primitive interventricular septum to the definitive interventricular septum, at stage 17HH, placed a label in the incipient muscular ridge, located between the primordium of the apical trabeculated region of both ventricles. As noted above, this ridge is part of the primitive cardiac septum (8-shaped septum) (Fig. 1C). This label was subsequently found at stage 36HH when the pattern of the mature heart is completed, in the limit between the basal and the middle third of the definitive interventricular septum (Figs. 1D and 2D). These facts show that the middle and the apical two-thirds of the definitive interventricular septum originate from the primitive interventricular septum (de la Cruz et al 1997)(Figs. 1 and 2). These results are consistent with findings obtained by means of in vivo labeling of the inferior and superior endocardial AV cushions (de la Cruz et al 1982, 1983; García-Peláez et al 1984) in which the basal third of the definitive interventricular septum was found labeled (chapter VI, Fig. 4; chapter VII, Fig. 6). Also, for the inferior endocardial cushion of the AV canal, the region of the inlet (de la Cruz et al 1982, 1983) was labeled (chapter VI, Fig. 4). For the case of the superior endocardial cushion of the AV canal, the septal wall of the outlet of the left ventricle (de la Cruz et al 1982; García-Peláez et al 1984) was also found to be labeled (chapter VII, Fig. 6). Therefore, based on these experiments the embryological structures that constitute the definitive interventricular septum are (1) the inferior endocardial cushion of the AV canal, which gives origin to the basal third of the definitive interventricular septum in the region of the inlet (Fig. 3) (chapter VI, Fig. 4); (2) the superior endocardial cushion of the AV canal, which gives origin to the basal third of this septum in the region of the outlet (Fig. 3) (chapter VII, Fig. 6); and (3) the primitive interventricular septum, which forms the middle third and the apical third of the definitive interventricular septum, the greater bulk or part of this septum (Figs. 1D, 2D, and 3).

With respect to the closure of the primary interventricular foramen, it takes place in the chick embryo at stage 28HH. It is important to point out that the primary interventricular foramen at stage 17HH is much larger than at stage 24HH. Thus, when the label was placed in vivo at stage 17HH in the primitive interventricular septum it was found in the inferior border of the primary interventricular foramen of the heart at stage 24HH (de la Cruz et al 1997) (Fig. 4). This fact shows that the primitive interventricular septum grows toward the future basal third of the definitive interventricular septum (Figs. 1, C and D; and 4).

By means of in vivo labeling studies of the chick embryo heart, the primordium of the primitive interventricular septum was discovered (de la Cruz et al 1997), as

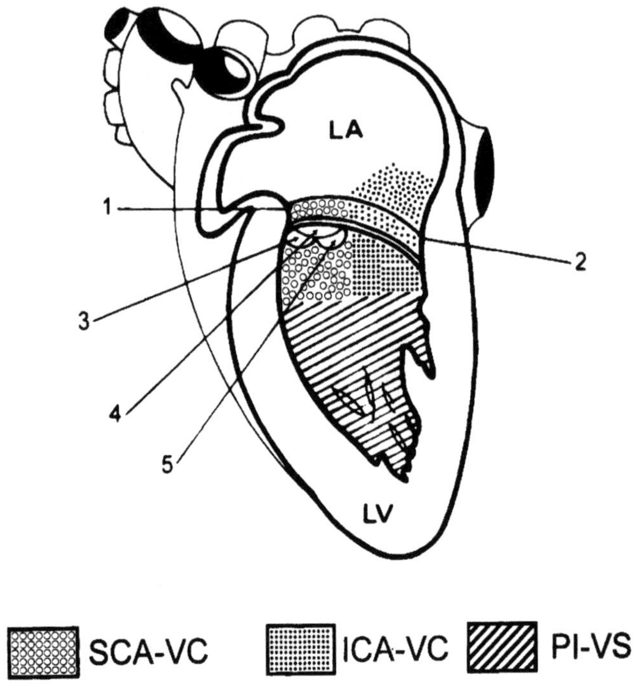

FIGURE 3. Diagram of a dissection of the left cavities of the mature heart showing a map of the embryological constitution of the definitive interventricular septum, from in vivo labeling experiments of the superior and inferior endocardial cushions of the atrioventricular canal and of the primitive interventricular septum in the chick embryo heart. LA = left atrium; LV = left ventricle; SCA-VC = superior endocardial cushion of the atrioventricular canal; ICA-VC = inferior endocardial cushion of the atrioventricular canal; PI-VS = primitive interventricular septum; 1 = portion of the anteroseptal leaflet of the mitral valve that constitutes the mitroaortic continuity; 2 = portion of the anteroseptal leaflet of the mitral valve that inserts into the septum; 3 = right anterior aortic cusp; 4 = left anterior aortic cusp; 5 = posterior aortic cusp. Reprinted with permission of from de la Cruz et al (1997) Anat Rec 247:512.

well as its contribution to the definitive interventricular septum (de la Cruz et al 1997). Also the important role of differential growth (cell multiplication) (Sissman 1966; Harh and Paul 1975) and movements of cell populations (Harh and Paul 1975; de la Cruz 1979) in the morphogenesis of this septum were revealed.

These new findings (Sissman 1966; Harh and Paul 1975; de la Cruz 1979; de la Cruz et al 1997) cast doubts on the concept concerning the development of the interventricular septum in man as proposed by Flank (1909), Frazer (1932), Streeter (1948), Grant (1962), Van Mierop and associates (1962), Netter and Van Mierop (1969), and Van Mierop and Kutsche (1985). These authors believed it was caused by the folding and coalescence of trabeculated pouches, whereas DeVries and Saunders (1962) proposed the theory that the trabeculated pouches undergo a rotation process. Gittenberger-de Groot and coworkers (1994) have recently suggested that the ventricular infundibular fold gives partial origin to the interventricular septum. However, this is questionable, because at no stage of its development does the ventricular infundibular fold separate both ventricular cavities; furthermore, from in vivo labeling, the role of the ventricular infundibular fold in the development of the heart is linked to the processes that occur at

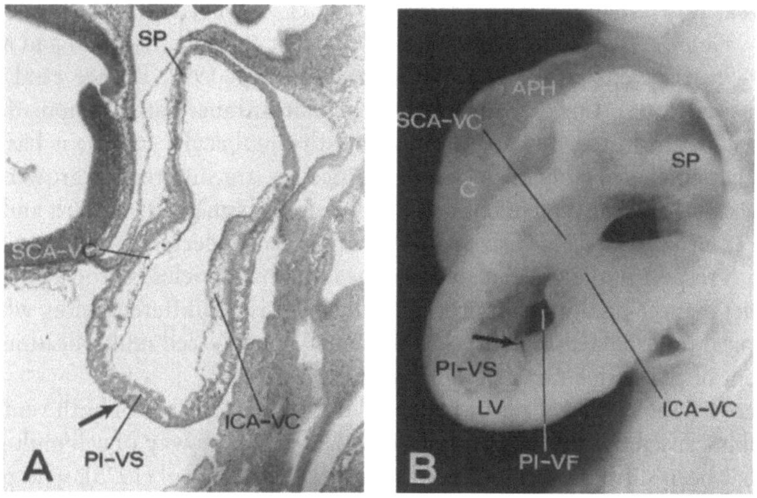

FIGURE 4. Photographs of in vivo labeling experiment in the chick embryo in which the label was placed at stage 17HH in the ventricular apical trabeculated region of the first cardiac septum and is traced up to stage 24HH. **A.** Sagittal histological section of the heart (stage 17HH) after placing the label (arrow) in the ventricular apical trabeculated region of the first cardiac septum (8-shaped septum). **B.** Photograph of a dissection of the left cavities at stage 24HH, showing the same label (arrow) at the inferior border of the primary interventricular foramen (PI-VF). SCA-VC = superior endocardial cushion of the atriventricular canal; ICA-VC = inferior endocardial cushion of the atrioventricular canal; SP = septum primum; PI-VS = primitive interventricular septum; LV = left ventricle; APH = arterial pole of the heart; C = conus. Reprinted with permission of from de la Cruz et al (1997) Anat Rec 247:512.

the base of the heart, specifically, participating in the formation of the tricuspid ring (chapter VI, Fig. 9), probably in the development of the anterior leaflet of the tricuspid valve (chapter VI) and in the formation of the supraventricular crest (chapter VII).

The apical trabeculated regions of both ventricles and the primitive interventricular septum at stage 17HH are very small, whereas the primordium of the inlet constitutes almost the entirety of the ventricles (Fig. 1C). The same description is made by Wenink and Gittenberger de Groot (1985) and Wenink (1992) in human embryos at horizon XIV of similar cardiac morphology. At later developmental stages, the apical trabeculated region of both ventricles and the primitive interventricular septum increase in size, and the inlet becomes relatively smaller; the same takes place in man (Wenink and Gittenberger-de Groot 1985; Wenink 1992).

Histological studies of both ventricular inlets and of the outlet of the chick embryo heart at stage 17HH show a large amount of mesenchymal tissue with abundant extracellular matrix (Fig. 1C). In addition, at later developmental stages in the region of the ventricular inlet, important processes of histodifferentiation take place, as is apparent in the morphogenesis of the atrioventricular valve apparatus (chapter VI), the atrioventricular septum (chapter VI), and the inlet region of the interventricular septum, and in the presence of a highly specialized tissue such as the conduction tissue. Because of the important morphological changes that occur in the embryological development of the ventricular inlet, this region has been the subject of studies at the molecular level for the purpose of investigating the mechanisms that determine them (Markwald et al 1977; Bernanke and Markwald 1982; Runyan and Markwald 1983; Krug et al 1985, 1987; Markwald et al 1990a, 1990b; Markwald and Lepera 1987; Sinning et al 1988; Mjaatvedt and Markwald 1989; Mjaatvedt et al 1991; McGuire and Orkin 1992; Rezaee et al 1993; Isokawa et al 1994). On the other hand, the apical trabeculated region of both ventricles is constituted by cardiac muscle with a trabecular aspect; it has been shown that in this region the dominant processes are differential growth (cell multiplication) and movements of cell populations (Sissman 1966; Harh and Paul 1975; de la Cruz 1979; de la Cruz et al 1997). The relative decrease in the size of the inlets with respect to the trabeculated regions of both ventricles is probably caused by the fact that the predominant process in the inlets is cell differentiation, whereas in the apical trabeculated regions, the differential growth (cell multiplication) and movement of cell populations are the dominant processes.

The growth of the free walls of the apical trabeculated region of both ventricles is probably caused by the process of differential growth by way of cell multiplication as has been substantiated by the results of Harh and Paul (1975), who placed two labels in the free wall of each ventricle in the chick embryo and subsequently found that in the course of development both marks became separated from each other. It is highly probable that labeling experiments with a replication-defective retrovirus could give us more precise information on this point.

CONCLUSIONS

Owing to the similarity of the embryological development of the apical trabeculated region of each ventricle and the primitive interventricular septum in man and in the chick, the information obtained by means of the in vivo labeling studies in the chick embryo is important and probably applicable for the evaluation of postmortem studies in both species.

1. The primordium of the primitive interventricular septum appears in the straight tube heart (stage 9+HH) in the ventral fusion line of both cardiac primordia, at the level of the right and left interventricular grooves.
2. The primitive interventricular septum is expressed morphologically at stage 17HH in which it is both incipient and muscular; it separates the rudimentary apical trabeculated region of both ventricles. This rudimentary septum forms part of the primitive cardiac septum (8-shaped septum), which is also constituted by the superior and inferior cushions of the AV canal and the septum primum.
3. The primitive interventricular septum gives origin to the middle and apical two-thirds of the definitive interventricular septum.
4. The processes of differential growth (cell multiplication) and movement of cell populations play a most important role in the development of the apical trabeculated segment of both ventricles and of the primitive interventricular septum.

REFERENCES

Bernanke DH, Markwald RR. 1982. Migratory behavior of cardiac cushion tissue cells in collagen lattice culture system. Dev Biol 91:235–45.

de la Cruz MV. 1979. Different concepts of univentricular heart. Experimental embryological approach. Herz 4:67–72.

de la Cruz MV, Castillo MM, Villavicencio L, Valencia A, Moreno-Rodriguez RA. 1997. Primitive interventricular septum, its primordium, and its contribution in the definitive interventricular septum: in vivo labelling study in the chick embryo heart. Anat Rec 247:512–20.

de la Cruz MV, Giménez-Ribotta M, Saravalli O, Cayré R. 1983. The contribution of the inferior endocardial cushion of the atrioventricular canal to cardiac septation and to the development of the atrioventricular valves: study in the chick embryo. Am J Anat 166:63–72.

de la Cruz MV, Quero-Jiménez M, Arteaga M, Cayré R. 1982. Morphogénèse du septum interventriculaire. Coeur 13:443–8.

de la Cruz MV, Sánchez-Gómez C, Cayré R. 1991. The developmental components of the ventricles: their significance in congenital cardiac malformations. Cardiol Young 1:123–8.

de la Cruz MV, Sánchez-Gómez C, Palomino MA. 1989. The primitive cardiac regions in the straight tube heart (Stage 9^{-}) and their anatomical expression in the mature heart: an experimental study in the chick embryo. J Anat 165:121–31.

DeVries PA, Saunders JB. 1962. Development of the ventricles and spiral outflow tract in the human heart. A contribution of the development of the human heart from age group IX to age group XV. Carnegie Contrib Embryol 256:89–114.

Flank M. 1909. The heart. In Hill LE, editor. Further advances in physiology. Longmans Green. New York: p 34–71.

Frazer JE. 1932. Development of the heart, and vessels of the anterior part of the embryo. In Manual of Embryology. New York: William Wood and Co. p 306–26.

García-Peláez I, Díaz-Góngora G, Arteaga M. 1984. Contribution of the superior atrioventricular cushion to the left ventricular infundibulum. Experimental study on the chick embryo. Acta Anat 118:224–30.

Gittenberger-de Groot A, Bartelings MM, Polemann RE. 1994. Overview: cardiac morphogenesis. In Clark EB, Markwald RR, Takao A, editors. Developmental mechanisms of heart disease. Armonk, NY: Futura Publishing Co Inc. p 157–68.

Grant RP. 1962. The embryology of ventricular flow pathways in man. Circulation 25:756–79.

Harh JY, Paul MH. 1975. Experimental cardiac morphogenesis. I. Development of the ventricular septum in the chick. J Embryol Exp Morphol 33:13–28.

Isokawa K, Rezaee M, Wunsch A, Markwald RR, Krug EL. 1994. Identification of transferrin as one of multiple EDTA-extractable extracellular proteins in early chick heart inductive interactions. J Cell Biochem 54:207–18.

Krug EL, Mjaatvedt CH, Markwald RR. 1987. Extracellular matrix from embryonic myocardium elicits an early morphogenetic event in cardiac endothelial differentiation. Dev Biol 120:348–55.

Krug EL, Runyan RB, Markwald RR. 1985. Protein extracts from early embryonic hearts initiate cardiac endothelial differentiation. Deb Biol 112:414–26.

Markwald RR, Fitzharris TP, Manasek FJ. 1977. Structural development of endocardial cushions. Am J Anat 148:85–120.

Markwald RR, Lepera RC. 1987. The temporal and site restricted expression of cell adhesion and substrate associated molecules during endothelial transformation to mesenchyme in the embryonic chick heart. Anat Rec 218:87A.

Markwald RR, Mjaatvedt CH, Krug EL. 1990a. Induction of endocardial cushion tissue formation by adheron-like molecular complexes derived from the myocardial basement membrane. In Clark EB, Takao A, editors. Developmental cardiology: morphogenesis and function. Mount Kisco, NY. Futura Publishing Co Inc. p 191–204.

Markwald RR, Mjaatvedt CH, Krug El, Sinning AR. 1990b. Inductive interactions in heart development: role of cardiac adherons in cushion tissue formation. Ann N Y Acad Sci 558:13–25.

McGuire PG, Orkin RW. 1992. Urokinase activity in the developing avian heart: a spatial and temporal analysis. Dev Dyn 193:24–33.

Mjaatvedt CH, Krug EL, Markwald RR. 1991. An antiserum (ES1) against a particulate form of extracellular matrix blocks the transformation of cardiac endothelium into mesenchyme in culture. Dev Biol 145:219–30.

Mjaatvedt CH, Markwald RR. 1989. Induction of an epithelial-mesenchymal transition by an in vivo adheron-like complex. Dev Biol 136:118–28.

Netter FH, Van Mierop LHS. 1969. Embryology. In Netter FH, editor. CIBA Collection of Medical Illustrations. Ardsley, New Jersey. CIBA Pharmaceutical Co. Vol. 5, p. 119–25.

Rezaee M, Isokawa K, Halligan N, Markwald RR, Krug EL. 1993. Identification of an extracellular 130-kDa protein involved in early cardiac morphogenesis. J Biol Chem 268:14404–11.

Runyan RB, Markwald RR. 1983. Invasion of mesenchyme into three-dimensional gels: a regional and temporal analysis of interaction in embryonic heart tissue. Dev Biol 95:108–14.

Sinning AR, Lepera RC, Markwald RR. 1988. Initial expression of type I procollagen in chick cardiac mesenchyme is dependent upon myocardial stimulation. Dev Biol 130:167–74.

Sissman NJ. 1966. Cell multiplication rates during development of the primitive cardiac tube in the chick embryo. Nature (Lond) 210:154–7.

Streeter GL. 1948. Development horizons in human embryos. Description of age group XV, XVI, XVII, and XVIII, being the third issue of the Carnegie Collection. Carnegie Contrib Embryol 32:133–203.

Van Mierop LHS, Alley RD, Kausel HW, Stranahan A. 1962. The anatomy and embryology of endocardial cushion defects. J Thorac Cardiovasc Surg 43:71–83.

Van Mierop LHS, Kutsche LM. 1985. Development of the ventricular septum of the heart. Heart Vessels 1:114–9.

Wenink ACG. 1992. Quantitative morphology of the embryonic heart: an approach to development of the atrioventricular valves. Anat Rec 234:129–35.

Wenink ACG, Gittenberger-de Groot AC. 1985. The role of atrioventricular endocardial cushions in the septation of the heart. Int J Cardiol 8:25–44.

CHAPTER 6

Embryological Development of the Ventricular Inlets. Septation and Atrioventricular Valve Apparatus

María V. de la Cruz and Roger R. Markwald

A ventricular inlet is characterized anatomically by the presence of an atrioventricular valve apparatus, the tricuspid on the right side and the mitral on the left side. The atrial limit of the right ventricular inlet is the tricuspid valve ring and that of the left ventricular inlet is the mitral valve ring. The limit of the inlets of both ventricles with their apical trabeculated region correspond with the base of the papillary muscles. Furthermore, in the left ventricle one more anatomical reference is the limit between its smooth region (inlet) and its apical trabeculated region (chapter X).

The study of the embryological development of the inlets will be divided into three sections for the sake of didactic clarity: (1) septation of the primitive inlet and acquisition of the inlet of the right ventricle, (2) development of the atrioventricular valve apparatus, and (3) how cushions become leaflets.

SEPTATION OF THE PRIMITIVE INLET AND ACQUISITION OF THE INLET OF THE RIGHT VENTRICLE

By means of in vivo labeling experiments in the chick embryo heart, de la Cruz and associates (1987, 1989, 1991) demonstrated that the inlet of both ventricles originates from a single primordium (primitive inlet) that appears at stage 12HH; it corresponds to the segment adjacent to the right atrioventricular groove of the caudal limb of the loop and it connects both primitive atria with the primordium of the apical trabeculated region of the left ventricle (de la Cruz et al 1987, 1989, 1991) (chapter IV, Fig. 7). It is for this reason that it has been called the inlet of the left ventricle (chapter IV). Thus, the primordium of the apical trabeculated region of the right ventricle is not initially connected to the primitive right atrium; therefore, this ventricle lacks an inlet (Fig. 1) (chapter IV) and receives its blood supply from the primordium of the left ventricle during early heart development.

The primitive inlet and the primordium of the primitive atria, from their initial

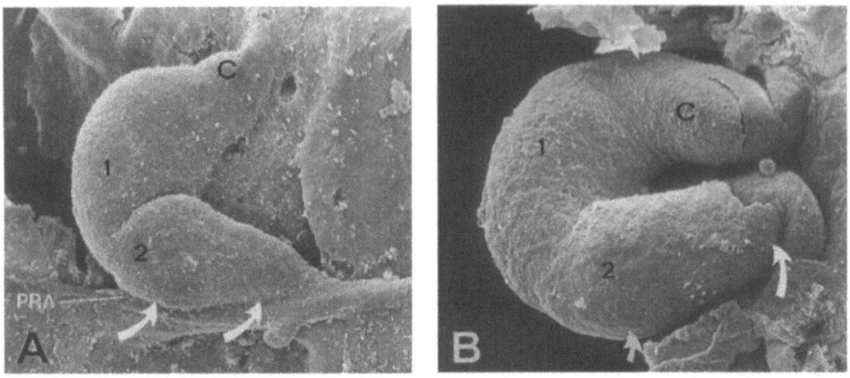

FIGURE 1. Photomicrographs obtained with the scanning electron microscope of the chick embryo heart at stage 12HH and 14HH showing that the primitive inlet and both primitive atria have a caudal position with respect to the primordium of the apical trabeculated region of the right ventricle, which is cephalic. **A.** Frontal view of the heart at stage 12HH. **B.** Left lateral view of the heart at stage 14HH. 1 = primordium of the apical trabeculated region of the right ventricle; 2 = primordium of the apical trabeculated region of the left ventricle; C = primitive outlet or conus; PRA = primitive right atrium. The segment between the two arrows is the primitive inlet.

appearance in the C-shaped looped heart at stage 12HH (de la Cruz et al 1987, 1989, 1991) in the chick and in man, horizon X (embryo 3707 of 4 somites) (DeVries and Saunders 1962), are caudal and distal to the primordium of the apical trabeculated region of the right ventricle, which is cephalic (Fig. 1A). This relationship persists during the S-shaped loop period, which in the chick corresponds to stage 14HH (Fig. 1B) and in man to horizon XI (embryo 6344 of 13 to 14 somites) (Streeter 1942). At the end of the torsion of the cardiac tube, i.e., stage 16HH in the chick and horizon XI (embryo 2053 of 20 somites) (Streeter 1942) in man, the primordia of the apical trabeculated region of the right and left ventricles are situated side by side and adjacent to each other; simultaneously both primitive atria have a dorsal position with respect to those primordia (chapter IV). In this manner, there is a relationship of proximity between the primordia of the apical trabeculated region of the right ventricle, the primitive inlet, and the future right atrium (chapter IV, Fig. 3). Although there is still no connection between the future right atrium and the primordium of the apical trabeculated region of the right ventricle by way of the inlet, a new spatial relationship of proximity has taken place among these three primordia, which will permit that connection in subsequent stages of development.

Our studies of in vivo microcinematography of the chick embryo heart (de la Cruz et al 1983), as well as microdissections examined by scanning electron microscopy or histological section, all show that in the heart of the chick embryo at stage 17HH two masses of cushion tissue appear in the atrioventricular (AV) canal: the dorsal or inferior AV endocardial cushion (associated with the greater curvature of the looped heart) and the ventral or superior AV endocardial cushion (Sissman 1970; de la Cruz et al 1983) associated with the inner curvature (Fig. 2, B and C). These cushion will eventually fuse to divide the AV canal into two orifices at later stages of development: a right one that gives origin to the tricuspid orifice and a left one giving origin to the mitral orifice. Van Mierop and coworkers (1962), DeVries and Saunders (1962), Netter and Van Mierop (1969), and Magovern and associates (1986) described

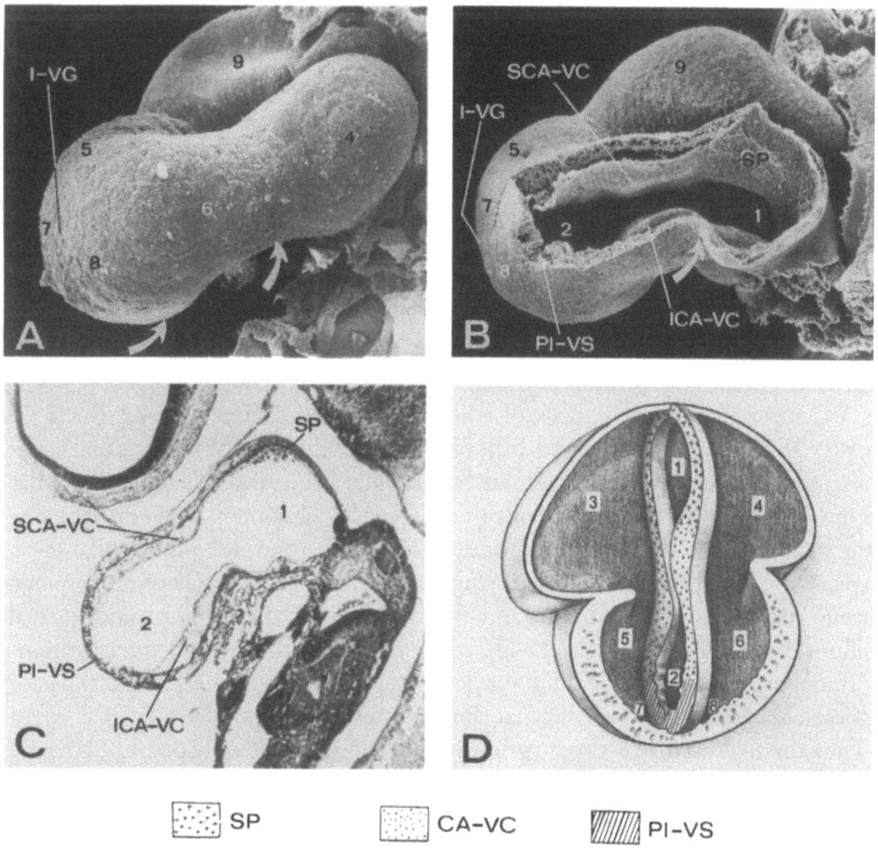

FIGURE 2. Anatomic and histological studies of the 8-shaped cardiac septum or primitive cardiac septum, when it appears at stage 17HH in the chick embryo and divides the heart into four chambers. **A.** Left lateral external aspect of the heart. The segment between the two arrows is the left ventricular inlet. **B.** Left lateral aspect in which the free wall of the left atrium, the inlet, and the apical trabecular region of the left ventricle have been removed. Notice the atrioventricular groove (arrow), the superior endocardial atrioventricular cushion (SCA-VC), and the inferior endocardial atrioventricular cushion (ICA-VC), which are continuous with the septum primum (SP) at the atrial level and with the primitive interventricular septum (PI-VS) in the ventricular apical trabecular region. **C.** Left lateral view of the sagittal histological section showing the 8-shaped septum or primitive cardiac septum. The primitive cardiac septum is almost entirely constituted at the ventricular level by cushion tissue (inlet), by muscular tissue at the apex, which corresponds to the incipient primitive interventricular septum, and at the atrial level by the septum primum, which is also small. Notice that at first the 8-shaped septum or primtive cardiac septum is formed mainly by tissue of the atrioventricular cushions. **D.** Schematic representation of four-chambered cavity showing the embryological components of the 8-shaped septum or primitive cardiac septum. 1 = foramen primum; 2 = primary interventricular foramen; 3 = primitive right atrium; 4 = primitive left atrium; 5 = inlet of the right ventricle; 6 = inlet of the left ventricle; 7 = primordium of the apical trabeculated region of the right ventricle; 8 = primordium of the apical trabeculated region of the left ventricle; 9 = primitive outlet or conus; I-VG = interventricular groove; SP = septum primum; CA-VC = cushion of the atrioventricular canal; PI-VS = primitive interventricular septum. Figure 2, A, B, and D reprinted with permission of from de la Cruz et al (1997) Anat Rec 247:512.

the appearance of these two endocardial cushions in the AV canal in the heart of the human embryo at horizon XIV (Streeter 1945), a stage similar in morphology to that of the chick embryo heart at stage 17HH. Wenink and Gittenberger-de Groot (1985) described the appearance of AV endocardial cushions in the 3.6-mm human embryo whose cardiac morphology also corresponds to horizon XIV (Streeter 1945).

The superior and the inferior endocardial cushions of the AV canal from their initial appearance in the chick embryo heart at stage 17HH develop in a plane aligned directly with the septum primum, which in the external aspect of the atrial wall corresponds to the interatrial groove (de la Cruz et al 1983) and to the primitive very incipient muscular interventricular septum at the level of the apex, where it separates the primordium of the apical trabeculated region of the right ventricle from the primordium of the apical trabeculated region of the left ventricle (de la Cruz et al 1983, 1997) both of which are still rudimentary (Fig. 2, B and C) (chapter V, Fig. 1C). Consequently, the superior and the inferior endocardial cushions of the AV canal were never situated to the left of the primitive interventricular septum. This first cardiac septum or primitive cardiac septum has two orifices, one at the atrial level, i.e., the foramen primum, and another one at the ventricular level, the primary interventricular foramen (Fig. 2, B and D). The borders of the foramen primum are the septum primum and the superior and the inferior endocardial cushions of the AV canal (Fig. 2, B–D), whereas those of the primary interventricular foramen are the primitive interventricular septum and the inferior and superior endocardial cushions of the AV canal (Fig. 2, B–D).

Thus the first cardiac septum (primitive cardiac septum) is shaped like a figure 8. It is constituted by the septum primum, the inferior and superior endocardial cushions of the AV canal, and the primitive interventricular septum (de la Cruz et al 1983, 1997). It separates simultaneously both primitive atria and the apical trabeculated region of both ventricles, and it divides the single inlet (primitive inlet) into a right and left inlet (de la Cruz et al 1983, 1997) (Fig. 2, B–D). Thus each ventricle connects with its corresponding atrium (de la Cruz et al 1983). Obviously, the right ventricular inlet originates from the single original common inlet (primitive inlet) or left ventricular inlet.

DeVries and Saunders (1962) studied the heart in human embryo 6502 of horizon XIV when the superior and inferior endocardial cushions of the AV canal appear. They point out, as in the chick, that those two endocardial cushions are in continuity without boundaries with the primitive interventricular septum; therefore the right primitive atrium communicates with the right ventricle and the left primitive atrium with the left ventricle. Wenink and Gittenberger-de Groot (1985) similarly describe a human embryonic heart in which the superior and the inferior endocardial cushions of the AV canal are aligned and in direct continuity with the primitive interventricular septum as observed by de la Cruz and colleagues (1983, 1997) in the chick embryo. In contrast, Van Mierop and associates (1962) and Netter and Van Mierop (1969), studying human embryos similar in age (horizon XIV) and cardiac morphology to those described by both DeVries and Saunders (1962) and by Wenink and Gittenberger-de Groot (1985), concluded that both the superior and the inferior AV endocardial cushions were located to the left of the primitive interventricular septum and that the right ventricle acquired its inlet when these two cushions became aligned with the primitive interventricular septum. Work in the chick (de la Cruz et al 1983, 1997) strongly supports the descriptions of DeVries and Saunders (1962) and Wenink and Gittenberger-de Groot (1985).

When the 8-shaped septum divides the chick embryo heart at stage 17HH into four cavities, the inlets of both ventricles are larger than their apical trabeculated regions (Fig. 2C). At later developmental stages, the inlets become smaller relative to the apical trabeculated regions because of differential growth and the movements of cellular populations (chapter V). Wenink and Gittenberger-de Groot (1985), Lamers and coworkers (1992), and Wenink (1992) describe in human embryos similar cardiac morphology to the stage 17HH chick embryo heart, namely that both inlets are originally larger than the trabeculated apical regions.

Cinematographic studies of the atrioventricular canal in the chick embryo heart (de la Cruz et al 1983) show that during the developmental stages in which the superior and inferior endocardial cushions of the AV canal have not yet fused the cushions function as valves to divide the blood flow into two currents, a small one that flows into the right ventricle through a narrow right atrioventricular orifice and another much larger flow that fills the left ventricle through a large left atrioventricular orifice.

The inferior and superior endocardial cushions of the AV canal begin to fuse in the chick embryo heart (de la Cruz et al 1983) at stage 26HH and in man (DeVries and Saunders 1962; Van Mierop et al 1962; Netter and Van Mierop 1969) at horizon XVI (Streeter 1948), at which time the hearts are morphologically similar in both species. Fusion takes place in the chick concurrent with the closure of the foramen primum. It begins in the region adjacent to that foramen and it progresses toward the ventricle (de la Cruz et al 1983) (Fig. 3). The in vivo labeling experiments

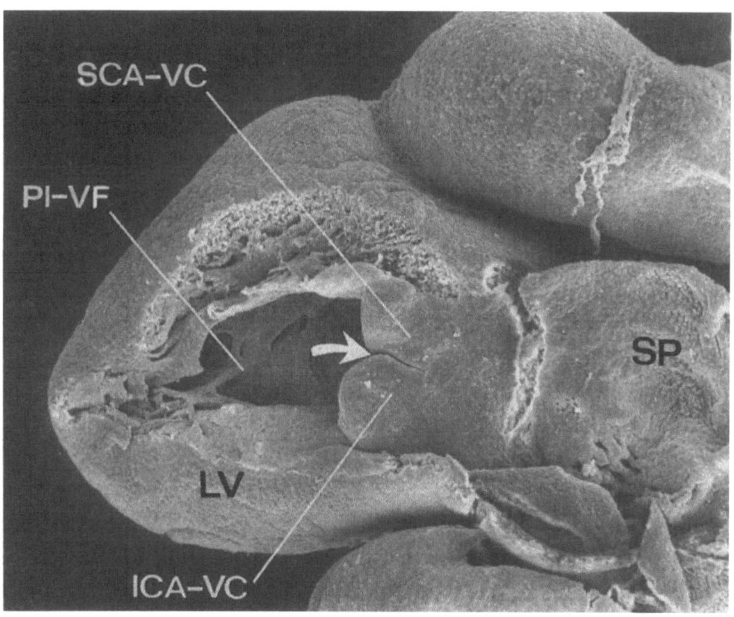

FIGURE 3. Photograph obtained with the scanning electron microscope of a dissection that has opened the left cardiac chambers of the chick embryo at stage 27HH. Notice the progress of the fusion of the superior endocardial cushion (SCA-VC) with the inferior endocardial cushion (ICA-VC) of the atrioventricular canal, which began at stage 26HH. The arrow points to the fusion line of both cushions. SP = septum primum; LV = left ventricle; PI-VF = primitive interventricular foramen.

indicate that the inferior endocardial cushion of the AV canal in the chick embryo (de la Cruz et al 1983) contributes to the closure of the foramen primum (Fig. 4D). These data suggest that the cushion tissue, which forms the borders of the foramen primum in man (Van Mierop et al 1962; Netter and Van Mierop 1969; Wenink and Gittenberger-de Groot 1985), also originates from the inferior endocardial cushion of the AV canal and serves to facilitate closure of this foramen.

As development proceeds, the inferior and superior endocardial cushions of the AV canal in both chick and man change their shape (Van Mierop et al 1962; Netter and Van Mierop 1969; de la Cruz et al 1983), their dimensions, and their histological constitution (Markwald et al 1975, 1977; Kinsella and Fitzharris 1980; Argüello et al 1988; Icardo 1989a, 1989b). The fused endocardial cushions resemble an arch-shaped septum whose convex surface faces the right atrium while the concave aspect faces the left ventricle (Van Mierop et al 1962; Netter and Van Mierop 1969; de la Cruz et al 1983) (Fig. 5). The cephalic limb of the arch gives origin to a left evagination (Fig. 5), which contributes to the development of that portion of the anteroseptal leaflet of the mitral valve that inserts into the junction between the interatrial and AV septa (Van Mierop et al 1962; Netter and Van Mierop 1969; de la Cruz et al 1983). On the other hand, a right evagination originates from the caudal limb (Fig. 5) and participates in the development of the septal leaflet of the tricuspid valve in man (Van Mierop et al 1962; Netter and Van Mierop 1969) and in the development of numerous homologous microleaflets in the chick (de la Cruz et al 1983; Cayré et al 1993). The arch-shaped cushion septum, limited by these two evaginations, participates in the development of the definitive atrioventricular septum. In both species the AV septum separates the right atrium from the inlet of the left ventricle (Van Mierop et al 1962; Netter and Van Mierop 1969; de la Cruz et al 1982, 1983; Van Mierop and Kutsche 1985; Cayré et al 1993) (Fig. 5).

de la Cruz and associates (1983) showed that the inferior endocardial cushion of the AV canal gives origin to both the atrioventricular septum and the immediately adjacent region of the interventricular septum. When the inferior endocardial cushion was labeled in vivo in the chick embryo, both of these septa appeared marked in the mature heart (Fig. 4). However when de la Cruz and coworkers (1997) labeled in vivo the primitive interventricular septum of the chick embryo, label was found in the limit between the basal and the middle third of the definitive interventricular septum. This shows that the primitive interventricular septum gives origin to the middle and apical two-thirds of the definitive interventricular septum (chapter V, Figs. 2D and 3).

The contribution of the inferior endocardial cushion to the development of the atrioventricular septum and the adjacent region of the interventricular septum has been shown not only by in vivo labeling of this cushion (de la Cruz et al 1983), but also by studying four-chamber views in histological sections of the chick embryo heart at stages 30HH, 37HH, and 39HH. At stage 30HH the atrioventricular septum is entirely composed of cushion mesenchyme (Fig. 6). At stage 37HH, muscular cells from the interventricular septum begin to invade the atrioventricular septum (Fig. 7), and at stage 39HH, the atrioventricular septum has become muscularized (Fig. 8) or myocardialized (see chapter II). A similar process in man also results in myocardialization or "muscularization" of the fused AV cushions.

The in vivo labeling experiments and the histological studies show that the presence of the inferior endocardial cushion of the AV canal is indispensable to the process of septation of the ventricular inlets. In chapter II, the molecular regulation

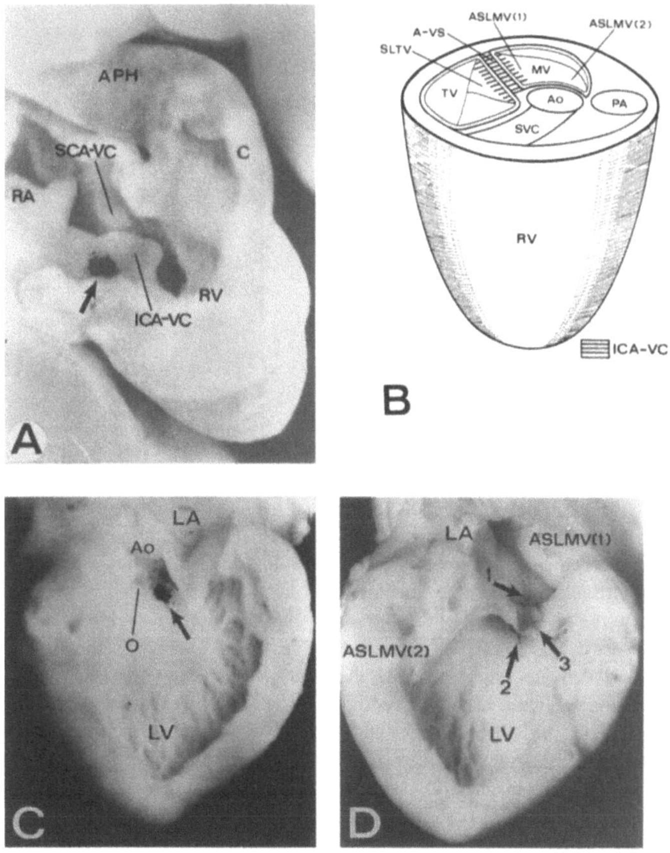

FIGURE 4. Photographs and diagram of the in vivo labeling of the inferior endocardial cushion of the AV canal in the chick embryo heart at stage 18HH showing the contribution of this cushion in cardiac septation and the development of the atrioventricular leaflets. **A.** Microdissection of the right cavities of a chick embryo heart at stage 23HH, 24 hours after labeling the inferior endocardial cushion of the atrioventricular canal, showing the label (arrow) in the inferior cushion of the atrioventricular canal (ICA-VC). **B.** Diagram of a transverse section at the level of the atrioventricular orifices and the great arteries. The striped areas show the contribution of the inferior cushion of the atrioventricular canal to the septal leaflet of the tricuspid valve, to the atrioventricular septum, and to that region of the anteroseptal leaflet of the mitral valve that has inserted into the AV septum. **C, D.** Dissection of the mature heart (stage 35HH) showing the left cavities. **C.** The anteroseptal leaflet of the mitral valve was lifted and an arrow points to the atrioventricular septum and to the adjacent region of the interventricular septum, both of which have been labeled. **D.** The same embryo before the anteroseptal leaflet of the mitral valve was lifted. Notice the label in the interatrial (arrow 1) and interventricular septa (arrow 2) and in the region of the anteroseptal leaflet of the mitral valve that inserts into the septum (arrow 3). RA = right atrium; LV = left ventricle; C = conus; Ao = aorta; TV = tricuspid valve; MV = mitral valve; O = outlet of the anatomical left ventricle; SCA-VC = superior cushion of the atrioventricular canal; ICA-VC = inferior cushion of the atrioventricular canal; ASLMV (2) = region of the anteroseptal leaflet of the mitral valve that constitutes the mitroaortic continuity; ASLMV (1) = region of the anteroseptal leaflet of the mitral valve that inserts into the septum; APH = arterial pole of the heart; RV = right ventricle; A-VS = atrioventricular septum; SLTV = septal leaflet of the tricuspid valve; SVC = supraventricular crest; PA = pulmonary artery. Reprinted with permission of from de la Cruz et al (1983) Am J Anat 166:63.

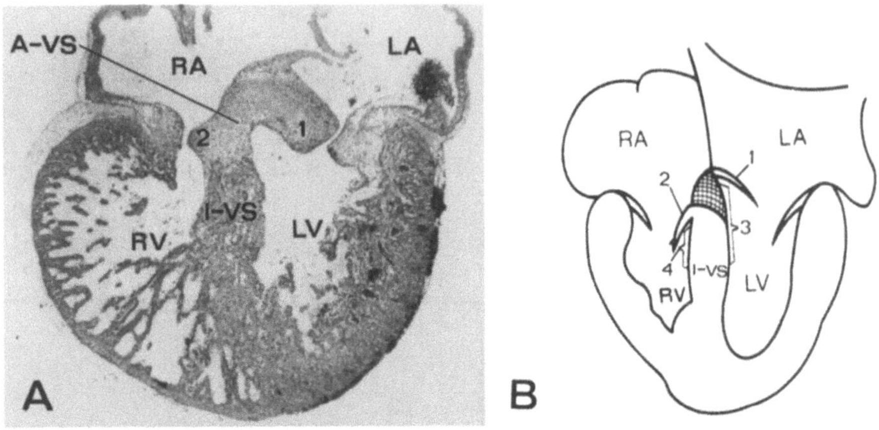

FIGURE 5. Photomicrograph and diagram showing that the atrioventricular septum originates from the inferior cushion of the atrioventricular canal and forms part of the septal wall of the right atrium and part of the septal wall of the inlet of the left ventricle. **A.** Photomicrograph of a traditional frontal view of a four-chamber chick embryo heart in histological section at stage 29HH showing the arch-shaped atrioventricular septum (A-VS) whose cephalic limit is the left cephalic evagination (1), which contributes to the development of the anteroseptal leaflet of the mitral valve that inserts into the septum, and whose caudal limit is the right caudal evagination (2), which is the future septal leaflet of the tricuspid valve in man (microleaflets in the chick). Its convex surface faces the right atrium (RA) and its concave surface faces to the left ventricle (LV). Notice that the atrioventricular septum separates the right atrium from the inlet of the left ventricle. It is also important to point out that the region of the septal wall of the right atrium adjacent to the insertion of the septal leaflet of the tricuspid valve in man, microleaflets in chick (2), is the atrioventricular septum (inferior cushion of the atrioventricular canal). **B.** Schematic representation of a four-chamber section of the mature heart, showing the atrioventricular septum and its anatomical relations. RA = right atrium; LA = left atrium; RV = right ventricle; LV = left ventricle; I-VS = interventricular septum; 1 = anteroseptal leaflet of the mitral valve that inserts into the septum; 2 = septal leaflet of the tricuspid valve; 3 = septal wall of the inlet of the left ventricle (atrioventricular septum plus interventricular septum); 4 = septal wall of the inlet of the right ventricle; cross-hatched area = atrioventricular septum.

of cushion tissue formation is presented, including the important contribution of these cushions to the septation process of the inlets and to valvulogenesis.

DEVELOPMENT OF THE ATRIOVENTRICULAR VALVE APPARATUS

The atrioventricular valve apparatus is composed of several structures: the ring or annulus, the leaflets or cusps, the chordae tendinae, and the papillary muscles, which appear developmentally in this sequence.

From its onset, the mitral ring is cephalic to the tricuspid ring. This is caused by the fact that the anteroseptal leaflet of the mitral valve (which inserts into the AV septum) originates from the left cephalic evagination of the inferior endocardial cushion of the AV canal, whereas the septal leaflet of the tricuspid valve (microleaflets in the chick) originates from the right caudal evagination of this endocardial cushion (Van Mierop et al 1962; Netter and Van Mierop 1969; de la Cruz et al 1983) (Fig. 5).

Importantly the ring of each atrioventricular valve has different embryological

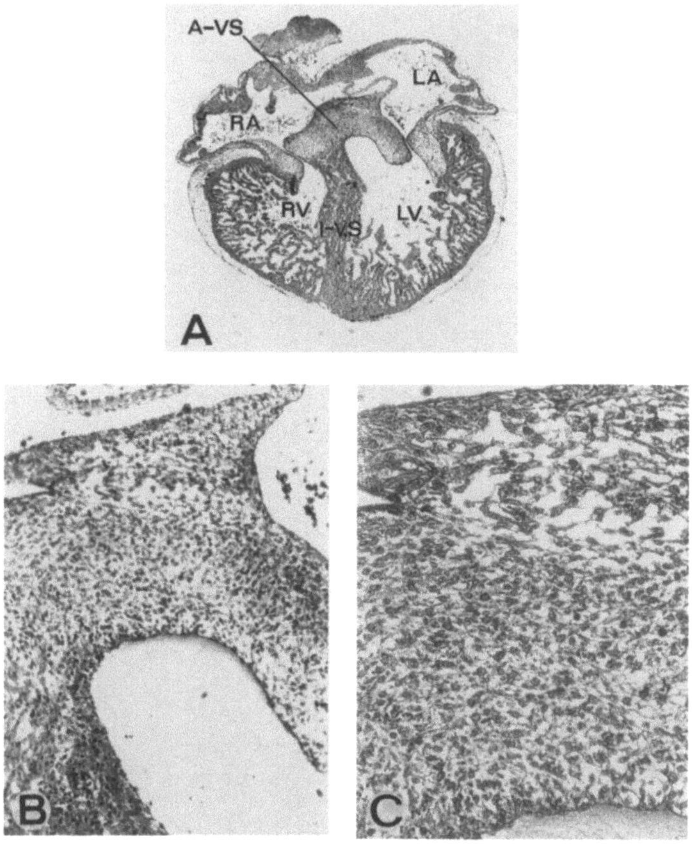

FIGURE 6. Photographs of the four chambers in histological sections of the chick embryo heart at stage 30HH. Notice that the atrioventricular septum (A-VS) is constituted by mesenchymal tissue. A. Complete heart. B, C. Higher magnifications of the atrioventricular septum. I-VS = interventricular septum; RV = right ventricle; LV = left ventricle; RA = right atrium; LA = left atrium.

components that determine the different size of each ring. The right orifice is quite small at the beginning of its development with respect to the left orifice, which is large. The small size of the right atrioventricular ring compared with the left one is probably caused in part by the fact that the right atrioventricular groove is deep, whereas the left atrioventricular groove is shallow, almost nonexistent. Consequently when the heart becomes divided into four chambers by the 8-shaped septum, the right orifice is smaller than the left one. It is of interest to point out, as had been suspected in man (Van Mierop et al 1962; Netter and Van Mierop 1969; Wenink and Gittenberger-de Groot 1985), that the increase in size of the right atrioventricular ring, i.e., the tricuspid ring, is closely linked to the prospective fate of the ventricular infundibular fold. We suppose it is also closely linked to the fate of the right atrioventricular groove.

The differences in size between the tricuspid and the mitral rings are alike in hearts of similar morphology as was shown in the human embryo (DeVries and Saunders 1962; Van Mierop et al 1962; Netter and Van Mierop 1969; Wenink and Gittenberger-de Groot 1985) and in the chick embryo (de la Cruz et al 1983). The

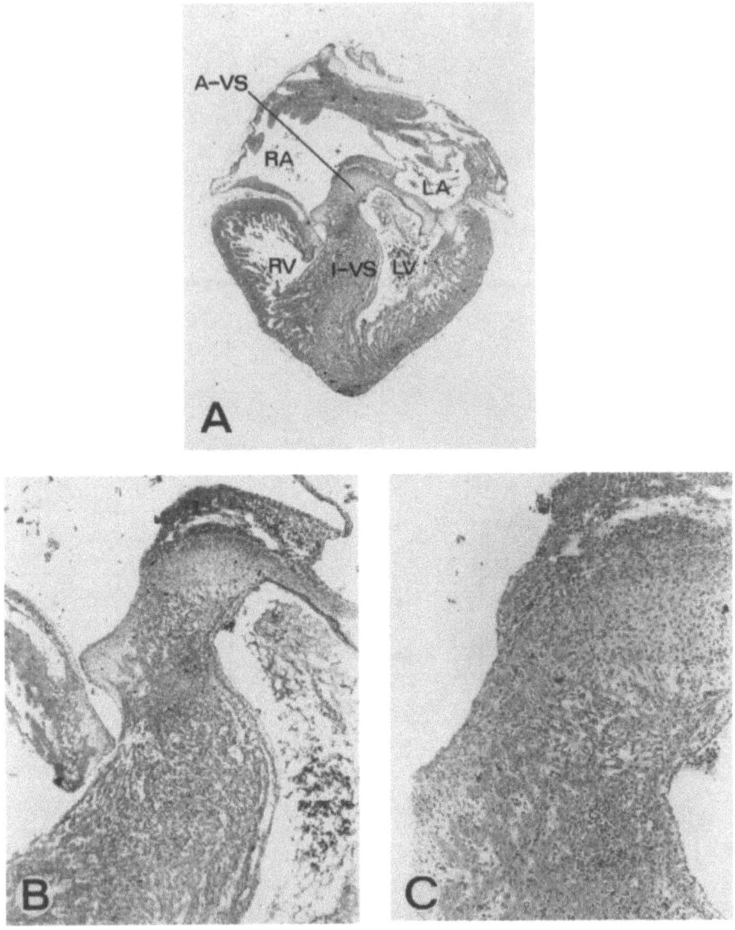

FIGURE 7. Photographs of the four chambers in histological sections of the chick embryo heart at stage 37HH. Notice the beginning of the invasion of the atrioventricular septum (A-VS) by muscular cells originating from the interventricular septum. **A.** Complete heart. **B, C.** Higher magnifications of the atrioventricular septum. I-VS = interventricular septum; RV = right ventricle; LV = left ventricle; RA = right atrium; LA = left atrium.

right atrioventricular ring in both species is constituted by three embryological components (Van Mierop et al 1962; Netter and Van Mierop 1969; de la Cruz et al 1983; Wenink and Gittenberger-de Groot 1985): (1) the right atrioventricular groove, which is quite deep from its inception at the stage of C-shaped loop (chapter IV, Fig. 1 A and C) and forms its right posterior border (Fig. 9D); (2) the inferior or dorsal endocardial cushion of the AV canal, which constitutes the medial region of this ring (Figs. 4 and 9D); and (3) the ventricular infundibular fold, which forms its anterior region (Fig. 9 A, C, and D).

The ventricular infundibular fold is a muscular structure whose free inner border is formed by cushion tissue (Fig. 9B); it is located at the base of the heart and it extends from the right border of the right atrioventricular orifice to the superior endocardial cushion of the AV canal, which it joins in the proximity of its base (Fig.

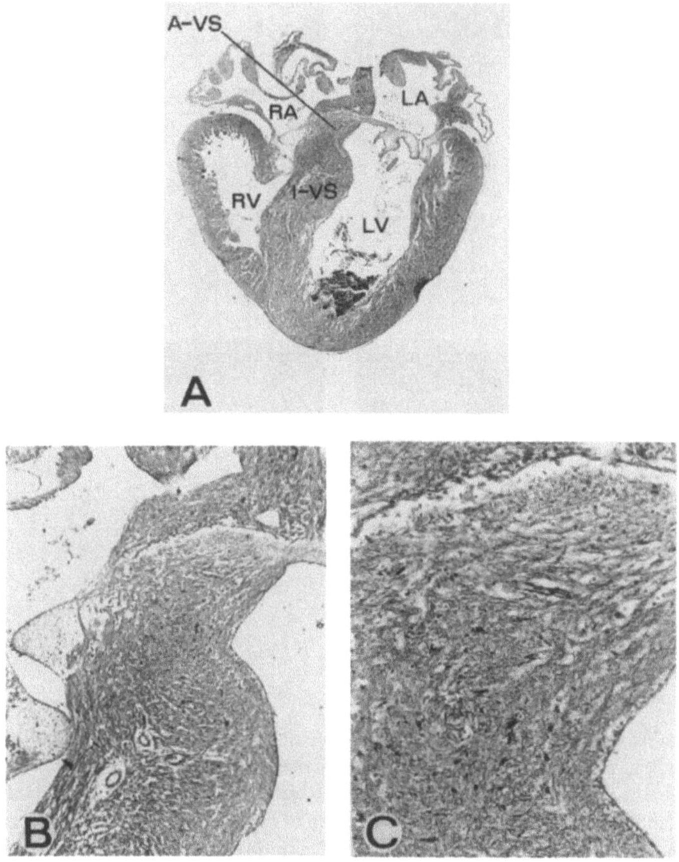

FIGURE 8. Photographs of the four chambers in histological sections of the chick embryo heart at stage 39HH. Notice that the atrioventricular septum (A-VS) is entirely muscular. **A.** Complete heart. **B, C.** Higher magnifications of the atrioventricular septum. I-VS = interventricular septum; RV = right ventricle; LV = left ventricle; RA = right atrium; LA = left atrium.

9). This fold forms part of the posterior wall of the conus or outlet of both ventricles, which is connected to the apical trabeculated region of the right ventricle because at this stage of the development, the left ventricle still lacks an outlet (Fig. 9, A, C, and D). This fold has been designated the bulboventricular flange (Netter and Van Mierop 1969); primary fold (Wenink and Gittenberger-de Groot 1985); conoventricular flange (Kramer 1942); atrioventricular infundibular fold (Anderson et al 1977) and ventriculo-infundibular fold (de la Cruz et al 1992). Taking into consideration the embryological constitution of this fold, the correct designation is the one given by Anderson and colleagues (1977).

The left atrioventricular ring in the chick is constituted by three embryological components: (1) the inferior or dorsal endocardial cushion of the AV canal which forms the medial region of this ring (de la Cruz et al 1983) (Fig. 4); (2) the left atrioventricular groove, which gives origin to the posterior and left border of the ring; and (3) the superior or ventral endocardial cushion, which forms its anterior border and subsequently contributes to the development of the aortic root (de la

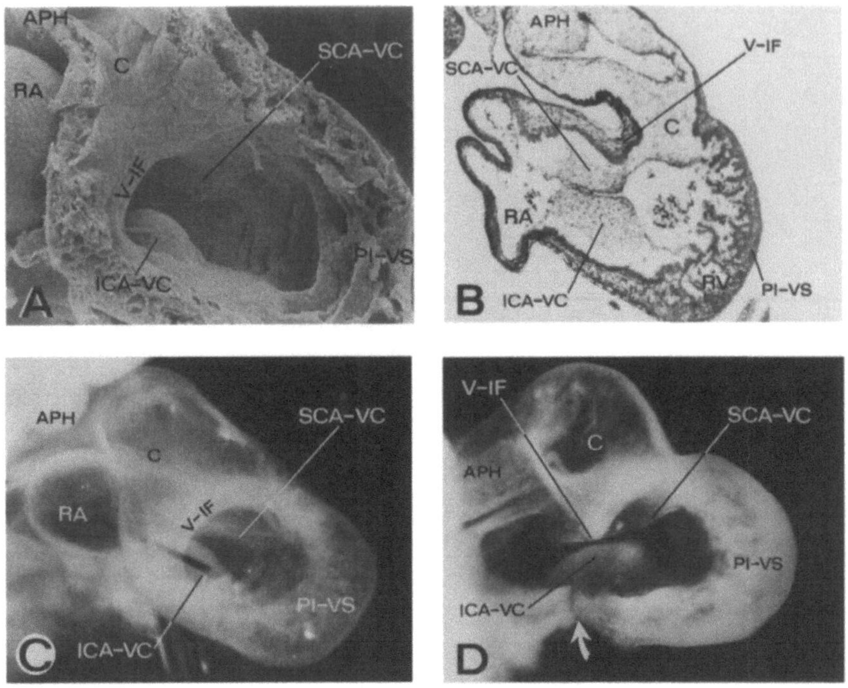

FIGURE 9. Anatomic study and histological section of the ventricular-infundibular fold of the chick embryo heart at stage 20HH. **A.** Photograph obtained with the scanning electron microscope of the dissection of the right ventricle in which the free wall has been removed. Notice the ventricular-infundibular fold (V-IF) forming the anterior region of the right atrioventricular ring and also its insertion in the basal zone of the superior endocardial cushion of the atrioventricular canal (SCA-VC). **B.** Sagittal histological section parallel to the endocardial cushions of the atrioventricular canal, right aspect. Notice the ventricular-infundibular fold (V-IF), inserting into the basal zone of the superior endocardial cushion of the atrioventricular canal (SCA-VC) and its inner border constituted by cushion tissue. **C.** Right view of the heart. The free wall of the right ventricle was removed and a hair was introduced between the ventricular-infundibular fold (V-IF) and the inferior cushion of the AV canal (ICA-VC). Observe this hair inside of the right atrium. This shows that the ventricular-infundibular fold forms the anterior region of the right atrioventricular ring and the inferior cushion of the AV canal (ICA-VC) forms the medial region of this ring. **D.** The same heart in which the ventricular-infundibular fold (V-IF) was partially removed. Notice the inferior cushion of the AV canal (ICA-VC), which forms the medial region of the right atrioventricular ring and the right atrioventricular groove (arrow), is the right posterior border of this ring. RA = right atrium; C = conus or primitive outlet; PI-VS = primitive interventricular septum; RV = right ventricle; APH = arterial pole of the heart or truncus. Figure 9D reprinted with permission of, from de la Cruz et al (1983) Am J Anat 166:63.

Cruz et al 1982, Garcáa-Peláez et al 1984) (chapter VII, Fig. 6). These embryological structures that constitute the mitral valve orifice in the chick (de la Cruz et al 1982, 1983; García-Peláez et al 1984) have also been described in man, in morphologically similar hearts (Van Mierop et al 1962; Netter and Van Mierop 1969; Wenink and Gittenberger-de Groot 1985).

A comparative embryological study of the leaflets, the chordae tendinae, and the papillary muscles in the chick and in man merits a brief anatomical description of these structures in the mature heart of both species.

The mitral valve in the chick (Romanoff 1960; de la Cruz et al 1972, 1982, 1983) is quite similar to that of man (Lam et al 1970; Ranganathan et al 1970). It has a posterolateral or mural leaflet and an anteroseptal leaflet that exhibits two portions, one which is inserted into the septum and a free portion which constitutes the mitroaortic continuity (Ranganathan et al 1970) (Fig. 4, B and D) (chapter X). The commissural leaflets are exceptional in the chick. Papillary muscles are always present in two groups, one posterior, close to the interventricular septum, and the other anterior, distant from the septum. In addition there are three types of chordae tendinae that Lam and coworkers (1970) described in the human mitral valve.

The septal leaflet of the tricuspid valve in humans corresponds in the chick to multiple microleaflets that are directly inserted into the septum by means of chordae tendinae without any papillary muscles (Cayré et al 1993), as is the case with the septal leaflet of the tricuspid valve in man (Silver et al 1971). The great mural leaflet of the chick is muscular (Cayré et al 1993), and it is divided by the anterolateral papillary muscle into two regions: anterior and posterolateral (Cayré et al 1993), which are similar to the anterior and posterior leaflets of the tricuspid valve in man (Fig. 10).

In general there are two types of valves, i.e., those in which the contribution of the ventricular walls is very important and those in which the ventricular wall has a minimal participation (Van Mierop et al 1962; Wenink and Gittenberger-de Groot 1985). The studies of Wenink (1992) and Wenink and Gittenberger-de Groot (1985, 1986) in human embryos show that the contribution of the ventricular walls is minimal in the anterior leaflets, i.e., in the anterior leaflet of the tricuspid valve and

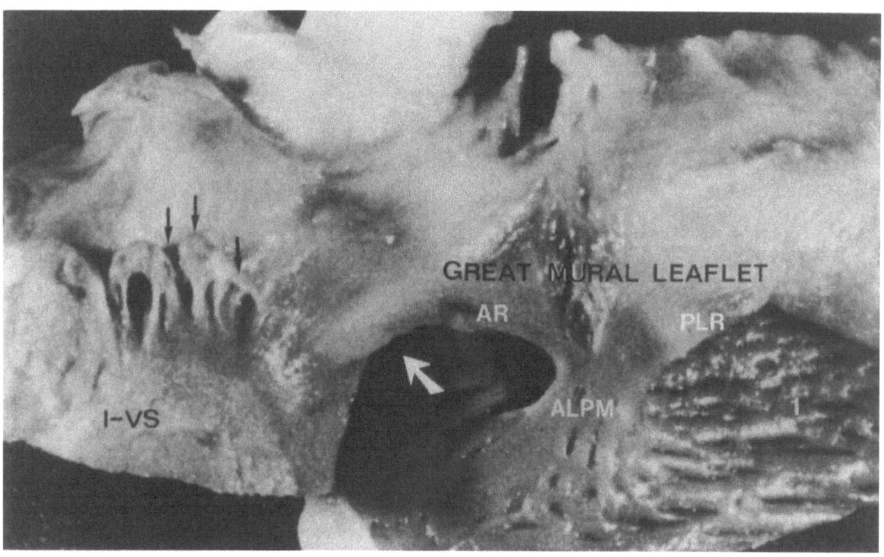

FIGURE 10. The right atrioventricular valvular apparatus in the adult chick heart showing its different components. The anterolateral papillary muscle (ALPM) divides the great mural leaflet into an anterior (AR) and posterolateral (PLR) region. Arrows point to the microleaflets in the right ventricular septal surface. IVS = interventricular septum; 1 = right ventricular free wall. White arrow points to the outlet of the anatomical right ventricle. Reprinted with permission of, from Cayré et al (1993) Acta Anat 148:27.

in the portion of the anteroseptal leaflet of the mitral valve that forms the mitroaortic continuity. Van Mierop and associates (1962) and Netter and Van Mierop (1969) found the same in human embryos and de la Cruz and colleagues (1982, 1983) in the chick embryo heart.

In general, the leaflets in the chick and in man have a dual embryological origin: the endocardial cushions of the AV canal and the muscular ventricular walls (Van Mierop et al 1962; Netter and Van Mierop 1969; de la Cruz et al 1983; Van Mierop and Kutsche 1985; Wenink and Gittenberger-de Groot 1985).

We will begin our study in both species by referring first to the AV endocardial cushions. The superior or ventral endocardial cushion and the inferior or dorsal endocardial cushion of the AV canal have been studied in this chapter. Likewise both species (man and chick) also develop lateral cushions: the right lateral endocardial cushion and the left lateral endocardial cushion of the AV canal. These appear at stage 26HH in the chick (Fig. 11) and at horizon XVI in man (Van Mierop et al 1962; Netter and Van Mierop 1969) with similar cardiac morphology.

The contribution of the AV endocardial cushions in the development of the atrioventricular leaflets in man was studied by Van Mierop and associates (1962) and Netter and Van Mierop (1969). According to these authors, the superior and inferior endocardial cushions of the AV canal contribute to the development of the

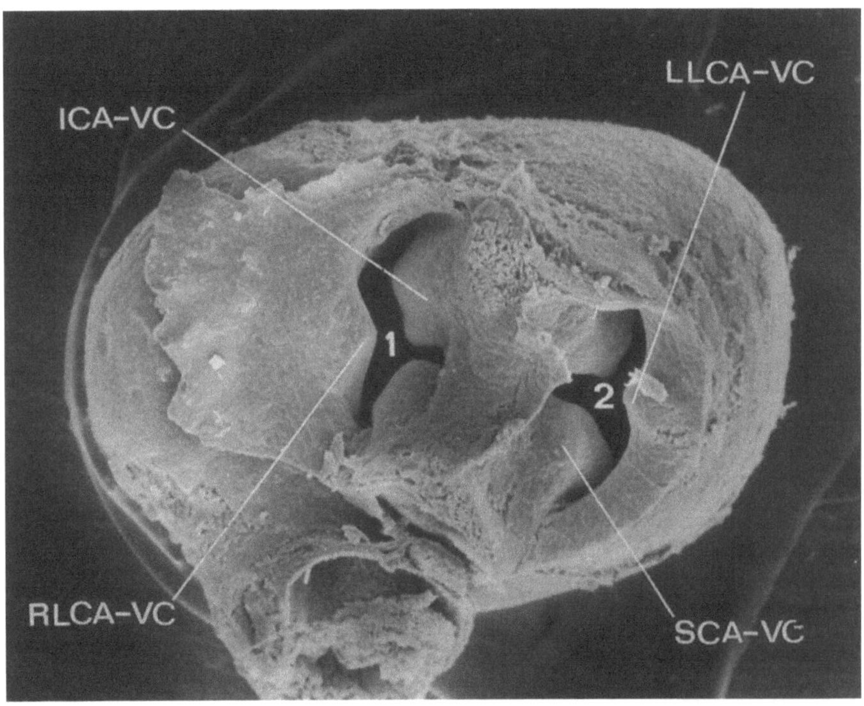

FIGURE 11. Study with scanning electron microscopy of a transverse section at the level of the atrioventricular orifices of the chick embryo heart at stage 26HH. Notice the left lateral endocardial cushion of the atrioventricular canal (LLCA-VC) and the right lateral endocardial cushion of the atrioventricular canal (RLCA-VC), which appear at this developmental stage. ICA-VC = inferior cushion of the atrioventricular canal; SCA-VC = superior cushion of the atrioventricular canal; 1 = right atrioventricular orifice; 2 = left atrioventricular orifice.

anteroseptal leaflet of the mitral valve, and the left lateral cushion of the AV canal contributes to the development of the mural leaflet. As concerns the commissural leaflets, the superior and left lateral endocardial cushions participate in the constitution of the anterior commissural leaflet, and the inferior and left lateral endocardial cushions participate in the constitution of the posterior commissural leaflet.

Netter and Van Mierop (1969) published a diagram showing the contribution of the different endocardial cushions of the AV canal in each of the tricuspid leaflets. Thus, in the septal or medial leaflet, the superior, inferior, and right lateral endocardial cushions participate, whereas in the posterior leaflet it is the right lateral endocardial cushion that participates. With respect to the anterior leaflet of the tricuspid valve, Netter and Van Mierop (1969) propose that the right lateral endocardial cushion and the dextrodorsal conus ridge contribute to its development.

In vivo labeling experiments of the inferior endocardial cushion of the AV canal in the chick embryo show that this endocardial cushion contributes to the formation of the basal region of the portion of the anteroseptal leaflet of the mitral valve that is inserted into the septum (de la Cruz et al 1983) and to the formation of the septal microleaflets of the tricuspid valve in the chick heart (de la Cruz et al 1983) (Fig. 4, B and D), homologous to the septal leaflet of the tricuspid valve in man (Cayré et al 1993). The in vivo labeling of the superior endocardial cushion of the AV canal provides evidence that the region of the anteroseptal leaflet of the mitral valve, which forms the mitroaortic continuity, originates from this endocardial cushion (de la Cruz et al 1982; García-Peláez et al 1984). This new information provided by the in vivo labeling experiments in the chick embryo heart (de la Cruz et al 1982, 1983; García-Peláez et al 1984) supports the ideas of Van Mierop and coworkers (1962) and Netter and Van Mierop (1969) concerning the contribution of the inferior and superior endocardial cushions of the AV canal in the development of the anteroseptal leaflet of the mitral valve and the participation of the inferior endocardial cushion of the AV canal in the septal leaflet of the tricuspid valve in the human heart. However, it disagrees with the view of Netter and Van Mierop (1969) concerning the contribution of the superior and right lateral endocardial cushions of the AV canal in the development of the septal leaflet of the tricuspid valve. With respect to the mural or posterior leaflet of the mitral valve in the chick, it seems that the left lateral endocardial cushion contributes to its development; however, this must be substantiated by in vivo labeling experiments of this cushion, which would also clarify the position (Netter and Van Mierop 1969) on the development of this leaflet in man.

It is important to point out that the posterolateral and anterior tricuspid leaflets in the chick (Cayré et al 1993), which are homologous with the posterior and anterior tricuspid leaflets in man, are originally constituted by cushion tissue in the chick embryo (Figs. 6A and 12A) although they are muscular in the mature heart (Fig. 12E). The in vivo labeling experiments of the inferior and superior endocardial cushions of the AV canal in the chick embryo (de la Cruz et al 1982, 1983; García-Peléez et al 1984) show that they do not participate in the development of the posterolateral leaflet nor the anterior tricuspid leaflets. However, the contribution of the right lateral endocardial cushion to the development of both leaflets has not yet been established because this endocardial cushion has not been studied with in vivo labeling techniques. Therefore, the contribution of the right lateral endocardial cushion to the posterior, septal, and anterior leaflets of the human tricuspid valve as pointed out by Netter and Van Mierop (1969) is still unknown. Moreover,

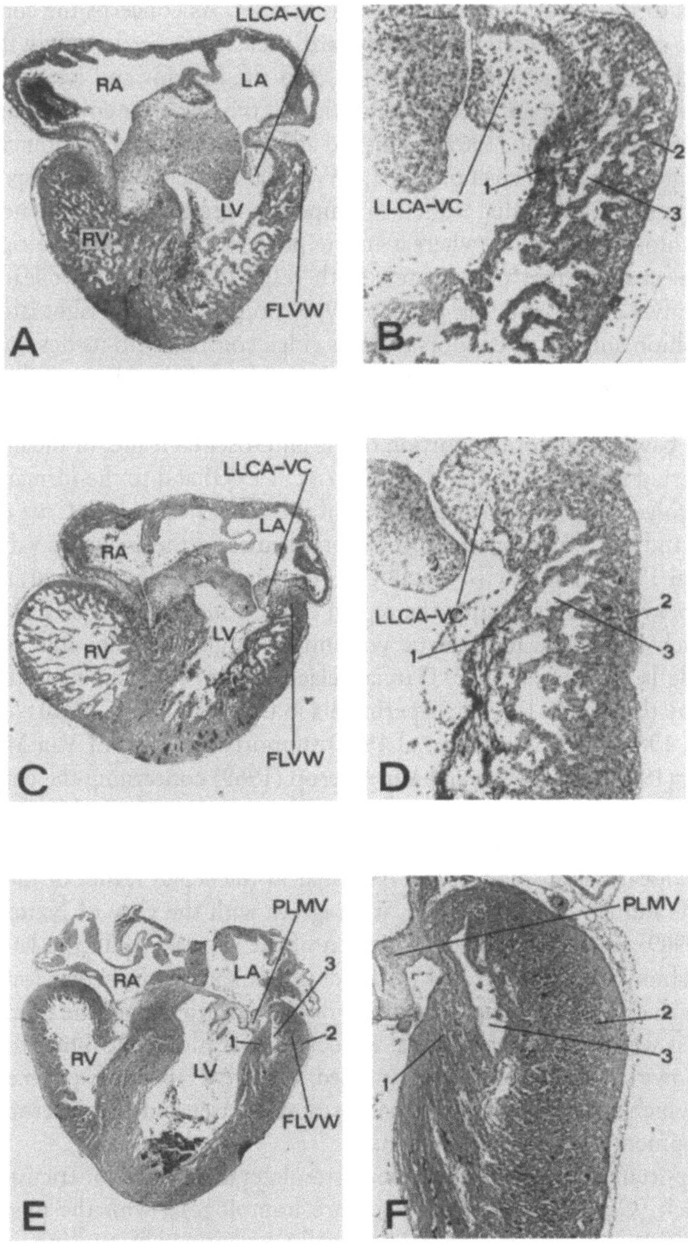

FIGURE 12. Photographs of the four chambers in histological sections of the chick embryo heart at stages 28HH, 30HH, and 39HH showing the participation of the free left ventricular wall (FLVW) and the adjacent region to the left lateral endocardial cushion of the atrioventricular canal (LLCA-VC) in the development of the posterior leaflet of the mitral valve (PLMV). **A, B.** Stage 28HH. Notice the intercellular spaces (3) within the free wall of the left ventricle in relation to the left lateral endocardial cushion of the atrioventricular canal. **C, D.** Stage 30HH. The intercellular spaces (3) become larger. **E, F.** Stage 39HH. Notice the large intercellular space (3), which separated the free ventricular wall of the left ventricule into a thin subendocardial muscular layer (1) and a thick compact subepicardial muscular layer (2). RA = right atrium; LA = left atrium; RV = right ventricle; LV = left ventricle.

Netter and Van Mierop (1969) maintain that in man, the dextrodorsal conus ridge also participates in the development of the anterior leaflet of the tricuspid valve. This view is open to discussion, because when the dextrodorsal conal ridge in the chick is labeled in vivo, the label never appears in the anterior leaflet of the tricuspid valve (de la Cruz et al 1982) (chapter VII). Instead we believe the ventricular infundibular fold contributes to the development of this leaflet, because that structure (the ventricular infundibular fold) forms the anterior region of the tricuspid ring and its inner free border is formed by cushion tissue (Fig. 9B).

One of the most important aspects of which we have little information concerns the contribution of the ventricular muscular walls in the development of the leaflets, the chordae tendinae, and the papillary muscles. Our knowledge is based on postmortem studies, which are both meager and incomplete.

During stage 28HH intercellular spaces appear within the myocardium of the free wall of the left ventricle, adjacent to the left lateral cushion of the AV canal (Fig. 12). In subsequent stages, these intercellular spaces coalesce and divide the myocardial free wall into a thick subepicardial layer and a thin subendocardial layer (Fig. 12). The subepicardial layer remains as the free wall of the left ventricle, and the subendocardial layer participates in the formation of the medial and apical region of the posterior leaflets of the mitral valve because their basal region is derived from the left lateral cushion of the AV canal (Fig. 12, E and F). This subendocardial layer also participates in the development of its chordae tendinae and its papillary muscles (Fig. 12, E and F). This space between the posterior leaflets of the mitral valve and the free wall of the left ventricle is covered by epithelial cells whose origin is still unknown.

The developmental process of the atrioventricular valve apparatus in terms of the contribution of the cardiac muscle is still unknown; key questions include how these intercellular spaces are formed, how they coalesce, where the epithelial cells lining them come from, and how they divide the myocardium into two layers, a subepicardial layer and a subendocardial layer, which gives origin to the medial and apical regions of the atrioventricular leaflets, the chordae tendinae, and the papillary muscles. Other unresolved questions come to mind: Why do these intercellular spaces not appear in the ventricular cardiac muscle whose prospective fate is to form the free walls of the apical trabeculated region of the ventricles? Why do these intercellular spaces not appear in the muscular walls of the conus lined by cushion tissue?

HOW DO CUSHIONS BECOME LEAFLETS?

Valve or leaflets form in both the inlets (AV canal) and great arterial root (truncus) for each ventricle. As noted above, mature AV leaflets are composed of a core of mesenchyme that differentiates into connective tissue and myocardial fibers of ventricular origin. The association of leaflets with ventricular myocardium is mostly a characteristic of the AV inlet valves and may be linked to the formation of papillary muscles. The association with muscle is only one of potentially several differences between valves formed in the AV canal versus great arterial root (truncus). For example, *Sox-4* is expressed in cushion-forming cells of both regions, yet mutations in this gene only affected formation of the great arterial root (truncus) (Ya et al 1997). Although even more differences in gene expression are likely to be found, the central defining event of valvulogenesis—either AV or arterial cuff (truncus)—is the formation of a mesenchymal core covered by endocardial endothelium.

Although in vivo labeling strongly supports the traditional view that the endocardial cushions form this core of prevalvular mesenchyme, there remains a need to establish this concept more fully, particularly if molecular mechanisms are to be understood. Wenink (1987) proposed a radically different origin for valves, which is presented in Fig. 13. From histological similarities, Wenink (1987) introduced the option that "sulcus" tissue, not cushions, is the progenitor of the inlet valves. Sulcus tissue is that part of the overall epicardial mesenchyme that fills the grooves or sulci that encircle the AV canal. On the right side, these mesenchymal grooves cut deeply into the AV inlet where, if the criterion of "guilt by association" is to be used, a case for a sulcus origin can be made (Fig. 13B) Indeed, much of Wenink's proposal derives from the argument that cushion mesenchyme does not look like mature valve tissue. This serves to underscore the need to use in vivo labeling or molecular markers to study a dynamic process that occurs over time. As described below, such experiments consistently point to the cushion alternative (Fig. 13C). For example, a cushion origin for leaflets can be reasoned from the expression pattern of an antigen, JB3, that is associated with heart development from its earliest stages. JB3 antigens are first seen as the tracks left behind by mesodermal cells between stages 3 and 4 as they migrate from the primitive streak to the heart-forming fields (Wunsch et al 1994) Later, during formation of the tubular heart, the JB3 antibody

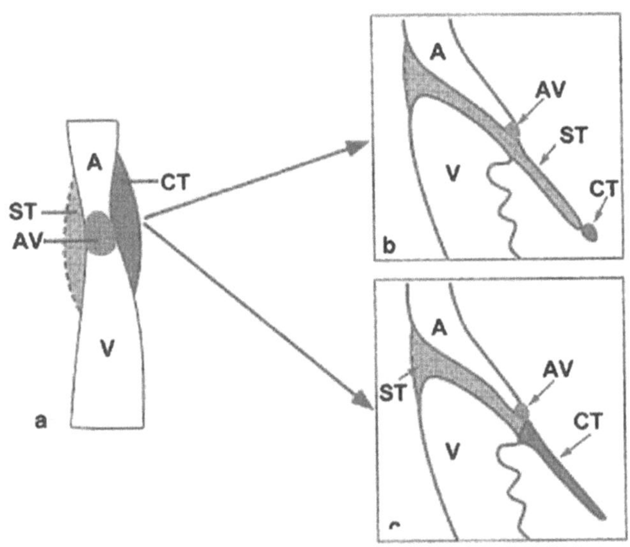

FIGURE 13. Hypothetical model of the atrioventricular junction illustrating two hypothetical and historical options for the origin of the inlet leaflets. In (**a**), sulcus tissue (ST) on the surface of the heart and cushion tissue (CT) on the inside are separated by the atrioventricular myocardium (denoted as the circle labeled AV). In (**b**), after Wenink (1987), expansion of sulcus tissue is presented as one option for the origin of the leaflet, whereas in (**c**) cushion tissue is envisioned as the progenitor of the leaflet. In both options, the continuity of the AV myocardium with atrium (A) or ventricle (V) is broken as sulcus and cushion mesenchymes come into direct contact. Antibody and in vivo marking experiments support the cushion option depicted in (**c**). (Courtesy of Dr. Andy Wessels, Medical University of South Carolina).

uniquely marks the precursors of a subset of endothelial cells that specifically transform into cushion mesenchymal cells and reveals their origin to be from the heart fields (Eisenberg and Markwald 1995).

Finally, within fully mesenchymalized cushions, JB3 is distributed as fine microfibrils, prompting the suggestion that JB3 proteins form a transitional scaffolding on which the extracellular proteins of the future valve leaflets are assembled and integrated. What, then, is JB3 antigen? Using the JB3 antibody to immunopurify and eventually microsequence the JB3 antigen, it appears that JB3 is a fibrillin (specifically, fibrillin-2) (Brenda Rongish, Robert Meecham, and Charles Little, personal communication). This has relevance to the topic at hand because mutations in fibrillin genes result in Marfan's syndrome, a connective tissue disorder affecting the cardiac inlet valves (McKusick 1992). In support of the JB3 data, Wessels and associates (1996), using monoclonal antibodies developed to specifically recognize either cushion or sulcus mesenchyme, found that the leaflets expressed only cushion tissue antigens. They also showed that the sulcus mesenchyme eventually fused with cushion mesenchyme, disrupting the continuity of the myocardium between atrium and ventricle at the level of the AV canal. If not serving to form leaflets, then the role of the sulcus mesenchyme may be to form a part of the skeletal framework that stabilizes the valvular tissues derived from the AV cushions.

Given the critical, life-dependent, hemodynamic role played by the heart valves, it is surprising that so little is known about the processes by which cushions become valve or leaflets and by what regulatory mechanisms. As shown in Figs. 5, 6, and 11, after the fusion of the superior and inferior cushions to form the AV septum, the lumen of each ventricular inlet is encircled by a rim of cushion mesenchyme (derived from a lateral cushion + the AV cushion). Between stages 26 and 30, bulges or "buds" of AV mesenchyme emerge, which continue to expand into the lumen through stage 39 (Figs. 5 and 12). As a starting point to resolve molecular mechanisms, we have proposed a hypothesis that cushion "buds" become leaflets using developmental mechanisms similar to those observed for other expansions of mesenchyme, as in the limb bud. In obvious analogy to the limb apical ectodermal ridge, a "ridge hypothesis" is conceptualized in Fig. 14. This hypothesis is, in reality, part of the hypothesis originally proposed for remodeling of the inner curvature, described in chapter II (chapter II, Fig. 16). The ridge hypothesis proposes that the thickened endocardium that lines the fully mesenchymalized AV cushions secretes factors (e.g., growth factors) that promote proliferation and eventual expansion of the mesenchyme closest to the endocardial ridge. In the limb bud, the apical ridge secretes isoforms of basic fibroblast growth factor, e.g., FGF-2, FGF-4, and FGF-8, which serve to upregulate and sustain expression of *Msx-1* in the mesenchyme immediately beneath the apical ridge, the so-called progressive zone (Fallon et al 1994). Maintaining expression of *Msx-1* correlated with proliferation and distal elongation of the progressive zone (Fallon et al 1994; Szebenyi et al 1995; Wang and Sassoon 1995). Thus, FGF signaling through *Msx-1* is proposed as the mechanism used by the endocardium to regulate outgrowth of cushion buds into prevalvular, fan-shaped leaflets.

However, before seriously proposing the above hypothesis, we initiated preliminary experiments to test certain assumptions predicted by the hypothesis. We found that (1) the mitotic cells within the superior cushion are nonrandomly distributed, more being associated with the endocardium than centrally or in the

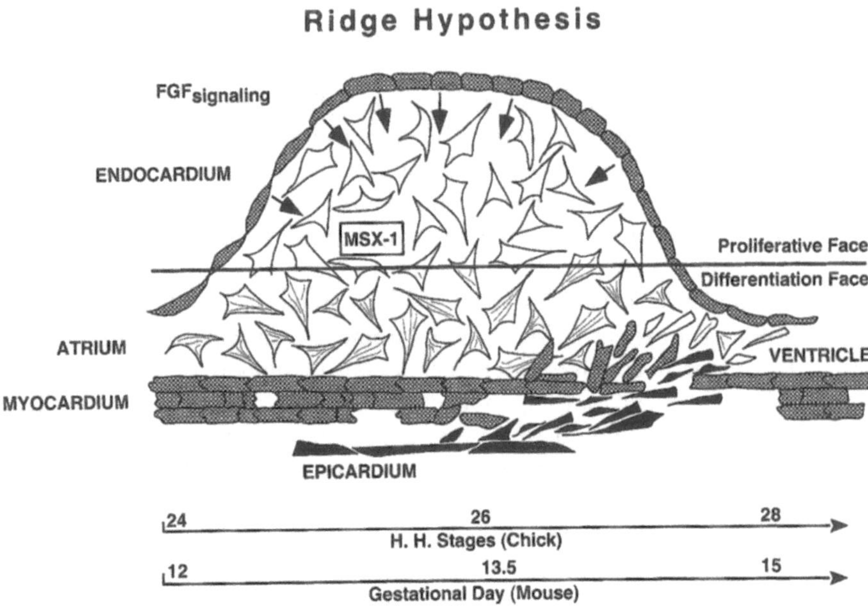

FIGURE 14. "The Ridge Hypothesis" is a molecular model that seeks to explain how the outer half or proliferative face of a mesenchymalized AV cushion becomes a leaflet. It is proposed that by stage 26, a mesenchymal "bud" develops, which over time (stages 28 to 40) will continue to expand distally into the lumen. Growth is induced by the "ridge" of endocardial endothelium that constitutes the epithelial lining of the cushion. The ridge induces proliferation of the underlying mesenchyme, as in the limb, by secreting fibroblast growth factors (FGF). Interaction of the ligand with receptors on target mesenchyme is envisioned as signaling proliferation by upregulating and sustaining expression of a homeodomain, transcription factor, *Msx-1*, which is present in cushion cells adjacent to the lumen and, in the limb, has been correlated with proliferation and growth. As described in more detail in chapter II (see Fig. 16), cushion cells that escape the proliferative field (as defined by endocardial signaling) differentiate and participate in remodeling of the adjacent myocardium.

myocardial face (Fig. 15A); (2) the cushion endocardium expressed FGF-2 and FGF-4, both mRNA (Fig. 15B) and protein (Fig. 15C); (3) the receptors for FGF ligands were expressed by mesenchyme of the luminal face (Fig. 15D); and (4) the mesenchyme of cushions can respond in vivo to FGF ligands (Y. Sugi and R. Markwald, unpublished data). The latter was shown by in vivo microinjection of a retrovirus vector encoding FGF-4 into the conus region at stage 19, when ridges were just beginning to form. Normally, leaflets do not form in the conus, but in response to overexpression of FGF-4 ligands, the conal mesenchyme was "ignited". After 16 hours it formed a "bud" of mesenchyme (Fig. 16) that, if incubation was continued, grew until it completely occluded the lumen. Although preliminary, these findings are consistent with the precepts of the ridge hypothesis and indicate that the endocardial endothelium may not only be the progenitor of cushion mesenchyme but also functions to regulate directly or indirectly the fate of its cushion progeny.

Finally, in proposing the limb–heart analogy, we do so on the basis of emerging precedents in the literature that many of the genes expressed by either heart or limb were also expressed in the other (for a review, compare chapters 2 and 3 in Kavlock

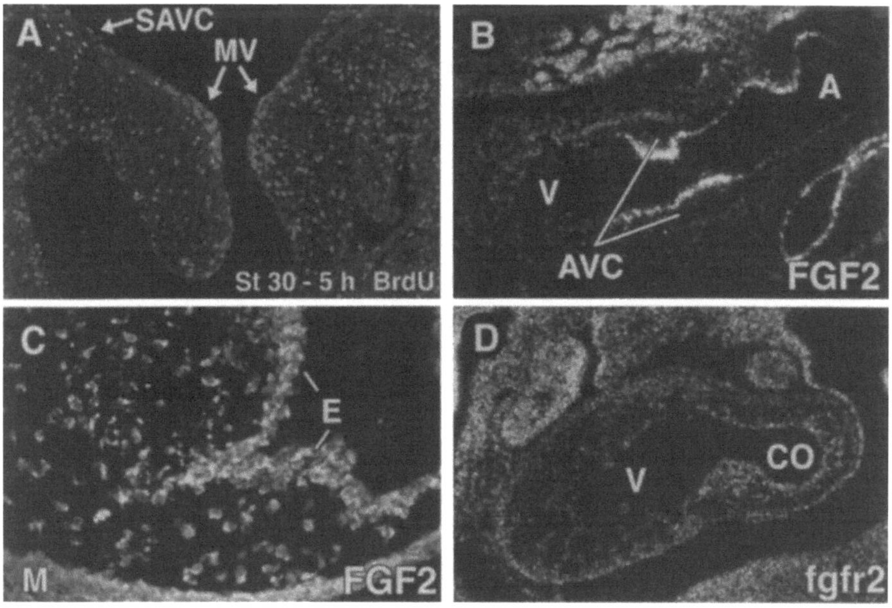

FIGURE 15. Experiments to test the ridge hypothesis. **A.** Developing leaflets of the mitral valve (MV) were labeled 5 hours with bromodeovyuridine (BrdU) at stage 30 to reveal sites of actively dividing cells. Note that in the superior AV cushion (SAVC) and the adjacent left lateral cushion proliferating cells (revealed by anti-BrdU antibodies) are clustered beneath the endocardium as would be predicted by the ridge hypothesis. 120×. **B.** In situ hybridization for fibroblast growth factor-2 (FGF-2) mRNA; note that endocardium of both the superior and inferior AV cushions (AVC) are intensely labeled; atrium (A), ventricle (V); similarly the endocardium of the conus/arterial root region (lower right) also expressed the gene. 90×. **C.** Fluorescein isothiocyanate immunostain for FGF-2 protein in the conus/arterial root junction. A similar expression pattern occurred in the AV cushions. Note the strongest expression for the FGF ligand is observed in the endocardium (E) and adjacent mesenchyme and diminishes on cells closer to the myocardium (M). 270×, **D.** In situ hydridization for message localization of FGF receptor-2 (fgfr2). Note expression in the mesenchyme of the conal (CO) cushion indicating potential of cushion mesenchyme to bind FGF ligands. Similar findings were observed for the AV cushions. 75×.

and Daston 1997). One example with clinical relevance is the Holt Oram syndrome, which is characterized by limb malformations and cardiac septal defects (Basson et al 1997). Positional cloning established that the defects derived from the mutation of a T-box transcription factor, *TBX-5*. This gene is expressed in both organs, although the specific tissue sites were not determined. However, early indications are that *TBX-5* is expressed in the AV canal and the mesodermal core of the limb (R. Schwartz, personal communication). This serves to demonstrate that development may proceed by generalized mechanisms in which the time and place of expression become the central regulatory issue.

CONCLUSIONS

The integration of postmortem and in vivo studies in the chick embryo with postmortem studies in the human embryo allow us to reach the following conclusions, which are valid for both species:

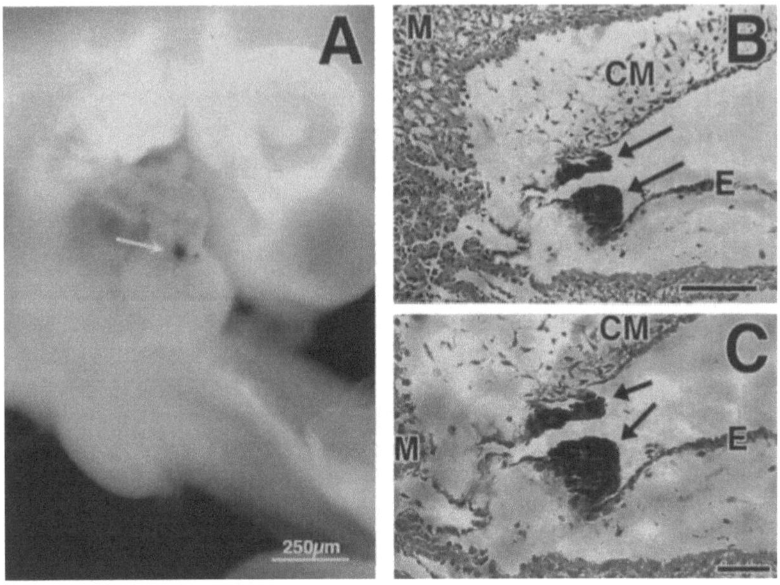

FIGURE 16. **A.** A replication-defective, SNZ retrovial construct overexpressing FGF-4 (gift of Takashi Mikawa, Cornell University) was microinjected into the conus region (arrow) of a stage 19 embyro. The retrovirus contained a full-length, sense cDNA for FGF-4 positioned downstream to a LacZ reporter that was used to visualize infected cells (dark spot indicated by the arrow). **B, C.** Low and high magnifications, respectively, of infected cells seen in a cross-section made at the level indicated by the arrow in A, 16 hours after microinjection. Note expansion of labeled cushion mesenchymal cells (CM) (arrows) into the lumen. Such "bud-like" outgrowths are not normally seen at this time or place in the outlet limb, indicating that cushion cells can respond in vivo to FGF ligands (Courtesy of Dr. Yukiko Sugi, Medical University of South Carolina).

1. The primordium of the ventricular inlet (the primitive inlet or AV canal) appears in the chick embryo at stage 12HH and is the segment adjacent to the right atrioventricular groove in the caudal limb of the loop. It connects both primitive atria with the primordium of the apical trabeculated region of the left ventricle. Therefore, the primordium of the apical trabeculated region of the right ventricle is not yet connected with the right atrium.
2. The first cardiac septum is formed by the atrial septum primum, the superior and inferior cushions of the AV canal, and the primitive interventricular septum. It appears in the chick embryo at stage 17HH (horizon XIV in humans). Owing to the embryological constitution of this septum, it separates simultaneously both primitive atria and the apical trabeculated region of both ventricles, and it divides the single or common inlet (primitive inlet) into right and left inlets. Thereafter, each ventricle connects with its corresponding atrium through its own inlet.
3. The inferior endocardial cushion of the AV canal contributes to the development of the atrioventricular septum and to the adjacent region of the interatrial and interventricular septa. Muscular cells arising from the interventricular septum invade the cushion tissue that constitutes the atrioventricular septum.
4. The inferior and superior endocardial cushion's of the AV canal contribute to the development of the basal region of the anteroseptal leaflet of the mitral

valve; in addition, the inferior endocardial cushion contributes to the development of the septal leaflet of the tricuspid valve. We do not know beyond speculation what the contribution's of the right and left lateral endocardial cushions of the AV canal and of the mesenchymal tissue of the ventriculo-infundibular fold are in the constitution of the remaining atrioventricular leaflets.

5. Multiple intercellular spaces appear in the basal region of the AV myocardial ventricular walls of the left ventricle, which coalesce to divide the myocardium into two layers: a subepicardial and a subendocardial layer. The latter participates in the development of the middle and apical zones of the posterior leaflets of the mitral valve, its chordae tendinae, and its papillary muscles. We do not know what processes are involved in these morphological changes.
6. Leaflets derive from a cushion mesenchymal core (not sulcus tissue). It is proposed that, in analogy to the limb, expansion and outgrowth of the mesenchymal core into the lumen of the AV canal is the outcome of an inductive interaction between endocardium and the underlying mesenchyme. The interaction may be mediated through FGF signaling and the homeobox gene, *Msx-1*. Expression of JB3/fibrillin defines sites where valves will develop and constitutes a major extracellular component of their mesenchymal core.

REFERENCES

Anderson RH, Becker AE, VanMierop LHS. 1997. What should we call the crista? Br Heart J 39:856–9.

Argüello C, Servín M, Arciniegas E, Valenzuela B. 1988. Fusion mechanisms of endocardial atrioventricular cushions. In: Quero-Jiménez M, Arteaga M, editors. Pediatric cardiology. Atrioventricular septal defect. Madrid: Doyma. p 64–75.

Basson TT, Bachinsky DR, Lin RC, Levi T, Elkins JA, Soults J, Grayzel D, Kroumpouzou E, Traill TA, Leblanc-Straceski J, Renault b, Kucherlapati R, Seidman JG, Seidman CE. 1997. Mutation in human cause limb and cardiac malformation in Holt-Gram syndrome. Nat Genet 15:30–5.

Cayré R, Valencia-Mayoral P, Coffe-Ramírez V, Sánchez Gómez C, Angelini P, De la Cruz MV. 1993. The right atrioventricular valvular apparatus in the chick heart. Acta Anat 148:27–33.

de la Cruz MV, Castillo MM, Villavicencio L, Valencia A, Moreno-Rodriguez RA. 1997. Primitive interventricular septum, its primordium, and its contribution in the definitive interventricular septum: in vivo labelling study in the chick embryo heart. Anat Rec 247:512–20.

de la Cruz MV, Cayré R, Arista-Salado O, Sadowinski S, Serrano A. 1992. The infundibular interrelationships and the ventriculoarterial connection in doublet outlet right ventricle. Clinical and surgical implications. Int J Cardiol 35:153–64.

de la Cruz MV, Giménez-Ribotta M, Saravalli O, Cayré R. 1983. The contribution of the inferior endocardial cushion of the atrioventricular canal to cardiac septation and to the development of the atrioventricular valves: study in the chick embryo. Am J Anat 166:63–72.

de la Cruz MV, Muñoz-Armas S, Muñoz-Castellanos L. 1972. Development of the Chick Heart. Baltimore, MD: Johns Hopkins University Press.

de la Cruz MV, Quero-Jiménez M, Arteaga M, Cayré R. 1982. Morphogénèse du septum interventriculaire. Coeur 13:443–8.

de la Cruz MV, Sánchez-Gómez C, Cayré R. 1991. The developmental components of the ventricles: their significance in congenital cardiac malformations. Cardiol Young 1:123–8.

de la Cruz MV, Sánchez-Gómez C, Palomino MA. 1989. The primitive cardiac regions in the straight tube heart (Stage 9–) and their anatomical expression in the mature heart: an experimental study in the chick embryo. J Anat 165:121–31.
de la Cruz MV, Sánchez-Gómez C, Robledo Tovi JL. 1987. Experimental study of the development of the ventricular inlets in the chick embryo. Embryologische Hefte. 1:25–37.
DeVries PA, Saunders JB. 1962. Development of the ventricles and spiral outflow tract in the human heart. A contribution of the development of the human heart from age group IX to age group XV. Carnegie Contrib Embryol 256:89–114.
Eisenberg LM, Markwald RR. 1995. Molecular regulation of atrioventricular valvuloseptal morphogenesis. Circ Res 77:1–6.
Fallon JF, Lopez A, et al. 1994. FGF-2: apical ectodermal ridge growth signal for chick limb development. Science (Wash DC) 264:104–7.
García-Peláez I, Díaz-Góngora G, Arteaga-Martínez M. 1984 Contribution of the superior atrioventricular cushion to the left ventricular infundibulum. Experimental study on the chick embryo. Acta Anat 118:224–30.
Icardo JM. 1989a. Changes in endocardial cell morphology during development of the endocardial cushions. Anat Embryol 179:443–8.
Icardo JM. 1989b. Endocardial cell arrangement: role of hemodynamics. Anat Rec 225:150–5.
Kavlock RJ, Daston GP. 1997. Drug Toxicity in Embryonic Development. I. Advances in Understanding Mechanisms of Birth Defects, Handbook of Experimental Pharmacology, Vol 124/1, Berlin: Springer. (see chapter 2, p 11–40; chapter 3, p 41–76)
Kinsella MK, Fitzharris TP. 1980. Origin of cushion tissue in the developing chick heart: cinematographic recordings of in situ formation. Science (Wash DC) 207:1359–1360.
Kramer TC. 1942. The partitioning of the truncus and conus and the formation of the membranous portion of the interventricular septum in the human heart. Am J Anat 71:343–70.
Lam JHC, Ranganathan N, Wigle DE, Silver MD. 1970. Morphology of the human mitral valve. I. Chordae tendinae: a new classification. Circulation 41:449–58.
Lamers WH, Wessels A, Verbeek FJ, Moorman AFM, Virágh S, Wenink ACG, Gittenberger-de Groot AC, Anderson RH. 1992. New findings concerning ventricular septation in the human heart. Implications for maldevelopment. Circulation 86:1194–205.
Magovern JH, Moore GW, Hutchins GM. 1986. Development of the atrioventricular valve region in the human embryo. Anat Rec 215:167–81.
Markwald, RR, Fitzharris TP, Adams Smith WN. 1975. Structural analysis of endocardial cytodifferentiation. Dev Biol 42:160–80.
Markwald RR, Fitzharris TP, Manasek FJ. 1977. Structural development of endocardial cushions. Am J Anat 148:85–120.
McKusick VA. 1991. The defect in Marfan syndrome. Nature 352:279–81.
Netter FH, Van Mierop LHS. 1969. Embryology. In: Netter FH, editor. CIBA Collection of Medical Illustrations. Ardsley, New Jersey: CIBA Pharmaceutical Co. Vol. 5, p 119–25.
Ranganathan N, Lam JHC, Wigle DE, Silver MD. 1970. Morphology of the human mitral valve. II. The valve leaflets. Circulation 41:459–67.
Romanoff AR. 1960. The Avian Embryo. New York: MacMillan. p 680–780.
Rongish BJ, Little CD. 1995. Extracellular matrix in heart development. Experentia 51:873–82.
Silver MD, Lam JHC, Ranganathan N, Wigle ED. 1971. Morphology of the human tricuspid valve. Circulation 43:333–48.
Sissman NJ. 1970. Developmental landmarks in cardiac morphogenesis: comparative chronology. Am J Cardiol 25:141–8.
Streeter GL. 1942. Development horizons in human embryos. Description of age group XI, 13 to 20 somites and age group XII, 21 to 29 somites. Carnegie Contrib Embryol 30:211–45.

Streeter GL. 1945. Development horizons in human embryos. Description of age group XIII, embryos about 4 or 5 millimeters long and age group XIV, period of indentation of the lens vesicle. Carnegie Contrib Embryol 31:27–63.
Streeter GL. 1948. Development horizons in human embryos. Description of age group XV, XVI, XVII, and XVIII, being the third issue of the Carnegie Collection. Carnegie Contrib Embryol 32:133–203.
Szebenyi G, Savage MP, Olwin BB, Fallon JF. 1995. Changes in the expression of fibroblast growth factor receptors mark distinct stages of chondrogenesis in vitro and during chick limb skeletal patterning. Dev Dyn 204:446–56.
Van Mierop LHS, Alley RD, Kausel HW, Stranahan A. 1962. The anatomy and embryology of endocardial cushion defects. J Thorac Cardiovasc Surg 43:71–83.
Van Mierop LHS, Kutsche LM. 1985. Development of the ventricular septum of the heart. Heart Vessels 1:114–9.
Wang Y, Sassoon D. 1995. Ectoderm–mesenchyme and mesenchyme–mesenchyme interactions regulate *Msx-l* expression and cellular differentiation in the murine limb. Dev Biol 168:374–82.
Wenink ACG. 1992. Quantitative morphology of the embryonic heart: an approach to development of the atrioventricular valves. Anat Rec 234:129–35.
Wenink ACG. 1987. Embryology of the heart. In: Anderson RH, Macartney FJ, Shinebourne EA, Tynan M, editors. Pediatric cardiology. Edinburgh: Churchill Livingstone. p 83–107.
Wenink ACG, Gittenberger-de Groot AC. 1985. The role of atrioventricular endocardial cushions in the septation of the heart. Int J Cardiol 8:25–44.
Wenink ACG, Gittenberger-de Groot AC. 1986. Embryology of the mitral valve. Int J Cardiol 11:75–84.
Wessels A, Markman MWM, Vermeulen JLM, Anderson RH, Viragh St, Mooman AFM, Lamers WH. 1996. The development of the atrioventricular junction in the human heart: an immunohistochemical study. Circ Res 78:110–7.
Wunsch A, Markwald RR, Little CD. 1994. Cardiac endothelial heterogeneity defines valvular development as demonstrated by the diverse expression of JB3 antigen, a fibrillin-like protein of the endocardial cushion tissue. Dev Biol 165:585–601.
Ya J, Schilham MW, de Beer PAJ, Tesink-Taekema S, France D, Moorman AFM, Lamers WH. 1997. *Sox-4*-deficient mice provide an animal model for the development of common trunk. (submitted).

CHAPTER 7

Embryological Development of the Outlet of Each Ventricle

María V. de la Cruz

The outlet is the subarterial segment of each of the ventricles. The arterial limit of the outlet of the anatomical right ventricle is the pulmonary valve and its limit with the apical trabeculated region of the right ventricle corresponds to a tangential plane at the proximal border of the supraventricular crest. The arterial limit of the outlet of the anatomical left ventricle is the aortic valve, and its limit with the apical trabeculated region of the left ventricle corresponds to a tangential plane at the free border of the portion of the anteroseptal leaflet of the mitral valve that constitutes the mitroaortic continuity.

Owing to the fact that the anatomical constitution of the outlet of each of the ventricles is complex, it is necessary and mandatory to study it to make a correct interpretation of the results obtained by means of the in vivo labeling experiments, whose objective is to know the anatomical manifestation of the embryological structures. Consequently, information is presented concerning the anatomical characteristics of each of the ventricular outlets, which precedes the description of their embryological development.

Because of the fact that the anatomical and embryological constitution of the outlet of each of the ventricles is different (de la Cruz et al 1977, 1982), we will divide this chapter into two sections: (1) the outlet of the anatomical right ventricle and (2) the outlet of the anatomical left ventricle.

OUTLET OF THE ANATOMICAL RIGHT VENTRICLE

Anatomical Introduction

The outlet of the anatomical right ventricle exhibits three walls: (1) the supraventricular crest, (2) the left wall (so-called septal wall), and (3) its anterior wall (Fig. 1A).

The supraventricular crest is muscular and it separates the outlet of the anatomical right ventricle from the tricuspid valve (Anderson et al 1977) (Fig. 1, A, C, and D). This crest is inserted by one of its ends into the interventricular septum, between the two limbs of the septomarginal trabeculation, and by the other end into the angle formed by the annulus of the tricuspid valve and the free wall of this ventricle (Fig. 1, A and D) (chapter X, Fig. 2B). It is important to point out that removal of the end of the supraventricular crest inserted into the interventricular

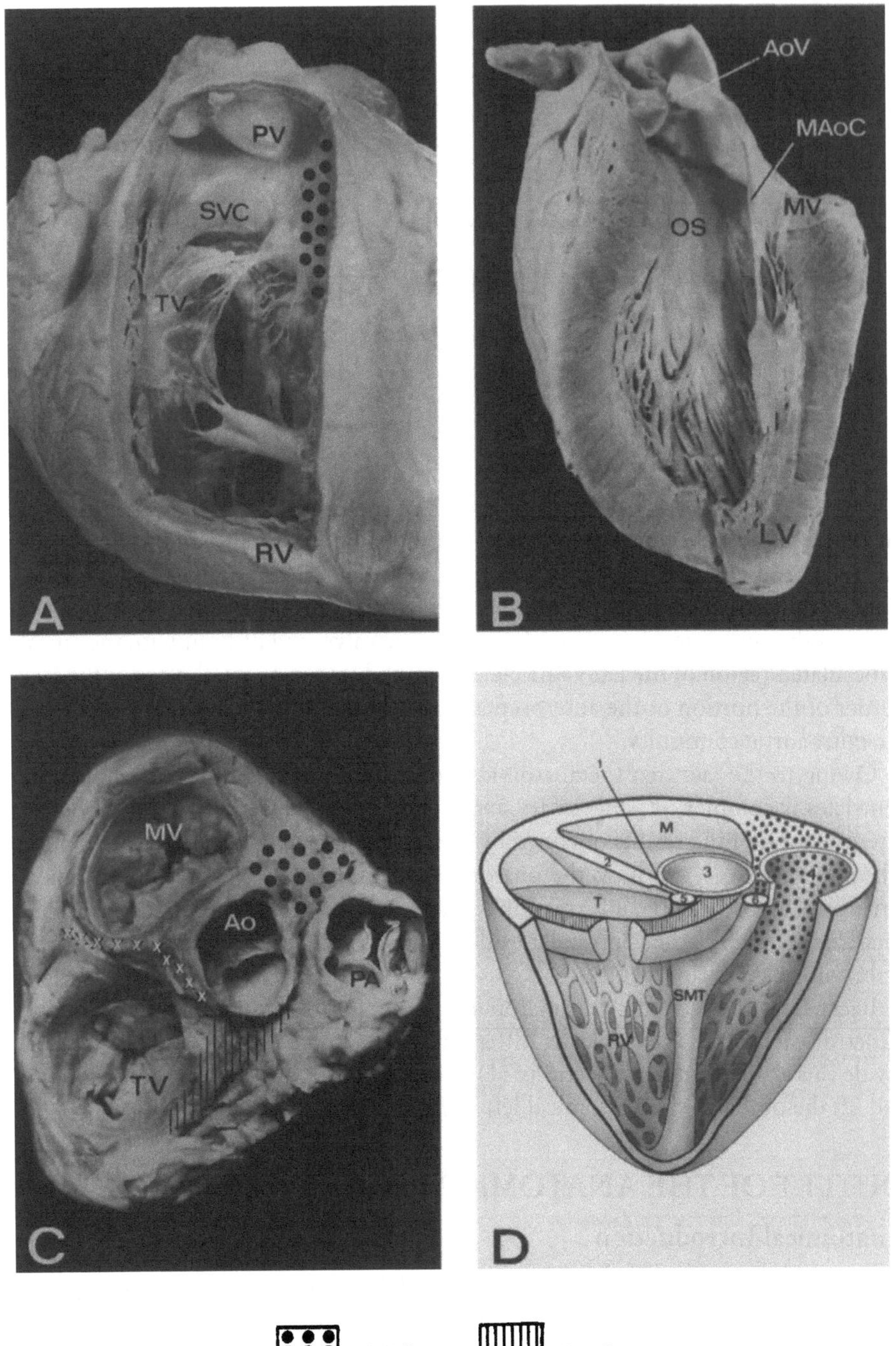

FIGURE 1. Photographs and diagram of dissections of human hearts exhibiting the anatomical features of the outlets of both ventricles and their relationship to each other and with the atrioventricular orifices. **A.** Dissection of the outlet of the anatomical right ventricle. The anterior wall has been removed showing the supraventricular crest (SVC) and the left wall of this outlet, or the so-called septal wall (dotted area). **B.** Dissections of the left ventricular cavity showing the two walls of its outlet, i.e., the septal wall or outlet septum (OS) and the free portion of the anteroseptal leaflet of

septum creates an orifice in the septal wall of the outlet of the anatomical left ventricle, beneath the anterior coronary cusps (Fig. 2, A, C, and D). The so-called septal wall is not a septum, because it does not separate two cavities from each other. This has been demonstrated by making an incision beginning under the pulmonary cusps and extending to the cardiac apex, parallel and adjacent to the septomarginal trabeculation (Fig. 2A). Separating the borders of this incision and observing from the left ventricular cavity, it was found that the so-called septal wall of the outlet of the anatomical right ventricle corresponds in the left ventricle to a muscular mass, which is part of the free ventricular wall (Fig. 2, A and B, and 1, C and D). Thus, it should not be designated as the septal wall of the outlet of the right ventricle, but rather, the left wall of the outlet of the right ventricle. The anterior wall of the outlet of the anatomical right ventricle is part of its free wall (Fig. 1, A and D).

Embryological Study de la Cruz and colleagues (1977), by means of in vivo labeling experiments, showed that the primitive outlet appears at stage 12HH, that it is the most cephalic segment of this heart and is frequently called the "conus", and that it is directly continuous with the primordium of the apical trabeculated region of the right ventricle (chapter IV, Fig. 5).

Using the in vivo labeling approches (de la Cruz et al 1977), a label was placed at the cephalic end of the primitive outlet segment or conus, at stage 12HH; at stage 22HH this label was found in the middle region of the conus (chapter IV, Fig. 6). The result of this experiment showed that (1) the original primitive outlet at stage 12HH corresponds, at stage 22HH, to the region of the primitive outlet or conus adjacent to the apical trabeculated region of the right ventricle (chapter IV, Figs. 6 and 5, C, C′, D, and D′) and (2) the arterial pole of the heart (truncus arteriosus) is not yet present at stage 12HH (chapter IV, Fig. 6).

Stage 22HH was chosen to study the prospective fate of the primitive outlet because at this stage the whole outlet is present (de la Cruz et al 1977), not as in stage 12HH (chapter IV, Figs. 6 and 5, C, C′, D, and D′); therefore it has well-defined boundaries, one cephalic, which corresponds to its union with the arterial pole of the heart (de la Cruz et al 1977) (chapter IV, Fig. 5, C and C′), and the other caudal, which corresponds to its union with the primordium of the apical trabeculated region of the right ventricle (de la Cruz et al 1977) (chapter IV, Fig. 5, C and C′). The aortic and pulmonary valves develop in the boundary between the arterial

the mitral valve or mitroaortic continuity (MAoC). **C.** Transverse section of the heart at the level of the atrioventricular grooves showing the relationship of the outlets with each other and with the atrioventricular orifices and the projection of the supraventricular crest (striped area), the interventricular septum (line of *x*'s), and the left wall of the outlet of the right ventricle (dotted area). **D.** Diagrammatic representation of the walls of the outlet of the anatomical right ventricle and of the relationship of both outlets, and also those of the inlets of both ventricles, with the outlet of the anatomical left ventricle (central fibrous body of the heart). The dotted area indicates the left wall of the outlet of the right ventricle. Striped area = supraventricular crest; Cross line = interventricular septum; PV = pulmonary valve; TV = tricuspid valve; MV = mitral valve; Ao = aorta; PA = pulmonary artery; SMT = septomarginal trabeculation; AoV = aortic valve; RV = right ventricle; LV = left ventricle; MAoC = mitroaortic continuity; 1 = membranous portion of the interventricular septum; 2 = muscular portion of the interventricular septum; 3 = outlet of the left ventricle; 4 = outlet of the right ventricle; 5 = inferior limb of the septomarginal traveculation; 6 = superior limb of the septomarginal trabeculation.

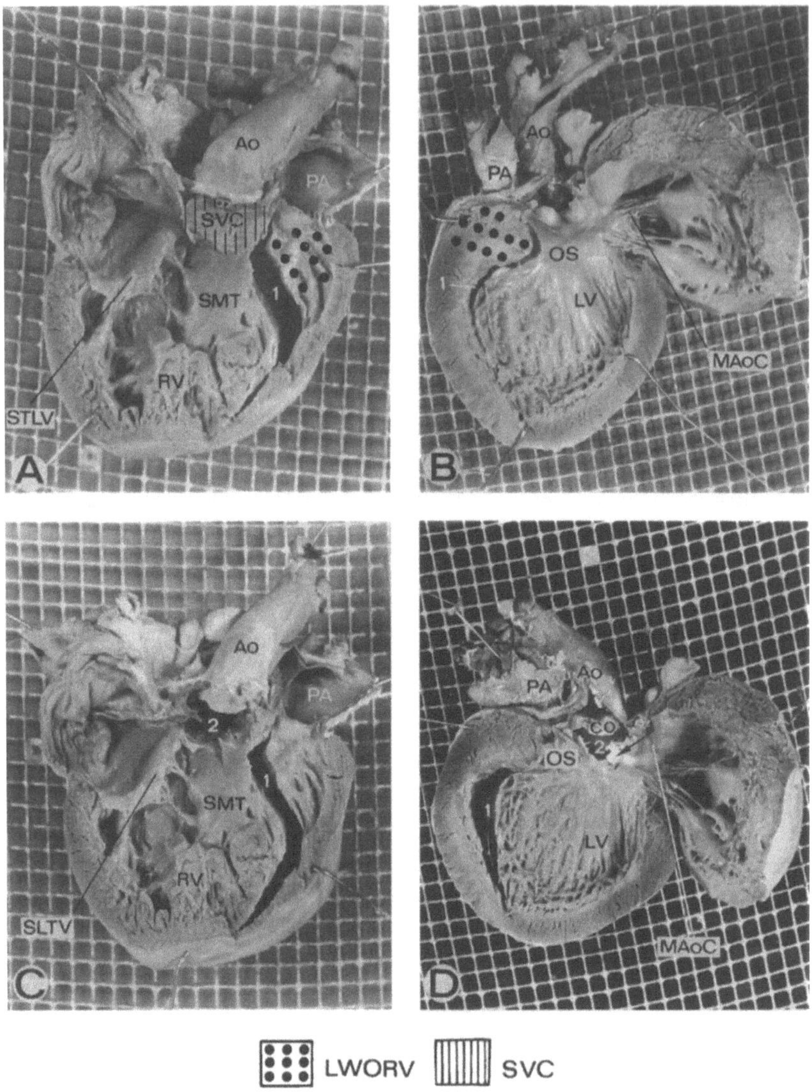

FIGURE 2. Photographs of dissections of the human heart showing the septal wall of each of the ventricles, for the purpose of demonstrating that the left wall of the outlet of the right ventricle, the so-called septal wall, is really the free ventricular wall, and also to show the projection of the insertion of the supraventricular crest (SVC) in the septal wall of the outlet of the left ventricle (OS). **A.** View of the septal wall of the right ventricle. Notice that the incision (1) separates the left wall of the outlet of the anatomical right ventricle, the so-called septal wall (dotted area), from the septal insertion of the supraventricular crest (SVC, striped area), and from the septomarginal trabeculation (SMT). **B.** View of the septal wall of the left ventricle. Notice that this same incision (1) is located immediately adjacent to the endocardium of the free wall of the anatomical left ventricle (dotted area), which corresponds in the right ventricle to the left wall of its outlet, the so-called septal wall of this outlet (dotted area). Furthermore the pulmonary artery (PA) is related to this zone. **C.** Right view (same as A) of the interventricular septum showing the orifice (2) that was produced by removing the supraventricular crest (SVC). **D.** View of the outlet septum of the left ventricle (OS) showing the orifice (2) in its muscular portion, beneath the anterior coronary cusps (CO); notice also its membranous portion (arrow). Ao = aorta; RV = right ventricle; LV = left ventricle; MAoC = mitroaortic continuity; SLTV = septal leaflet of the tricuspid valve; OS = outlet septum of the left ventricle; PA = pulmonary artery; CO = = coronary cusps; SMT = septomarginal trabeculation.

pole of the heart and the conus (the primitive outlet). By means of the in vivo labeling experiments in the chick embryo heart at stage 22HH, de la Cruz and associates (1977) showed that the cephalic boundary of the conus at this stage corresponds in the mature heart to the arterial boundary of the outlet of the anatomical right ventricle, which is the pulmonary valve (chapter IV, Fig. 5, C, C′, D, and D′), and its caudal boundary corresponds to the proximal border of the supraventricular crest, which is in the mature heart the limit between the outlet of the anatomical right ventricle and its apical trabeculated region (chapter IV, Fig. 5, C, C′, D, and D′). The results of these in vivo labeling experiments indicate that at stage 22HH, the limits of the primitive outlet or conus correspond to those of the outlet of the anatomical right ventricle in the mature heart (chapter IV, Fig. 5, C, C′, D, and D′).

At stage 22HH the septation of the primitive outlet (conus) begins with the formation of the dextrodorsal conus ridge (dextrodorsal ridge of the primitive outlet) and the sinistroventral conus ridge (sinistroventral ridge of the primitive outlet) (Fig. 3, A, and B). These ridges are straight (de la Cruz et al 1977; Thompson et al 1985) and their limits are those of the primitive outlet. Therefore, in the mature heart they will correspond to the boundary of the outlet of the anatomical right ventricle (chapter IV, Fig. 5, C, C′, D, and D′). Fusion of the ridges divides the primitive outlet (conus) into two distinct outlets, one anterior and to the right (anterior conus) and another one posterior and to the left (posterior conus) (Kramer 1942; DeVries and Saunders 1962; Van Mierop et al 1963; Asami 1969; Netter and Van Mierop 1969; de la Cruz et al 1972, 1977; Goor et al 1972; Pexieder 1978; Thompson et al 1985, 1987; Thompson and Fitzharris 1979) (Fig. 3B). The sinistroventral conus ridge in the chick is small; the same has been pointed out by DeVries and Saunders (1962) in man (Fig. 3A).

The in vivo labeling of each of these ridges has clarified the prospective fate of each ridge and consequently their contribution to the development of the outlet of each definitive ventricle. Three labels were placed in each conal ridge; one at the caudal end or limit with the apical trabeculated region of the right ventricle (de la Cruz et al 1982), another in the middle zone, and the third label at the cephalic end or limit with the arterial pole of the heart. All three labels of the dextrodorsal conus ridge were found in the mature heart in the supraventricular crest, which forms the right wall of the outlet of the right ventricle and separates it from the tricuspid orifice (Fig. 4, A and B). All three labels that were placed in the sinistroventral conus ridge (de la Cruz et al 1982) were found in the mature heart, in the left wall of the outlet of the right ventricle (Fig. 4, C and D) and some of them, in the adjacent zone of the anterior wall of this outlet. In addition, a label was also placed at stage 22HH in the middle zone of the anterior wall of the anterior conus, equally distant from the dextrodorsal and sinistroventral conus ridges. In the mature heart this label was found in the anterior wall of the outlet of the anatomical right ventricle (Fig. 5, A and B). Collectively, these results show that (1) the dextrodorsal conus ridge contributes to the development of the supraventricular crest (Fig. 4, A and B), (2) the sinistroventral conus ridge contributes to the development of the left wall of the outlet of the right ventricle (de la Cruz et al 1982), the so-called septal wall (Fig. 4, C and D), and (3) the zone of the anterior wall of the conus, equidistant from both conal ridges, contributes to the development of the anterior wall of the outlet of the anatomical right ventricle (Fig. 5, A and B).

The results of the in vivo labeling of the free wall of the anterior conus and of

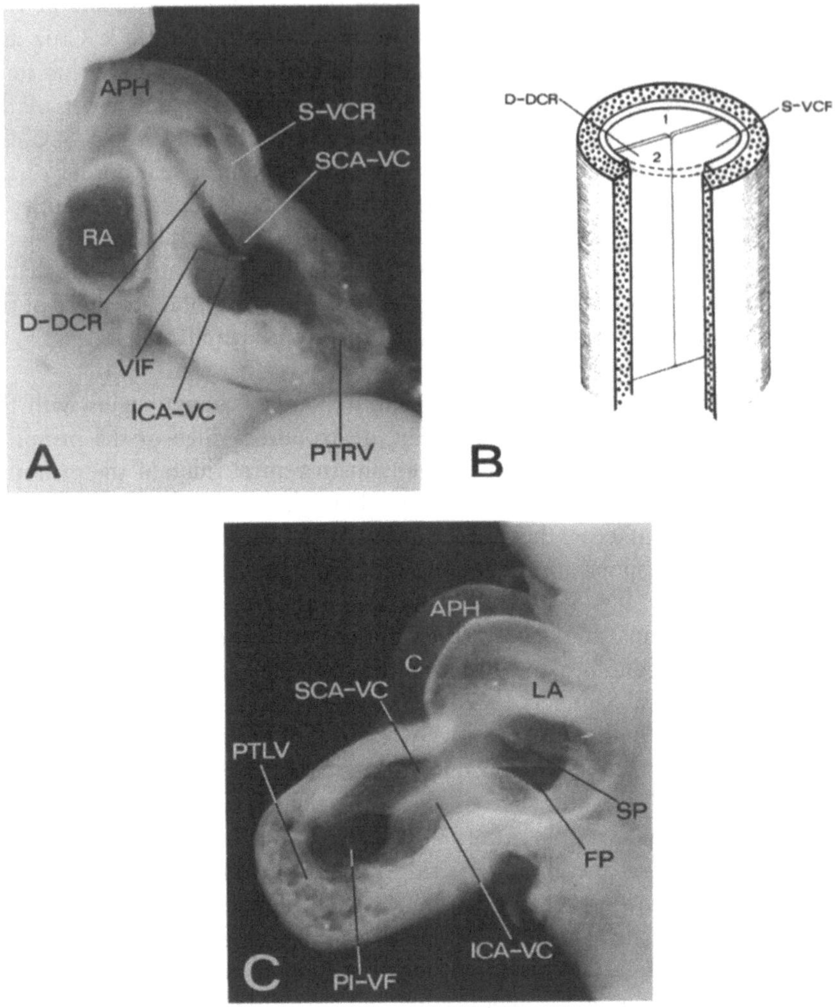

FIGURE 3. Photographs and diagram of the conal septation in the chick embryo at stage 22HH and its relationship with the superior cushion of the atrioventricular canal, which is part of the primitive cardiac septum. **A.** Dissection of the right anterior conus and apical trabeculated region of the right ventricle, showing the dextrodorsal (D-DCR) and sinistroventral conus ridges (S-VCR) that separate both conuses. Note that a hair has been introduced between the superior cushion of the atrioventricular canal (below) and the dextrodorsal conus ridge (D-DCR) together with the ventricular infundibular fold (VIF) (above); therefore, this hair is located in the posterior conus. **B.** Diagrammatic representation of both conal ridges, which divide the conus or primitive outlet into a right anterior conus (2) and a left posterior conus (1). **C.** Dissection of the left cardiac cavities of the same embryo showing the relationship of the superior cushion (SCA-VC) with the left posterior conus (C) and with the inferior cushion of the atrioventricular canal (ICA-VC). APH = arterial pole of the heart; RA = right atrium; LA = left atrium; PTRV = primordium of the apical trabeculated region of the right ventricle; PTLV = primordium of the apical trabeculated region of the left ventricle; C = conus; FP = foramen primum; SP = septum primum; PI-VF = primitive interventricular foramen.

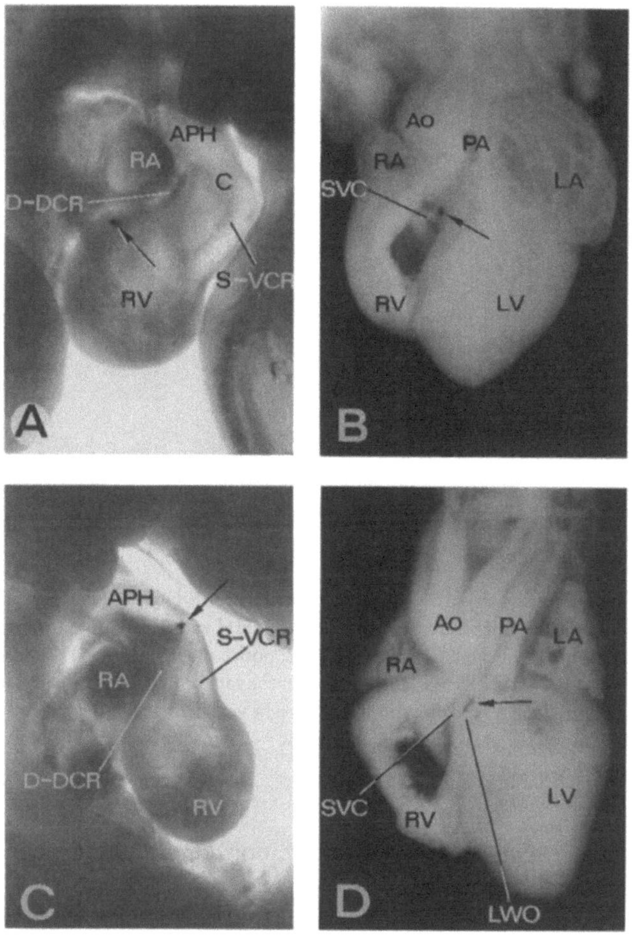

FIGURE 4. Photographs of in vivo labeling experiment in which labels were placed in the dextrodorsal conus ridge and the sinistroventral conus ridge at stage 22HH and were traced up to the mature heart. **A.** Right lateral view of the chick embryo heart at stage 22HH showing a label (arrow) placed in the caudal region of the dextrodorsal conus ridge. **B.** Dissection of the outlet of the right ventricle and the pulmonary artery in the mature heart, in the same embryo at stage 35HH, which shows the same label (arrow) in the proximal border of the supraventricular crest. **C.** Right lateral view of the chick embryo heart at stage 22HH. Notice the label (arrow) placed at the cephalic end of the sinistroventral conus ridge. **D.** Dissection of the outlet of the right ventricle in the mature heart of the same embryo, showing the same label (arrow) in its left wall (LWO). RA = right atrium; D-DCR = dextrodorsal conus ridge; S-VCR = sinistroventral conus ridge; C = conus; Ao = aorta; LA = left atrium; LV = left ventricle; APH = arterial pole of the heart or truncus; PA = pulmonary artery; LWO = left wall of the outlet of the right ventricle; RV = right ventricle; SVC = supraventricular crest.

the conal ridges permit us to conclude that the anterior conus contributes to the outlet of the anatomical right ventricle in the mature heart. Despite this valuable information concerning the prospective fate of the anterior conus, we do not know how it incorporates into the anatomical right ventricle.

It is important to point out that the dextrodorsal and the sinistroventral conus ridges, constituted by mesenchymal tissue, give origin to anatomical muscular structures in the mature heart. This fact may be caused by the invasion of the

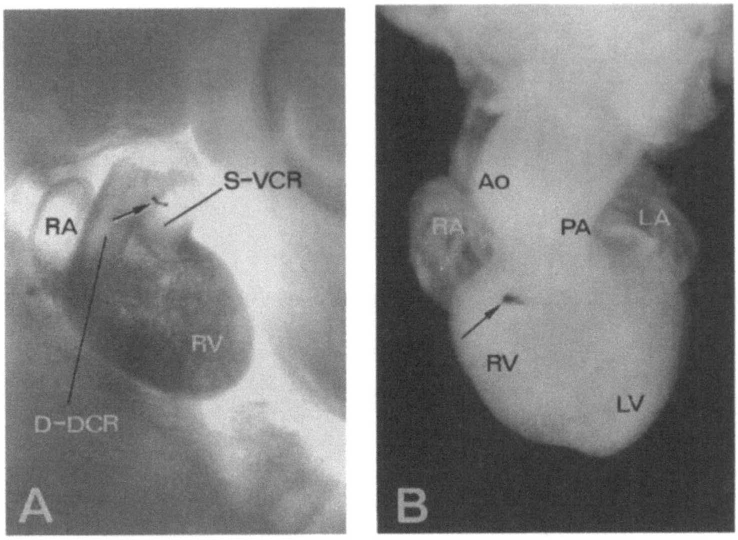

FIGURE 5. Photographs of the in vivo labeling experiment in which the label was placed in the anterior wall of the conus in chick embryo heart at stage 22HH and traced up to the mature heart. **A.** Right view of the chick embryo heart at stage 22HH; notice the label (arrow) placed in the anterior wall of the conus. **B.** Note the same label (arrow) in the same embryo in the anterior wall of the outlet of the right ventricle. RA = right atrium; RV = right ventricle; LA = left atrium; LV = left ventricle; S-VCR = sinistroventral conus ridge; D-DCR = dextrodorsal conus ridge; Ao = aorta; PA = pulmonary artery.

cardiac muscle as occurs in the muscularization of the inferior cushion of the atrioventricular canal (chapter VI).

We know that the ventricular infundibular fold is present at stage 17HH, when the first cardiac septum (primitive cardiac septum) appears and the right ventricle acquires its inflow tract (de la Cruz et al 1983). This embryological structure, the ventricular infundibular fold, separates the primitive outlet (conus) from the future tricuspid region of the primitive inlet (chapter VI, Fig. 9). When the septation of the primitive outlet begins at stage 22HH (de la Cruz et al 1977), the dextrodorsal conus ridge, which contributes to the development of the supraventricular crest, is in close proximity with the ventricular infundibular fold (Fig. 3A). This fact prompts the following question: Does the ventricular infundibular fold participate in the development of the supraventricular crest? To answer this question it is necessary to label in vivo the ventricular infundibular fold.

Because of the similarity in the embryological development of the conus in man and in the chick and the anatomical characteristics of the outlet in both species, the information obtained by means of the in vivo labeling in the chick is applicable to the study of the human heart.

OUTLET OF THE ANATOMICAL LEFT VENTRICLE

Anatomical Introduction

The anatomical studies of the walls of the outlet of the anatomical left ventricle of the mature heart show that it is constituted by two walls. One is the free portion of the anteroseptal leaflet of the mitral valve that constitutes the mitroaortic continuity; therefore, it separates the outlet of this ventricle from its inlet. The other wall is the interventricular septum or septal wall of this outlet (Fig. 1B). The septal wall has two portions, one located beneath the noncoronary cusp or posterior cusp and the right anterior coronary cusp, which separates this outlet from the inlet of the anatomical right ventricle (Figs. 1D and 2D); the other portion is located beneath the right and left anterior coronary cusp. It is important to point out that when one removes the end of the supraventricular crest that is inserted into the interventricular septum, an orifice is created in the septal wall of the outlet of the left ventricle, beneath the right and left anterior coronary cusps (Fig. 2, A, C, and D). The portion of the septal wall of the outlet of the left ventricle that separates it from the inlet of the right ventricle is muscular in the chick and membranous in humans.

Embryological Study

By means of in vivo labeling experiments of the superior cushion of the atrioventricular canal, de la Cruz and coworkers (1982) and García-Peláez and colleagues (1984) found that all the labels placed in this cushion were found in the mature heart in the free portion of the anteroseptal leaflet of the mitral valve (mitroaortic continuity), the wall that separates the outlet of the anatomical left ventricle from its inlet; in addition, the septal wall of this outlet appeared labeled (Fig. 6). The portion of the septal wall of this outlet located beneath the right anterior coronary cusps and noncoronary cusp (posterior cup) is called the membranous portion (Fig. 2D) (chapter V, Fig. 3.) and corresponds to the fusion area of the superior and inferior cushions of the atrioventricular canal and of the primitive interventricular septum (Wenink and Gittenberger-de Groot 1985) (Chapter V, Fig. 3). The portion of the septal wall of this outlet located beneath the right and left anterior coronary cusps is called the muscular portion, and when it is made transparent using methyl salicylate, it is possible to observe the labels that were found in the septal insertion of the supraventricular crest when the cephalic end of the dextrodorsal conus ridge is labeled. Consequently, this muscular portion of the outlet septum has a double origin, by the superior cushion of the atrioventricular canal on its left side (de la Cruz et al 1982; García-Peláez et al 1984) and by the dextrodorsal conus ridge on the right side (Fig. 6B). These in vivo labeling experiments show the important contribution of the superior cushion of the atrioventricular canal in the development of the outlet of the anatomical left ventricle.

It is important to review the relevant roles of the inferior (de la Cruz et al 1983) and superior cushions (de la Cruz et al 1982) of the atrioventricular canal in cardiac septation; they form jointly with the septum primum at the atrial level and the primitive interventricular septum at the apical trabeculated region of both ventricles, the first cardiac septum or primitive cardiac septum, which divides the cardiac tube into four cavities (de la Cruz et al 1983) (chapter VI, Fig. 2). Furthermore both atrioventricular cushions, the superior and inferior, have a similar prospective fate. The inferior cushion gives origin to the atrioventricular septum and to the adjacent region of the interatrial and interventricular septum, and it contributes to the development of the septal leaflet of the tricuspid valve and the portion of the anteroseptal leaflet of the mitral valve that inserts into the septum (de la Cruz et al 1983) (chapter VI, Fig. 4). The superior cushion forms the septal wall of the outlet of the left ventricle, and it gives origin to the free portion of the anteroseptal leaflet

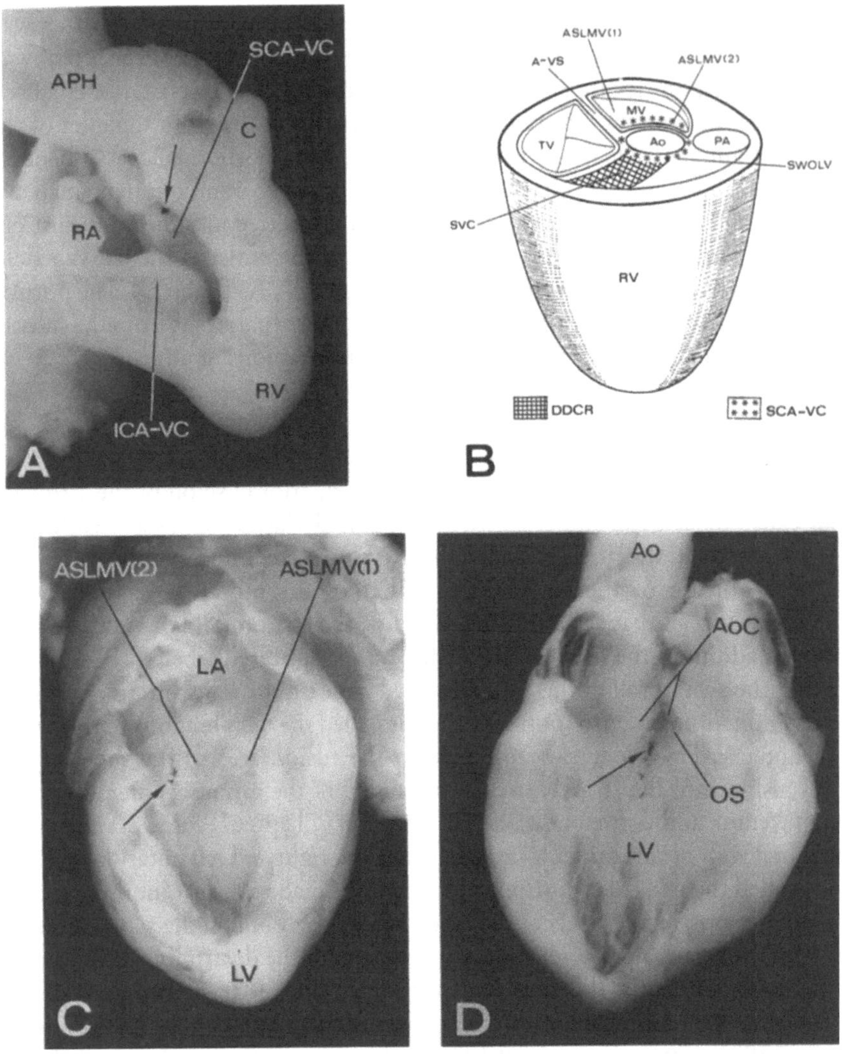

FIGURE 6. Photomicrographs and diagrammatic representation of the in vivo labeling experiment of the superior cushion of the atrioventricular canal in the chick embryo heart at stage 18HH, showing the contribution of this cushion to the development of the outlet of the left ventricle. **A.** Microdissection of the right cardiac cavities of the chick embryo at stage 23HH, 24 hours after the superior cushion was labeled. Notice the label (arrow) in the superior cushion of the AV canal. **B.** Schematic representation of a transverse section at the level of the atrioventricular orifices and the outlet of both ventricles. The asterisked area corresponds to the anatomical structures originating from the superior cushion of the AV canal at this level. **C.** Microdissection of the left ventricular cavity of the same embryo showing the label in the portion of the anteroseptal leaflet of the mitral valve or mitroaortic continuity before it was removed. **D.** Microdissection of the left ventricular cavity of the mature heart (stage 35HH). The anteroseptal leaflet of the mitral valve (mitroaortic continuity) was removed. Notice the label (arrow) in the septal wall of the outlet of the left ventricle. C = conus; APH = arterial pole of the heart; RV = right ventricle; RA = right atrium; SCA-VC = superior cushion of the atrioventricular canal; ICA-VC = inferior cushion of the atrioventricular canal; DDCR = dextrodorsal conus ridge; TV = tricuspid valve; MV = mitral valve; ASLMV (1) = portion of the anteroseptal leaflet of the mital valve that inserts into the septum; ASLMV (2) = free portion of the anteroseptal leaflet of the mitral valve or mitroaortic continuity; SWOLV = septal wall of the outlet of the left ventricle; SVC = supraventricular crest; A-VS = atrioventricular septum; Ao = aorta; PA = pulmonary artery; LV = left ventricle; AoC = aortic cusps; LA = left atrium; OS = outlet septum.

of the mitral valve (mitroaortic continuity), which is the other wall of the outlet of the anatomical left ventricle (de la Cruz et al 1982; García-Peláez et al 1984) (Fig. 6). Therefore this intimate embryological relationship between the inlet of both ventricles and the outlet of the left ventricle is expressed anatomically by the central fibrous body of the heart. On the other hand, owing to the embryologic origin of the walls of the outlet of the right ventricle, this anatomical structure does not constitute a part of the central fibrous body of the heart (Fig. 1, C and D).

Although the information obtained by in vivo labeling experiments for the superior cushion of the atrioventricular canal, the conal ridges, the anterior wall of the conus, and the primitive interventricular septum is coherent with the knowledge we possess on the normal anatomy of the outlet of each of the ventricles, there remains an important, key question: What is the prospective fate of the posterior wall of the posterior conus? I believe the pathway leading to the right answer will require in vivo labeling of this wall. The information thus obtained will also help us to know the process of incorporation of the conus.

CONCLUSIONS

The valuable information obtained, by means of in vivo labeling experiments in the chick, concerning the embryological development of the outlets of both ventricles, is indispensable for the evaluation of postmorten studies of this cardiac region, both in the chick and in man.

1. The conus, or primitive outlet, appears in the chick embryo at stage 12HH. It is the most cephalic segment of the heart and is connected with the primordium of the apical trabeculated region of the anatomical right ventricle. The septation of the conus or primitive outlet begins at stage 22HH by the formation of the dextrodorsal and the sinistroventral conus ridges, which fuse to form the conal septum. In this manner the conus or primitive outlet gives origin to the anterior conus and posterior conus, both of which are connected with the apical trabeculated region of the anatomical right ventricle caudally and with the arterial pole of the heart (truncus) cephalically.
2. The outlet of the anatomical right ventricle has three anatomical walls: the supraventricular crest, the left so-called septal wall, and the anterior wall. Each of these has its own primordium: the dextrodorsal conus ridge, the sinistroventral conus ridge, and the original anterior wall of the embryonic conus, respectively. Therefore, after septation by fused conus ridges, the anterior conus gives origin to the outlet of the anatomical right ventricle.
3. The wall of the outlet of the right ventricle, erroneously designated as septal wall, is the free ventricular wall, as has been shown by dissections of the outlet of the anatomical right ventricle in the mature heart of the chick and in man. This wall originates from the sinistroventral conus ridge and we designate it as the left wall of the outlet of the right ventricle.
4. The outlet of the anatomical left ventricle has two anatomical walls: the free portion of the anteroseptal leaflet of the mitral valve, or mitroaortic continuity, and its septal wall or outlet septum. The superior cushion of the atrioventricular canal contributes to the development of both walls. It is important to point out that the primitive interventricular septum and the inferior cushion of the atrioventricular canal also participate in formation of the membranous portion

of the outlet septum, and the dextrodorsal conus ridge by its right side participates in the muscular portion of the outlet septum.

5. We still do not know whether the ventricular infundibular fold participates in the development of the supraventricular crest nor do we know the prospective fate of the posterior wall of the left posterior conus. This information would clarify the question of the incorporation of the conus to the ventricles.

REFERENCES

Anderson RH, Becker AE, VanMierop LHS. 1977. What should we call the "crista"? Br Heart J 39:856–9.

Asami I. 1969. Beitrage zur Entwicklung des Kammerseptums in menschlichen Herzen mit besonderer Berucksichtigung der sogenannten Bulbusdrehung. Z Anat Entwicklungsgesch 128:1–17.

de la Cruz MV, Giménez-Ribotta M, Saravalli O, Cayr;e R. 1983. The contribution of the inferior endocardial cushion of the atrioventricular canal to cardiac septation and to the development of the atrioventricular valves: study in the chick embryo. Am J Anat 166:63–72.

de la Cruz MV, Munoz-Armas S, Munoz Castellanos L. 1972. Development of the chick heart. Baltimore, MD: Johns Hopkins University Press.

de la Cruz MV, Quero-Jiménez M, Arteaga M, Cayré R. 1982. Morphogénèse du septum interventriculaire. Coeur 13:443–8.

de la Cruz MV, Sánchez-Gómez C, Arteaga M, Argüello C. 1977. Experimental study of the development of the truncus and the conus in the chick embryo. J Anat 123:651–86.

DeVries PA, Saunders JB. 1962. Development of the ventricles and spiral outflow tract in the human heart. A contribution of the development of the human heart from age group IX to age group XV. Carnegie Contrib Embryol 256:89–114.

García-Peláez I, Díaz-Góngora G, Arteaga-Martínez M. 1984. Contribution of the superior atrioventricular cushion to the left ventricular infundibulum. Experimental study on the chick embryo. Acta Anat 118:224–30.

Goor DA, Dische R, Lillehei CW. 1972. The cono truncus. I. Its normal inversion and conus absorption. Circulation 46:375–84.

Kramer TC. 1942. The partitioning of the truncus and conus and the formation of the menbraneous portion of the interventricular septum in the human heart. Am J Anat 71:343–70.

Netter FH, Van Mierop LHS. 1969. Embryology. In: Netter FH, editor. CIBA Collection of Medical Illustrations, Ardsley, New Jersey: CIBA Pharmaceutical Co. Vol. 5, p 119–25.

Pexieder T. 1978. Development of the outflow tract of the embryonic heart. In: Resenquist GC, Bergsma D, editors. Morphogenesis and malformation of the cardiovascular system. birth defects: original article series. Vol. XIV, Number 7. New York: AR Liss.: p 29–68.

Thompson RP, Fitzharris TP. 1979. Morphogenesis of the truncus arteriosus of the chick embryo heart. II. Tissue reorganization during septation. Am J Anat 156:251–64.

Thompson RP, Sumida H, Abercrombie V, Satow Y, Fitzharris TP, Okamoto N. 1985. Morphogenesis of human cardiac outflow. Anat Rec 213:578–86.

Thompson RP, Abercrombie V, Wong M. 1987. Morphogenesis of the truncus arteriosus of the chick embryo heart: movements of autoradiographic tattoos during septation. Anat Rec 218:434–40.

Van Mierop LHS, Alley RD, Kausel HW, Stranahan A. 1963. Pathogenesis of transposition complexes. I. Embryology of the ventricles and great arteries. Am J Cardiol 12:216–25.

Wenink ACG, Gittenberger-de Groot AC. 1985. The role of atrioventricular endocardial cushions in the septation of the heart. Int J Cardiol 8:25–44.

CHAPTER 8

Embryological Development of the Atria. Septation and Visceroatrial Situs

Guillermo Anselmi and María V. de la Cruz

The anatomical right atrium in the chick is formed only by the primitive right atrium because of the fact that the sinus venosus is connected to this atrium but it is not incorporated into it. The anatomical right atrium in man is constituted embryologically by the primitive right atrium and by the sinus venosus. The anatomical left atrium in the chick is constituted only by the primitive left atrium and, in man, is formed by the primitive left atrium and the sinus of the pulmonary veins. By means of the septation process the atria acquire their septal wall. The primitive atria in both species are the only primitive cardiac segments that from their initial appearance are situated one to the right and the other to the left, according to the bilateral right and left symmetry of the organism; all other primitive cardiac segments are formed in series. As a result of this fact, the atria are the only cardiac cavities that can be used for the diagnosis of type of situs.

Because of the embryological constitution of each atrium, the peculiar features of their septation, and the fundamental role of the atria in the identification of the situs, we will divide this chapter into three sections: (1) embryological constitution of the atria, (2) septation, and (3) the atria in the context of the situs.

EMBRYOLOGICAL CONSTITUTION OF THE ATRIA

The in vivo labeling studies in the chick embryo heart by Stalsberg and De Haan (1969), Castro-Quezada and associates (1972), and de la Cruz and coworkers (1987, 1991) have shown that the primitive right and left atria do not appear at stage 9^{+}HH, that is, in the straight tube heart (chapter III, Fig. 5); they appear at stage 12HH (C-shaped loop), forming the caudal region of this heart, and both are connected with the primordium of the apical trabeculated region of the left ventricle by way of the primitive inlet (de la Cruz et al 1991) (chapters IV and VI) (chapter IV, Fig. 7) (Fig. 1). This heart corresponds morphologically to that of the human embryo 3707, 12 somites, horizon X (DeVries and Saunders 1962).

During the torsion process, at stage 14HH (S-shaped loop), both primitive atria acquire a dorsal and cephalic position because they have become displaced within the retrocardiac space; this space appears owing to the fact that the loop at this stage

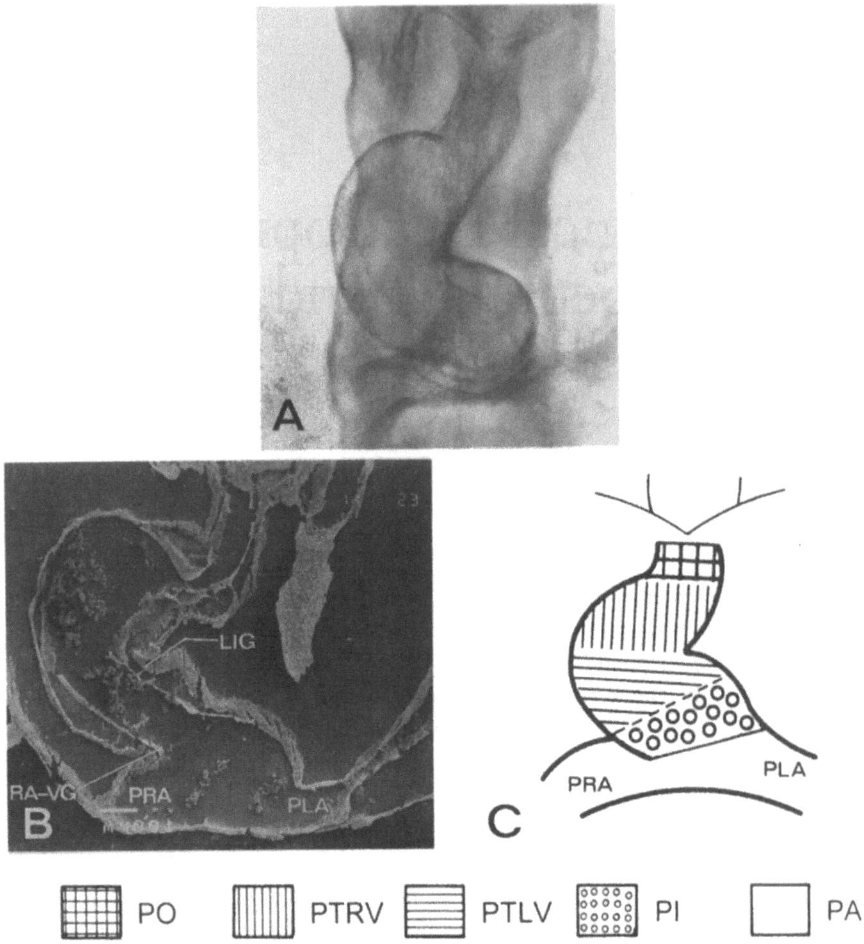

FIGURE 1. Photographs and diagram of the chick embryo heart at stage 12HH (C-shaped loop), showing the primitive atria, one situated on the right and the other on the left, caudal and connected by means of the primitive inlet with the primordium of the apical trabeculated region of the left ventricle. **A.** Ventral aspect of the heart. **B.** Frontal section of the heart. **C.** Diagram depicting the five primitive cardiac segments that constitute the heart at this stage of development. PO = primitive outlet; PTRV = primordium of the apical trabeculated region of the right ventricle; PTLV = primordium of the apical trabeculated region of the left ventricle; PI = primitive inlet; PRA = primitive right atrium; PLA = primitive left atrium; LIG = left interventricular groove; RA-VG = right atrioventricular groove.

of development is convex ventrally and concave dorsally (chapter IV, Fig. 2B). The chick embryo heart at stage 14HH is similar to that of the human embryo 6344, 14 somites, horizon XI (DeVries and Saunders 1962).

In the terminal stage of torsion, which corresponds to the chick embryo heart at stage 16HH and to the human embryo 2053, 20 somites, horizon XI (DeVries and Saunders 1962), a proximity relationship is established between the primordium of the apical trabeculated region of the right ventricle, the inlet of the left ventricle (primitive inlet), and the primitive right atrium (chapter IV, Fig. 3, B and F), an indispensable relationship for the normal septation of the heart at the next stage.

In the chick embryo at stage 17HH, heart septation begins with the appearance of the 8-shaped septum (de la Cruz et al 1983, 1997) (chapter VI), which separates simultaneously both primitive atria, the apical trabeculated region of each ventricle, and the primitive inlet into a right ventricular inlet and a left ventricular inlet (chapter VI). In this way, the primitive right atrium becomes connected through its own inlet with the apical trabeculated region of the right ventricle (de la Cruz et al 1983, 1997) (chapter VI, Fig. 2, B–D). The same is seen in human embryo 6502 of horizon XIV (Streeter 1945), of a similar cardiac morphology (chapter VI).

The sinus venosus in the chick appears between stages 14HH and 16HH (chapter IV, Fig. 2, D and E). Davis (1927) and Streeter (1942) describe the sinus venosus in the human embryo at horizon XI (embryo 2053) with the morphology similar to that of the chick embryo heart at stage 16HH. Therefore, in both species, the primitive atria, right and left, appear before the sinus venosus. However, the chick

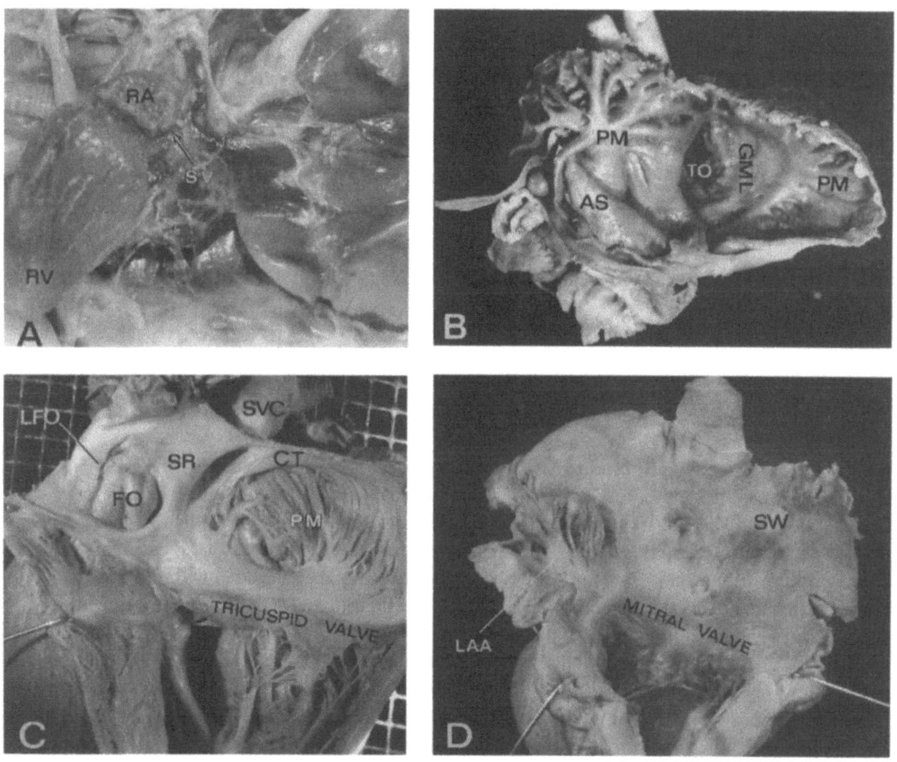

FIGURE 2. Photographs of the sinus venosus and the right atrium in the chick, and the right and left atria in man. **A.** External aspect of the sinus venosus (SV) of the chick. Notice that the sinus venosus (SV) is situated dorsally and is connected (arrow) with the anatomical right atrium (RA) situated on the right. **B.** Internal aspect of the anatomical right atrium of the chick. Notice that the atrial septal wall (AS) lacks a fossa ovalis and that the free walls only exhibit pectinate muscles (PM). **C.** Internal aspect of the anatomical right atrium in man showing in its septal wall the fossa ovalis (FO) and in its free walls: the sinus region (SR), the crista terminalis (CT), and the pectinate muscles (PM). **D.** Internal aspect of the anatomical left atrium of the man showing its septal wall (SW) and the internal aspect of the left atrial appendage (LAA). TO = tricuspid orifice; GML = great mural leaflet of the tricuspid valve; SVC = superior vena caval; LFO = limbus fossa ovalis.

embryo heart is not a good biological model to study the fate of the sinus venosus because, in the chick embryo, the sinus venosus is connected to the right atrium and it never becomes incorporated into either of the two atria (Fig. 2).

The description of the sinus venosus in the human embryo and its atrial incorporation has been the subject of numerous publications (Waterson 1921; Odgers 1935; Streeter 1942; Steding et al 1990). When the sinus venosus appears in the human embryo at horizon XI (embryo 2053), it is a vascular sac in a dorsocaudal position with respect to the dorsal wall of both atria; it is flat in the ventrodorsal axis and it is symmetrical (Streeter 1942). It is formed by a central region (transverse portion) and a pair of lateral horns: the right and left horn of the sinus venosus. The horns receive the right and left vitelline veins (omphalomesenteric veins) in its medial and caudal region, the right and left umbilical veins (allantoid veins) laterally and caudally (Fig. 3A). At horizon XII, the right and left common cardinal veins appear cephalically (Fig. 3B). The right common cardinal vein receives the anterior and posterior right cardinal veins; the left common cardinal vein receives the anterior and posterior left cardinal veins (Fig. 3B). The right and left sinoatrial sulc: form the borders of the sinoatrial office.

Likewise, at horizon XII, two processes begin that play a most important role in the incorporation of the sinus venosus in to the primitive right atrium: (1) The left sinoatrial sulcus begins to deepen, and for this reason, the left margin of the sinoatrial orifice becomes displaced toward the right atrium (Fig. 3, A and B). (2) The right horn of the sinus venosus at later horizons initiates a change in position from a more horizontal plane to a vertical one, thus placing itself into the dorsal wall of the right atrium (Fig. 3, A–C). In this horizon, the sinoatrial orifice has no valves, but it has muscular wall and cardiac jelly, which seem to have the purpose of preventing the retrograde blood flow during atrial contraction (Streeter 1942).

⟶

FIGURE 3. Diagrammatic representation of the embryological development of the sinus venosus in man, from its initial appearance at horizon XI up to its anatomical manifestation in the mature heart. **A, B, C** and **D,** ventral or anterior view. **E.** dorsal or posterior view of the mature heart. **A.** Notice that the right (2) and left (3) horns of the sinus venosus are symmetrical, that they have a dorsocaudal position with respect to the primitive atria, and that they are connected with the systemic venous system, which is also symmetrical. **B.** Notice that the left atriovenous groove begins to deepen (arrow) and that the right horn (2) of the sinus venosus becomes situated in a vertical position in the dorsal wall of the primitive right atrium. **C.** The dorsal wall of the sinus venosus, comprised between its two valves, forms the posterior wall of the anatomical right atrium, thus becoming incorporated. **D.** The zone marked with *x*'s indicates the region of the right atrium that originated from the sinus venosus, and the zone marked with small squares is the region originating from the primitive right atrium. **E.** Posterior or dorsal wall of the heart showing the contribution of the right horn of the sinus venosus (2) to the definitive right atrium and that of the left horn (3) into the coronary sinus (CS). SV = sinus venosus; PRA = primitive right atrium; PLA = primitive left atrium; PVS = pulmonary vein sinus; A-VO = atrioventricular orifice; 1 = transverse portion of the sinus venosus; VV = vitelline veins; RUV = right umbilical vein; LUV = left umbilical vein; S-AO = sinoatrial orifice; RACV = right anterior cardinal vein; LACV = left anterior cardinal vein; RCCV = right common cardinal vein; LCCV = left common cardinal vein; RPCV = right posterior cardinal vein; LPCV = left posterior cardinal vein; RVV = right vitelline vein; LVV = left vitelline vein; RSV = right sinus valve; LSV = left sinus valve; CPV = common pulmonary vein; SP = septum primum; FS = foramen secundum; SS = septum secundum; SVC = superior vena caval; IVC = inferior vena caval; RPV = right pulmonary vein; LPV = left pulmonary vein; MV = Marshall vein; RA = right atrium; LA = left atrium; RV = right ventricle; LV = left ventricle; PVs = pulmonary veins.

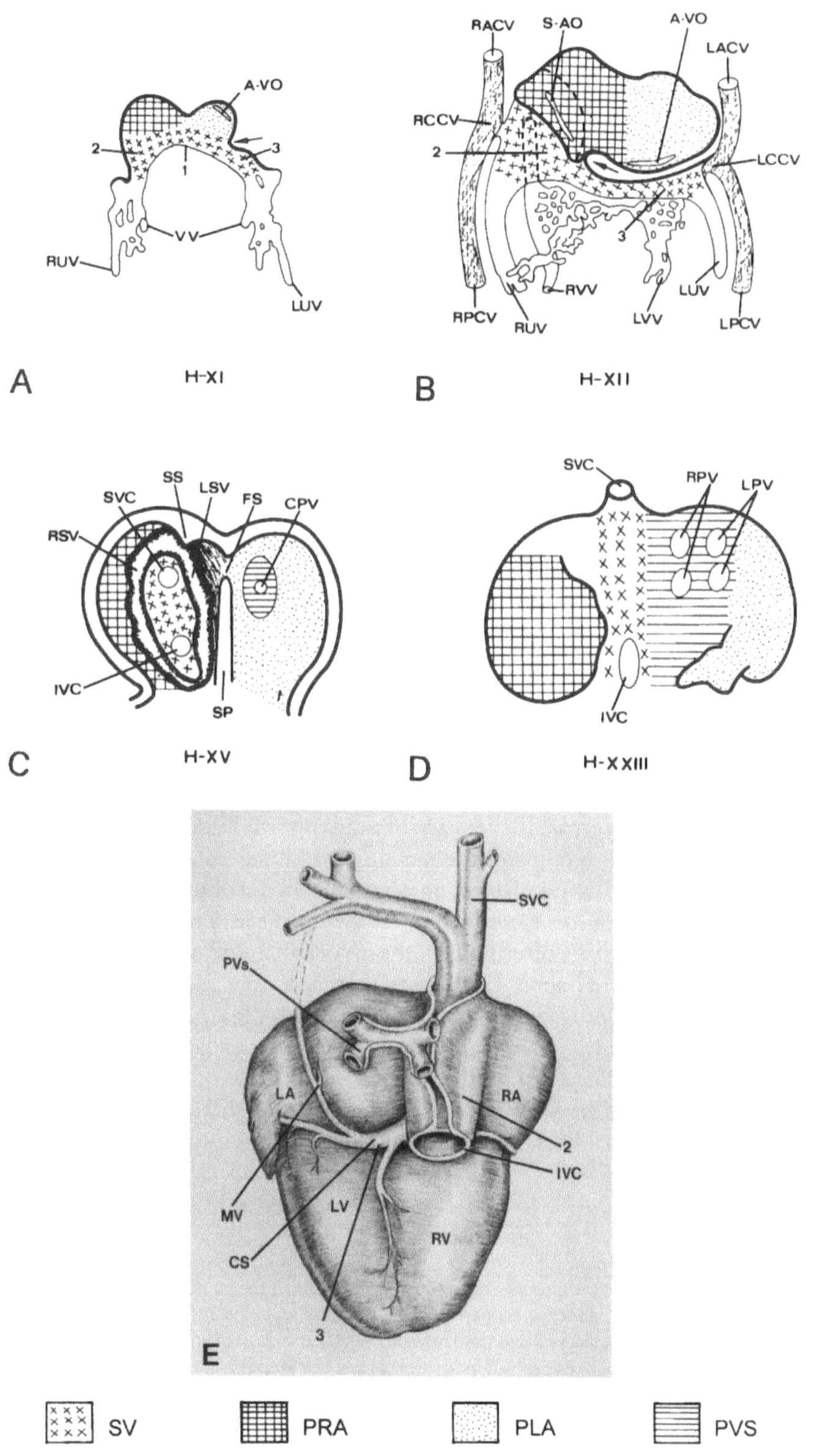
A-VO
2
1
3
VV
RUV
LUV
A
H-XI
RACV
S-AO
A-VO
LACV
RCCV
2
LCCV
3
RVV
LUV
RPCV
RUV
LVV
LPCV
B
H-XII
SS
LSV
SVC
FS
CPV
RSV
IVC
SP
C
H-XV
SVC
RPV
LPV
IVC
D
H-XXIII
SVC
PVs
LA
RA
2
IVC
MV
LV
RV
CS
3
E
SV
PRA
PLA
PVS

Odgers (1935) describes the appearance of the right sinus valve (right sinoatrial valve) and the left sinus valve (left sinoatrial valve), which grow from their onset into the right primitive atrium cavity in human embryos at horizon XIII. Steding and colleagues (1990), studying embryos of the same age, also point out that the sinus venosus opens into the right atrium between the right and left sinus valves, and the development of the septum primum also begins at this time. Steding and coworkers (1990) further describe in human embryos at horizon XIII that the proximal portion of the left horn of the sinus venosus has a tubular form, is situated in the left atrioventricular groove, and will give origin to the coronary sinus (Fig. 3E). The distal portion of the left horn and the left common cardinal veins are obliterated. This give rise to the ligament of Marshall, which sometimes persists as the oblique vein of Marshall in the wall of the left atrium (Fig. 3E).

Odgers (1935) describes in human embryos at horizon XIV and XV that the upper ends of both sinus valves fuse, forming a common superior fornix, which constitutes the prominent, albeit transient, septum spurium located in the cephalodorsal aspect of the right atrium (Fig. 4A).

According to the recent studies of Steding and associates (1990), the incorporation of the sinus venosus to the primitive right atrium begins in the human embryo of 9.5 mm (horizon XV). The more relevant facts of this process are (1) the right sinus valve, which is much larger than the left sinus valve, extends deep into the right atrium (Figs. 3C and 4); (2) the smaller left sinus valve also grows into the right atrium, leaving a space between it and the septum primum, called the interseptovalvular space (Licata 1954) (Fig. 3C); and (3) the dorsal wall of the sinus venosus, comprised between its right and left sinus valves, forms the posterior wall of the anatomical right atrium (Fig. 3C). In later horizons, the right sinus valve participates in the development of the crista terminalis, into which the pectinate muscles are inserted and which grows in the shape of a fan toward the apex of the right atrial appendage (Fig. 2C). It is of interest to mention that in the chick there are pectinate muscles in the right atrium similar in morphology and distribution to those in man although the sinus venosus is not incorporated into the atrium; consequently, the pectinate muscles originate directly from the myocardial wall of the primitive right atrium (Fig. 2). The left sinus valve fuses to the septum secundum, which has formed in the interseptovalvular space. The inferior vena cava and the tubular coronary sinus drain into the caudal region of the sinus venosus, between the two sinus valves (Fig. 4). The sinus septum (Steding et al 1990) or cavocoronary sinus septum (Licata 1954) develops between the orifices of these veins; this septum extends from the caudal base of the left sinus valve, to the caudal third of the base

⟶

FIGURE 4. Drawings of the internal views of the right atrium of the human embryo showing the different embryological components that participate in the atrial septation and in the formation of the Eustachian valve (inferior vena cava) and the Thebesius valve (coronary sinus). **A.** Notice the crescent-shaped septum secundum with its cephalodorsal arm (1) and the ventral arm (2) that are still not fused, and the cavocoronary sinus septum (CCSS), which together with the caudal part of the right sinus valve (RSV) forms the Eustachian valve, whereas the valve of Thebesius is formed exclusively by the caudal portion of the right sinus valve. **B.** The septum secundum (SS), with its two arms fused, constitutes the limbus of the foramen ovalis (FO); an arrow indicates the direction of blood flow through this foramen. SVC = superior vena cava; SSp = septum spurium; LSV = left sinus valve; IVC = inferior vena cava; SP = septum primum; CS = coronary sinus; TV = tricuspid valve.

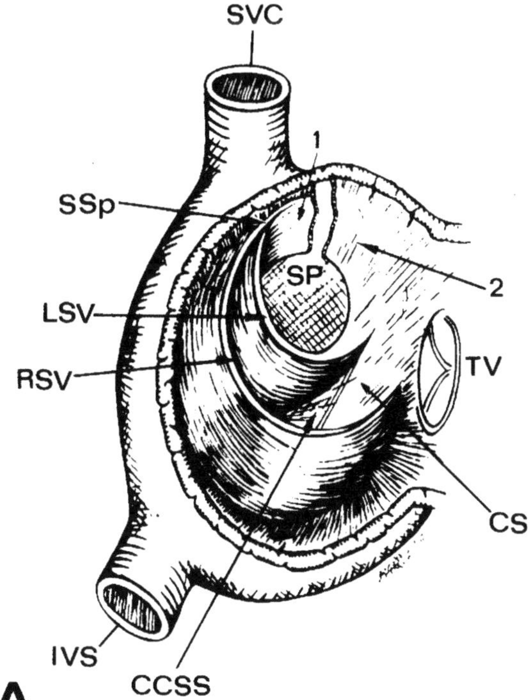
SVC
1
SSp
SP
2
LSV
RSV
TV
CS
IVS
CCSS

A

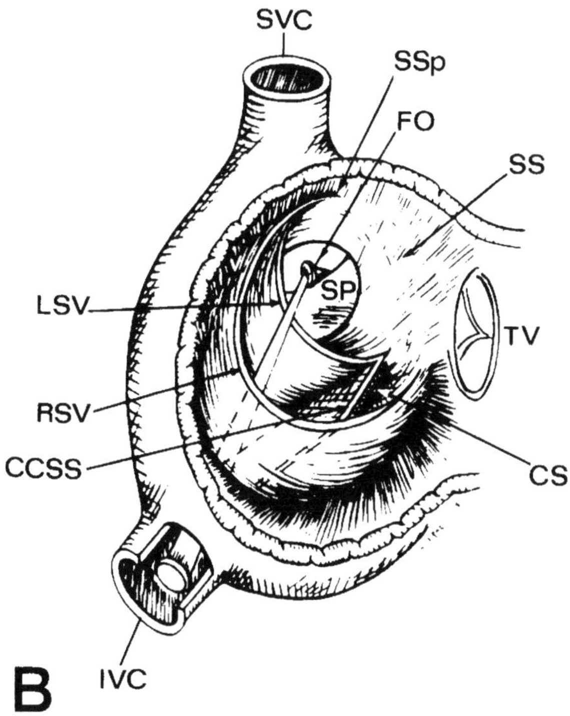
SVC
SSp
FO
SS
SP
LSV
TV
RSV
CCSS
CS
IVC

B

of the right sinus valve (Steding et al 1990) (Fig. 4B). Thus, the valve of the inferior vena cava (or Eustachian valve) is formed by the right sinus valve and the sinus septum (cavocoronary sinus septum) (Licata 1954) (Fig. 4B), whereas the Thebesian valve or coronary sinus valve is formed exclusively by the caudal part of the right sinus valve (Licata 1954; Steding et al 1990) (Fig. 4B). The superior part of the right sinus valve decreases in size and finally disappears because of numerous resorption areas, which form the net of Chiari.

In the mature heart, the anatomical limits of the sinus region of the right atrium are, cephalically, the orifice of the superior vena cava; caudally, the inferior vena cava and the coronary sinus orifices; to the right, the crista terminalis; and to the left, the septal wall of the right atrium (Figs. 2C and 5A). In summary, the anatomical right atrium has a sinus region that originates from the right horn of the sinus venosus and a region of fan-shaped pectinate muscles that originates from the primitive right atrial myocardium (Fig. 3). The limit between these two regions is the crista terminalis, which takes origin from the right sinus valve (Figs. 2C and 5A).

The definitive left atrium is constituted by the primitive left atrium and the pulmonary venosus sinus. The formation and eventual incorporation of the pulmonary veins into the primitive left atrium in the human embryo begin at horizon XIV (Streeter 1945). In this horizon there is a primitive right bronchus and a primitive left bronchus. The caudal end of each of these has a bulbus shape and is surrounded by mesenchymal tissue with numerous capillaries that constitute a venoarterial system (Streeter 1945). This pulmonary plexus drains through a short vessel that anastomoses to form common pulmonary veins that open into the dorsal wall of the left atrium (Streeter 1945). Later in development, the common pulmonary vein divides into two branches, each one of which in turn, branches into a pair of pulmonary veins. The incorporation or resorption of the common pulmonary vein and its two branches into the wall of the left atrium means that the four pulmonary veins will each have an individual opening into this chamber. Also the incorporated venous tissue constitutes a major portion of the smooth walled surface of this atrium. This is a gradual process. At horizon XXII (25 to 27 mm), Licata (1954) and Patten (1956) described an orifice for the right pair of pulmonary veins and one for the pair of left pul-

⟶

FIGURE 5. Diagrams representing that the situs solitus is characterized because the anatomical right atrium is placed on the right and the anatomical left atrium on the left. On the other hand the position of the ventricles depends on the type of ventricular loop; if it is convex to the right the anatomical right ventricle is situated to the right and the anatomical left ventricle to the left. Conversely, if the loop is convex to the left, the anatomical right ventricle is situated to the left and the anatomical left ventricle to the right; therefore the situation of the ventricles is an erroneous parameter for the diagnosis of the situs. **A.** The anatomical right atrium situated on the right and the anatomical left atrium on the left. **B.** Straight tube heart. The primordium of the apical trabeculated region of the right ventricle is cephalic and the primordium of the apical trabeculated region of the left ventricle is caudal. **C.** Convex loop to the right. **C′**. Its anatomical expression is an anatomical right ventricle to the right. **D.** Convex loop to the left. **D′**. Its anatomical expression is an anatomical right ventricle situated on the left. ARA = anatomical right atrium; ALA = anatomical left atrium; PM = pectinate muscle; CT = crista terminalis; SR = sinus region; AS = atrial septum; SVC = superior vena cava; IVC = inferior vena cava; PTRV = primordium of the apical trabeculated region of the right ventricle; PTLV = primordium of the apical trabeculated region of the left ventricle; PRA = primitive right atrium; PLA = primitive left atrium; ARV = anatomical right ventricle; ALV = anatomical left ventricle; PVs = pulmonary veins.

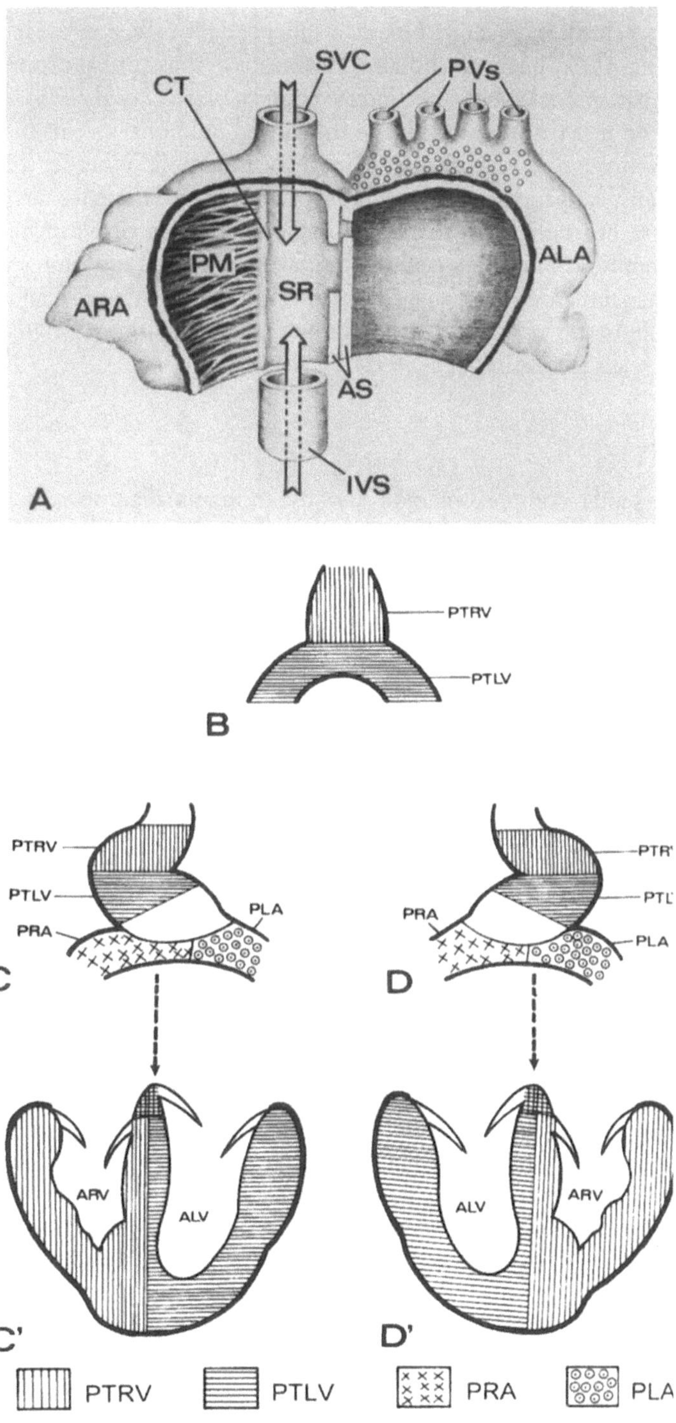
SVC
PVs
CT
PM
SR
ALA
ARA
AS
IVS
A
PTRV
PTLV
B
PTRV
PTLV
PLA
PRA
C
PTR
PTL
PRA
PLA
D
ARV
ALV
C'
ALV
ARV
D'
PTRV
PTLV
PRA
PLA

monary veins. Later in the 60-mm embryo (approximately 11 weeks), each of the four pulmonary veins has developed its own independent orifice in the left atrium (Patten 1956) (Fig. 3D). The results obtained by means of the use of appropriate fixatives in an adequate model such as the mouse embryo (Tasaka et al 1995) have provided information that the initial orifice of the central pulmonary veins may derive from the sinus venosus as with other vessels at the venous pole. Whether this applies also to the human awaits further study of appropriately staged human embryos.

In the mature heart there is no morphological structure that can be used as reference to establish a limit between a potential sinus region (pulmonary venous sinus) and the atrial region (primitive left atrium). In the chick, use of an antibody marker clearly indicates that the sinus venosus contributes to both right and left atrial posterior walls (DeRuiter et al 1995).

SEPTATION

The interatrial septal complex in man and other mammalian species has been considered to be constituted by different embryological components: the septum primum, the inferior and superior cushions of the atrioventricular AV canal, the septum secundum, the left sinus valve, and extracardiac mesenchyme called the spina vestibuli (Asami and Koizumi 1995). In the chick, it is formed by the septum primum and the inferior endocardial cushion of the AV canal.

The septum primum from its initial appearance, together with the superior and inferior endocardial cushions of the AV canal and the primitive interventricular septum, constitutes the primitive cardiac septum or 8-shaped septum (de la Cruz et al 1983, 1997) (chapter VI, Fig. 2, B–D). This primitive cardiac septum shows two orifices, one in the atrial region, the foramen primum, whose perimeter is formed by the free border of the septum primum and the superior and inferior endocardial cushions of the AV canal (de la Cruz et al 1983, 1997) (chapter VI, Fig. 2, B–D) (Fig. 6A). The other orifice, in the ventricular region, is the primary interventricular foramen (de la Cruz et al 1983, 1997) (chapters V and VI) (chapter VI, Fig. 2, B–D). The primitive cardiac septum (8-shaped septum) appears in the chick embryo heart at stage 17HH, with cardiac morphology similar to that of human embryo 6502 (horizon XIV) (chapters V and VI).

It is of interest to point out that despite the fact that the superior and inferior endocardial cushions of the AV canal are a part of the perimeter of the foramen primum, only the inferior endocardial cushion contributes to the closure of this foramen and in the development of the septal wall of the right atrium, as substantiated by the following facts: (1) When the superior endocardial cushion of the AV canal was labeled in vivo in the chick embryo, the label was never found in the atrial septum (de la Cruz et al 1982) (chapter VII, Fig. 6). (2) When the inferior endocardial cushion of the AV canal in the chick embryo was labeled in vivo, the following regions always appeared labeled: (a) the region of the atrial septum adjacent to the septal insertion of the anteroseptal leaflet of the mitral valve, i.e., the area of the foramen primum (de la Cruz et al 1983) (chapter VI, Fig. 4D), and (b) the septal wall of the right atrium, adjacent to the insertion of the septal leaflet of the tricuspid valve (de la Cruz et al 1983) (microleaflets in the chick). This fact casts doubt that the superior endocardial cushion of the AV canal contributes to atrial septation in man. Furthermore, it indicates that an embryological structure may form part of the border of an orifice but not contribute to its closure. The foramen

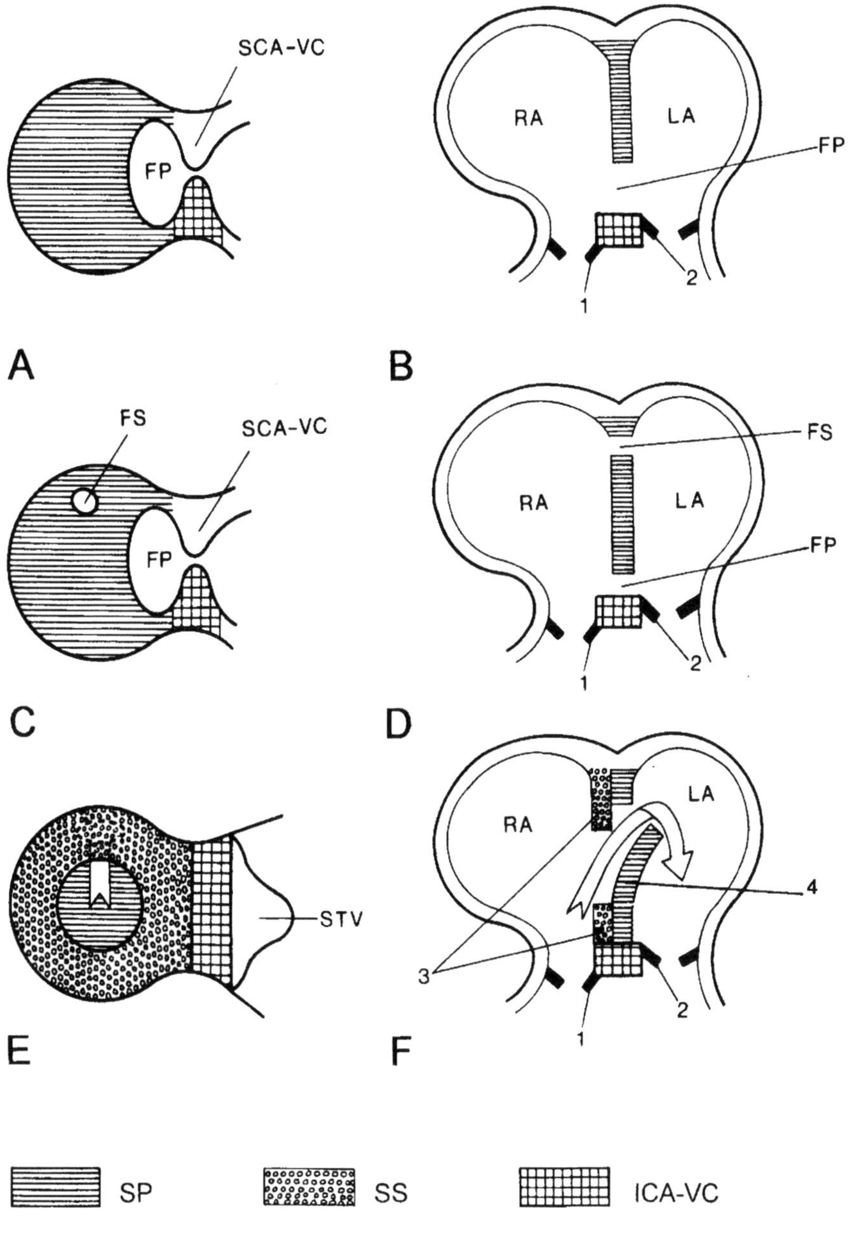

FIGURE 6. Diagrammatic representation of atrial septation in man. **A, C, E.** A view of the septal wall of the right atrium. **B, D, F.** Frontal section of both atria. SCA-VC = superior endocardial cushion of the AV canal; ICA-VC = inferior endocardial cushion of the AV canal; SP = septum primum; FP = foramen primum; RA = right atrium; LA = left atrium; FS = foramen secundum; SS = septum secundum (The arrow points the direction of the blood flow from the right atrium to the left atrium across the orifice of the foramen ovale in the fetus.); 1 = septal insertion of the septal leaflet of the tricuspid valve (STV); 2 = portion of the anteroseptal leaflet of the mitral valve, which inserts into the junction between the interatrial and atrioventricular septa; 3 = limbus foramen ovale; 4 = valve of the foramen ovale. Reprinted with the permission of from de la Cruz et al (1989) Bol Med Hosp Infant Mex 46(3):198.

primum is closed in the chick embryo heart at stage 26HH and in the human embryo of the same cardiac morphology at horizon XVI. The closure of this foramen is preceded in both species by the appearance in the septum primum of multiple orifices, in the chick embryo in the central zone of this septum and in man in the region adjacent to the future drainage of the superior vena caval and the right superior pulmonary vein. In man, these orifices coalesce to form the foramen secundum (Fig. 6, C and D).

It is important to establish the anatomical limits between the atrial septum and the atrioventricular septum, because the later forms part of both the septal wall of the right atrium and the septal wall of the left ventricular inlet and it separates the right atrium from the inlet of the left ventricle (chapter VI, Fig. 5) (Fig. 7, A and B). The definitive atrioventricular septum is located between the septal insertion of the anteroseptal leaflet of the mitral valve and the insertion of the septal leaflet of the human tricuspid valve or microleaflets in the chick (chapter VI, Fig. 5) (Fig. 7, A and B). This septum originates from the inferior cushion of the AV canal in both species (chapter VI, Fig. 5) (Fig. 7). The true atrial septum in the adult, which separates the right atrium from the left atrium, originates in the chick from the septum primum but in man from the septum primum plus the septum secundum and the left sinus valve (Figs. 6F and 7, B and C).

Another important component of the interatrial septal complex is the spina vestibuli, which in human is constituted by extracardiac mesenchyme that, according to Asami and Koizumi (1995), participates in the integration of the different components to form the definitive interatrial septal complex.

The septum secundum is a component of the interatrial septal complex in mammals. It appears in the spatium interseptovalvulare (Tandler 1912; Licata 1954) and, therefore, to the right of the septum primum (Figs. 4 and 6F). The septum secundum, according to Licata (1954) and Patten (1956), is a crescentic structure with one arm extending ventrally and the other cephalodorsally, thus forming the limbus foraminis ovalis (Licata 1954) (Figs. 4A and 6, E and F). The space limited by the limbus foraminis ovalis is covered by the septum primum (Fig. 6, E and F). It is also important to point out that the cephalodorsal arm of the septum secundum covers the foramen secundum like a curtain covers a window (Figs. 6, E and F; 7C). Furthermore, the left sinus valve fuses with the right aspect of the septum secundum. These embryological components are expressed anatomically by a valve apparatus in the fetus, the foramen ovale, whose annulus or limbus is the free border of the septum secundum and its valve, the septum primum. It provides one-way communication from the right atrium to the left atrium through the foramen secundum (Fig. 6, E and F). This valve apparatus can only open from right to left, thus fulfilling the requirements of the fetal hemodynamics in which the right atrial pressure is slightly higher than that of the left atrium (Castañeda et al 1994) (Fig. 6, E and F). After birth, the pressure in the left atrium is higher than that of the right atrium, and the septum primum or valve of the foramen ovalis (Botallo's foramen) applies itself to the free border of the septum secundum. Functional closure becomes anatomical closure during the neonatal period (Castañeda et al 1994). When anatomical closure takes place, this area is designated as the fossae ovalis, whose floor is the septum primum, and the limbus, the free border of the septum secundum (Fig. 7, B and C). In the chick, the orifices present in the septum primum become occluded soon after eclosion.

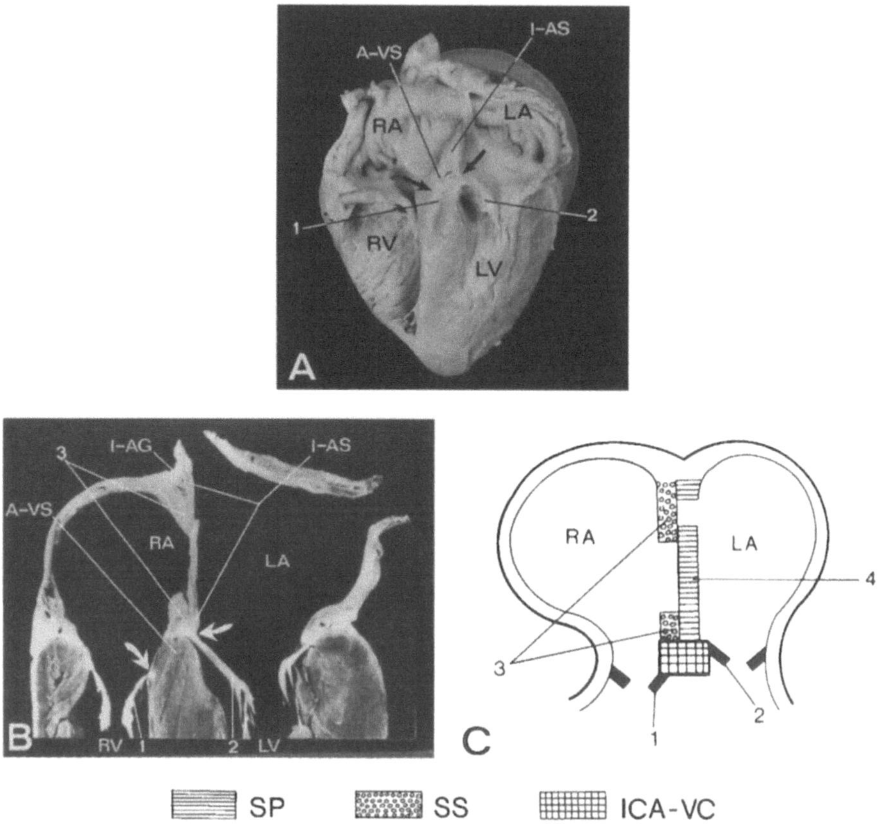

FIGURE 7. Photographs of a four-chamber section of the adult heart of the chick (**A**) and of man (**B**); diagram of the section in man (**C**). Notice that in both species the region of the septal wall of the right atrium adjacent to the insertion of the microleaflets in the chick and the septal tricuspid valve in man separates the anatomical right atrium from the inlet of the anatomical left ventricle; consequently it is the atrioventricular septum (A-VS). The arrows point its limits. Likewise in both species the region of the septal wall of both atria, comprised between the insertion of the anterior leaflet of the mitral valve and the interatrial groove (I-AG), separates both atria from each other and is the true interatrial septum (I-AS). RA = right atrium; LA = left atrium; RV = right ventricle; LV = left ventricle; A-VS = atrioventricular septum; 1 = septal tricuspid valve (microleaflets); 2 = portion of the anteroseptal leaflet of the mitral valve, which inserts into the junction between the interatrial and atrioventricular septa; 3 = limbus of the fossa ovalis (septum secundum); 4 = floor of the fossa ovalis (septum primum). Figure 7C reprinted with the permission of from de la Cruz et al (1989) Bol Med Hosp Infant Mex 46(3):198.

ATRIA IN THE CONTEXT OF THE SITUS

The atria are very important in the diagnosis of the three types of situs: (1) situs solitus is the most frequent one in which the anatomical right atrium is always situated on the right (Fig. 5A); (2) situs inversus, which is less frequent, is the mirror image of situs solitus, always with the anatomical right atrium situated on the left (Fig. 8A); the percentage of congenital cardiopathies in live newborns is the same as in situs solitus (8 to 10 per 1000) (Sanchez-Casco 1986); and (3) situs ambiguous (also called visceral heterotaxia), in which the atria are isomorphic

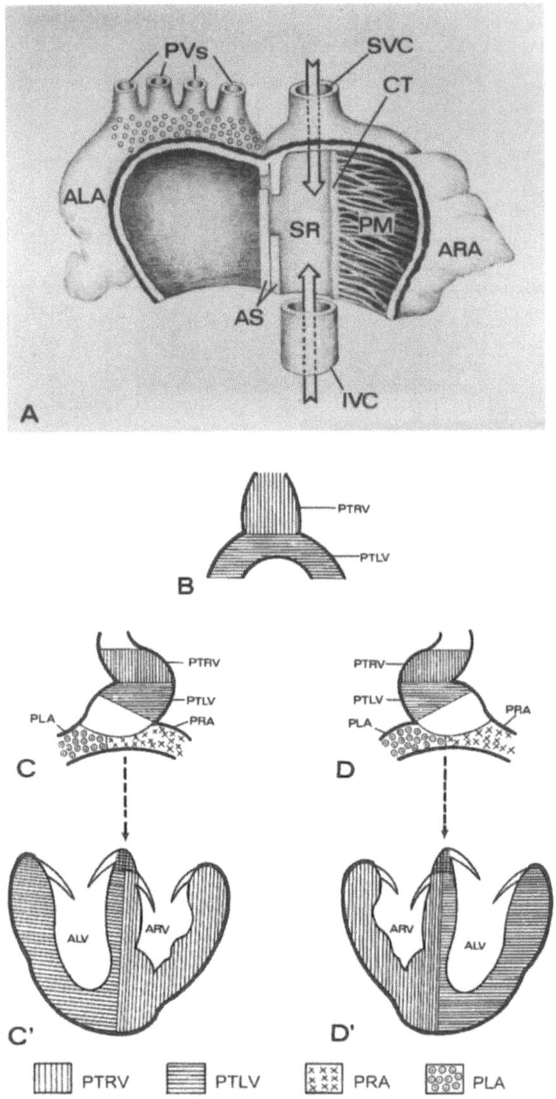

FIGURE 8. Diagrams showing that situs inversus is characterized because the anatomical right atrium is situated on the left and the anatomical left atrium is on the right, whereas the position of the ventricles depends on the type of loop; if it is convex to the left the anatomical right ventricle is situated to the left, and if it is convex to the right the anatomical right ventricle is on the right. Therefore the position of the ventricles is an erroneous parameter for the diagnosis of the situs. **A.** Anatomical right atrium situated on the left and anatomical left atrium situated to the right. **B.** Straight tube heart. The primordium of the apical trabeculated region of the right ventricle is cephalic and the primordium of the apical trabeculated region of the left ventricle is caudal. **C.** Convex loop to the left. **C′.** Its anatomical expression is an anatomical right ventricle to the left. **D.** Convex loop to the right. **D′.** Its anatomical manifestation is an anatomical right ventricle situated on the right. ARA = anatomical right atrium; ALA = anatomical left atrium; PM = pectinate muscle; CT = crista terminalis; SR = sinus region; AS = atrial septum; SVC = superior vena cava; IVC = inferior vena cava; PTRV = primordium of the apical trabeculated region of the right ventricle; PTLV = primordium of the apical trabeculated region of the left ventricle; PRA = primitive right atrium; PLA = primitive left atrium; ARV = anatomical right ventricle; ALV = anatomical left ventricle; PVs = pulmonary veins.

(atrial isomerism), is invariably associated with congenital cardiovascular pathology. This situs includes two varieties, i. e., dextroatrial isomerism, in which both atria exhibit the features pertaining to the anatomical right atrium; and levoatrial isomerism, in which both atria exhibit the features characteristic of the anatomical left atrium.

Owing to the presence of complex congenital cardiopathies in situs with atrial isomerism, the specialist in congenital cardiopathies appropriately uses the atria as the basis for their diagnosis. Atria are the only primitive cardiac cavities closely related to the visceral situs, because from the initial appearance the right primitive atrium is situated to the right and the left primitive atrium to the left (chapter IV, Fig. 7). The ventricles cannot be used to determine laterality, because the primordium of the apical trabeculated regions of each ventricle appear sequentially in the straight tube heart, i.e., they are cephalic and caudal (chapters III and IV) (chapter III, Figs. 4 and 5). The same is true also of the primitive outlet and the primitive inlet (chapters IV, VI, and VII) (chapter IV, Figs. 5 and 7). In addition, the right and left positions of the anatomical right ventricle and the anatomical left ventricle are also determined by the looping process. Thus in any of the three types of situs, the anatomical right ventricle may be situated to the right or to the left depending on whether the ventricular loop is convex to the right or to the left (de la Cruz et al 1959, 1971) (Figs. 5 and 8). Therefore, the position of the ventricles cannot be used as a parameter for the diagnosis of the situs (Figs. 5 and 8).

Knowledge of the unique morphological characteristics of the anatomical right atrium and the anatomical left atrium is indispensable to make the correct diagnosis of the different types of situs, which in turn implicitly includes the incidence or the complexity of the congenital cardiopathy. The characteristic morphological structures of the anatomical right atrium are fan-shaped patterns of the pectinate muscles, which originate from the primitive right atrium, and the crista terminalis and paramedial smooth or sinusal portion, which originate from the incorporation of the sinus venosus (Fig. 2C). The drainage of the inferior vena cava is also important in the diagnosis of the anatomical right atrium. This vessel drains into the anatomical right atrium situated on the right in the case of situs solitus (Fig. 5A) and into the anatomical right atrium situated on the left in situs inversus (Fig. 8A) as has been described by Anderson and colleagues (1987). Also, the right and left atrial appendages were considered as very important to distinguish between the anatomical right and left atria, however, the shape can be modified by flow (Macartney et al 1980).

In situs ambiguous with dextroatrial isomerism, both atria resemble the anatomical right atrium; the coronary sinus is absent and complex congenital cardiopathies are always present, the most important of which are the atrioventricular canal defect, plus transposition of the great arteries and sometimes an association with pulmonary stenosis or atresia (Van Mierop et al 1972).

Situs ambiguous with levoatrial isomerism is characterized by the fact that both atria lack a crista terminalis and pectinate muscles; therefore their walls are smooth. Furthermore, the coronary sinus is always present. With respect to systemic venous drainage, the suprahepatic segment of the inferior vena cava is absent and drainage into the heart takes place by way of the azygous or hemiazygous vein, which connects with the superior vena cava (Van Mierop et al 1972; Van Praagh and Van Praagh 1990). Drainage of the pulmonary veins is not a useful parameter for characterization of the anatomical left atrium, because totally anomalous pulmonary venous connections may occur in all three types of situs. The atrial septum is not useful either to identify any of the atria, because it may be absent in any of the three types of situs.

CONCLUSIONS

Results of in vivo labeling experiments in the chick embryo can yield significant insight with respect to the appearance of the atria and certain aspects of its septation in man. However, it is important to point out that the chick embryo, as a biological model, has limitations with respect to the contribution of the sinus venosus to the development of the definitive atria.

1. The anatomical right atrium in the chick exhibits pectinate muscles of similar morphology and distribution as in man; it lacks a smooth or sinusal region because the sinus venosus is connected but not incorporated into this atrium. Because the chick has pectinate muscle, without incorporation of the sinus venosus, it indicates that the pectinate muscles originate directly from the primitive right atrium. The anatomical right atrium in man exhibits, in addition to the pectinate muscles, the crista terminalis and the smooth sinus region. The anatomical left atrium in both species is smooth. Furthermore, the atrial septum is not a useful parameter for the diagnosis of each of the atria, because it may be absent.
2. The interatrial septal complex in the chick is constituted by the septum primum and the inferior endocardial cushion of the AV canal. In man, this complex is formed not only by similar components as in the chick, but also includes the spina vestibuli, the septum secundum, and the left sinoatrial valve. In both species the region of the septal wall of the right atrium adjacent to the insertion of the septal leaflet of the tricuspid valve and the microleaflets in the chick is the septal wall of the right atrium and the septal wall of the left ventricle. It is designated as the atrioventricular septum and it is formed by the inferior endocardial cushion of the AV canal.
3. The definitive atria are the cardiac chambers that serve to characterize the situs, because from the initial appearance of the primitive atria, one is right and the other is left. They form part of the bilateral symmetry of the organism; also important are the sinus venosus and the systemic venous system or venosus pole of the heart, which have a close relationship to atrial development. The three examples of situs are: situs solitus, in which the anatomical right atrium is situated on the right; situs inversus, in which the anatomical right atrium is on the left; and situs ambiguous, in which the atria are isomeric and there are two varieties: dextroatrial isomerism and levoatrial isomerism. These three types of situs may exhibit the anatomical right ventricle situated to the right or to the left depending on the type of loop, which is independent of the type of situs.
4. We do not yet understood the causal factors of bilateral right and left symmetry nor the exact developmental stage at which they appear (chapters I and II). Many questions remain. For example, why is it that situs ambiguous is always associated with complex congenital cardiopathies?

REFERENCES

Anderson RH, Macartney FJ, Shinebourne EA, Tynan M. 1987. Terminology. Paediatric cardiology. Edinburgh: Churchill Livingstone. Vol. 1, p 65–82.

Asami I, Koizumi K. 1995. Development of the atrial septal complex in the human heart: contribution of the spina vestibuli. In: Clark EB, Markwald RR, Takao A, editors. Developmental mechanisms of heart disease. Armonk, NY: Futura Publishing Co. p 255–260.

Castañeda AR, Jonas RA, Mayer JE, Hanley FL. 1994. Cardiac Surgery of the Neonate and Infant. Philadelphia: W.B. Saunders Co. p 255–60.

Castro-Quezada A, Nadal-Guinard B, de la Cruz MV. 1972. Experimental study of the formation of the bulboventricular loop in the chick. J Embryol Exp Morphol 27:623–37.

Davis CL. 1927. Development of the human heart from its first appearance to the stage found in embryos of twenty paired somites. Carnegie Contrib Embryol 19:245–84.

de la Cruz MV, Anselmi G, Cisneros F, Reinhold M, Portillo B, Espino-Vela J. 1959. An embryologic explanation for the corrected transposition of the great vessels: additional description of the main anatomic features of this malformation and its varieties. Am Heart J 57:104–17.

de la Cruz MV, Anselmi G, Munoz-Castellanos L, Nadal-Ginard B, Munoz-Armas S. 1971. Systematization and embryological and anatomical study of mirror-image dextrocardias, dextrotorsions and laevoversions. Br Heart J 33:841–53.

de la Cruz MV, Castillo MM, Villavicencio L, Valencia A, Moreno-Rodriguez RA. 1997. Primitive interventricular septum, its primordium, and its contribution in the definitive interventricular septum: in vivo labelling study in the chick embryo heart. Anat Rec 247:512–20.

de la Cruz MV, Gimenez-Ribotta M, Saravalli O, Cayré R. 1983. The contribution of the inferior endocardial cushion of the atrioventricular canal to cardiac septation and to the development of the atrioventricular valves: study in the chick embryo. Am J Anat 166:63–72.

de la Cruz MV, Quero-Jiménez M, Arteaga M, Cayré R. 1982. Morphogénèse du septum interventriculaire. Coeur 13:443–48.

de la Cruz MV, Sanchez-Gómez C, Cayré R. 1991. The developmental components of the ventricles: their significance in congenital cardiac malformations. Cardiol Young 1:123–8.

de la Cruz MV, Sanchez-Gómez C, Robledo-Tovi JL. 1987. Experimental study of the development of the ventricular inlets in the chick embryo. Embryologische Hefte 1:25–37.

DeRuiter MC, Gittenberger-de Groot AC, Wenink ACG, Poelmann RE, Mentink MMT. 1995. In normal development pulmonary veins are connected to the sinus venosus segment in the left atrium. Anat Rec 243:84–92.

DeVries PA, Saunders JB. 1962. Development of the ventricles and spiral outflow tract in the human heart. A contribution to the development of the human heart from age group IX to age group XV. Carnegie Contrib Embryol 256:89–114.

Licata RH. 1954. The human embryonic heart in the ninth week. Am J Anat 94:73–126.

Macartney FJ, Zuberbuhler JR, Anderson RH. 1980. Morphological considerations pertaining to recognition of atrial isomerism. Consequences for sequential chamber localisation. Br Heart J 44:657–67.

Odgers PNB. 1935. The formation of the venous valves, the foramen secundum and the septum secundum in the human heart. J Anat 69:412–25.

Patten BM. 1956. Desarrollo del sistema circulatorio: desarrollo del corazón. In: Embriología humana. Buenos Aires. Editorial "El Ateneo": p 655–71.

Sanchez-Casco. 1986. Etiología general e incidencia de las cardiopatías congénitas. In: Sanchez PA, editor. Cardiología pediátrica: Clínica y cirugía. Barcelona, Spain: Salvat Editores S.A. p 3–9.

Stalsberg H, DeHaan RL. 1969. The precardiac areas and formation of the tubular heart in the chick embryo. Dev Biol 19:128–59.

Steding G, Jinwen X, Seidl W, Männer J, Xia H. 1990. Developmental aspects of the sinus valves and the sinus venosus septum of the right atrium in human embryos. Anat Embryol 181:469–75.

Streeter GL. 1942. Development horizons in human embryos. Description of age group XI, 13 to 20 somites, and age group XII, 21 to 29 somites. Carnegie Contrib Embryol 30:211–45.

Streeter GL. 1945. Development horizons in human embryos. Description of age group XIII, embryos about 4–5 mm long, and age group XIV, period of indentation of the lens vesicle. Carnegie Contrib Embryol 31:27–63.

Tandler J. 1912. The development of the heart. In: Keibel F and Mall FP, editors. Manual of human Embryology. Philadelphia: J.B. Lippincott. 2:534–70.

Tasaka H, Krug EL, Markwald RR. 1995. Origin of the pulmonary vein in the mouse. In: Clark EB, Markwald RR, Takao A, editors. Developmental mechanisms of heart disease. Armonk, NY: Futura Publishing Co. p 347–50.

Van Mierop LHS, Gessner IH, Schiebler GL. 1972. Asplenia and polysplenia syndrome. Birth Defects, Editorial Original Article Series. Vol. VIII. 1:74–82.

Van Praagh R, Van Praagh S. 1990. Atrial isomerism in the heterotaxy syndromes with asplenia, or polysplenia, or normally formed spleen: an erroneous concept. Am J Cardiol 66:1504–6.

Waterson D. 1921. The development of the heart in man. Trans R Soc Edinburgh 52:257–304.

CHAPTER 9

Development of the Great Arteries

Karen Waldo and Margaret L. Kirby

Most information about the embryology of the great arteries in the human comes from elaborate descriptions by researchers such as Congdon (1922) and Padget (1948) earlier in this century. A broader understanding of the mechanisms behind vascular development has been gained more recently from animal models other than humans. Because avian embryos such as chick and quail are used extensively in developmental cardiovascular research, some of the major differences between human and chick will be mentioned as we discuss the development of the great arteries in humans. To avoid confusion in the ensuing discussion, "aortic arch" will refer to the definitive arch whereas "aortic arch artery" refers to one of the transient pharyngeal arch arteries that are precursors of all the adult great arteries.

ADULT CONFIGURATION OF THE GREAT ARTERIES

In the adult human, two great outflow vessels exit the heart to transport blood to the lungs, head, and body (Fig. 1). The pulmonary trunk leaves the right ventricle and divides under a left-sided aortic arch into the right and left pulmonary arteries that carry blood to the lungs. At birth, the patent ductus arteriosus extends from the left pulmonary artery near its origin from the pulmonary trunk to the inferior part of the aortic arch just beyond the base of the left subclavian artery (Gray 1973). Almost immediately after birth, it closes and is transformed into the ligamentum arteriosum. The aorta exits the left ventricle, crosses behind the pulmonary trunk, arches cranially leftward over the pulmonary arteries and atria, and descends posterior to the heart. Three major arteries branch from the superior part of the aortic arch (McVay 1984). The first branch, the brachiocephalic, or innominate, divides into the right common carotid artery medially and the right subclavian artery laterally. The second major vessel branching from the aorta is the left common carotid artery, and the third is the left subclavian artery (McVay 1984). A vertebral artery is the first branch from each subclavian to transport blood cranially (Gray 1973). The common carotids and the vertebral arteries carry blood to the neck and head while the subclavians transport blood to the shoulders and arms. The trunk and lower limbs are supplied by the thoracic and abdominal aorta (Gray 1973).

The configuration of the great arteries of the chicken differs from the human in several respects. The aorta is right-sided and has two rather than three major

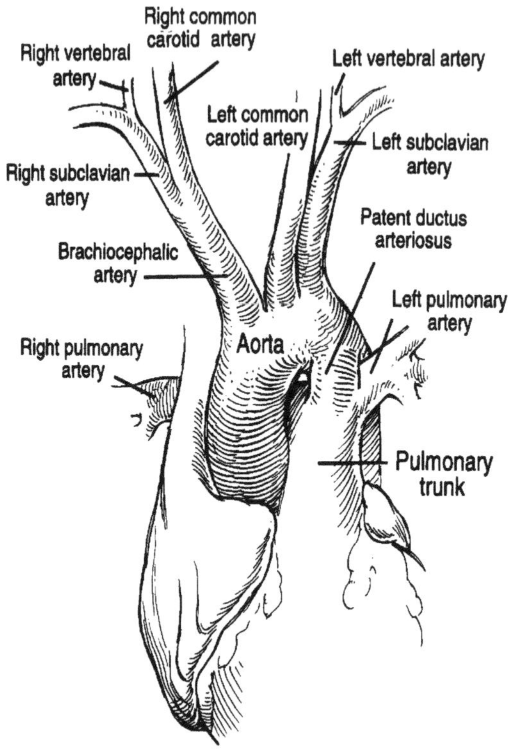

FIGURE 1. Configuration of the great arteries at birth. The patent ductus arteriosus joins the left pulmonary artery with the arch of the aorta just opposite the left subclavian artery. Closure of the ductus begins when breathing is initiated by the newborn.

branches that originate from the left side of the ascending aorta (Fig. 2). The left brachiocephalic artery is the first, most proximal branch, followed by a more superior right brachiocephalic artery. Both brachiocephalic arteries divide into a medial common carotid artery supplying the head and a lateral subclavian artery feeding the wings (Hughes 1934; Romanoff 1960; Getty 1975). At hatching, the chick has bilateral ductuses arteriosus that connect each pulmonary artery to the thoracic aorta dorsal to the heart (Romanoff 1960).

CONFIGURATION OF THE AORTIC ARCH ARTERIES

Aortic arch artery development has been described in detail in the early scientific literature (reviewed by Pexieder 1969). Some of the earliest descriptions date to the late 17th century (Malpighi 1672 as cited in Pexieder, 1969) and the early 19th century (Hueschke 1827 as cited by Pexieder, 1969). Kastschenko (1887) was one of the first investigators to use reconstructive techniques to describe the aortic arches in chick embryos (Pexieder 1969). Romanoff's (1960) and Lillie's (1952) texts of chick embryology rely heavily on Kastschenko's observations of the aortic arch arteries (Pexieder 1969). Lehman (1905) described the history of the aortic arches in mammals, whereas Congdon (1922) investigated the formation of the arch arteries in the human embryo. Pexieder (1969) and Bockman and associates (1987)

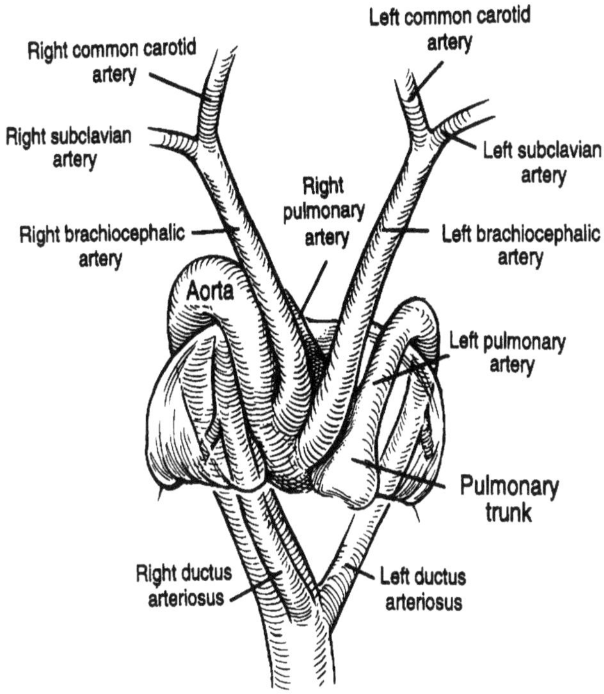

FIGURE 2. Configuration of the great arteries in the chick just before hatching. Both the right and left ductus arteriosus can be seen as patent vessels joining the descending aorta.

documented the appearance and disappearance of the arch arteries in the chick embryo and reported exhaustive measurements of the length, width, and height of the pharyngeal basket and of individual arch arteries.

The great arteries are derived from the aortic arch arteries and the truncoaortic sac of the embryonic pharyngeal basket. The pattern of the aortic arch arteries in higher vertebrates is derived from gill-bearing aquatic ancestors in which blood passed from a ventrally positioned heart, around the gut, and through the branchial arches where gas exchange occurred (Dohrn 1885; Skandalakis et al 1994). The branchial arch arteries in the gill region provide an afferent artery to an extensive oxygen-gathering capillary plexus. An efferent artery connects this plexus with the dorsal aorta so that the oxygen can be delivered systemically (Fig. 3). Two major changes occur in the vertebrate transition from early aquatic vertebrates to later land-living vertebrates: the development of a very complex head and face and the shift of oxygen and carbon dioxide exchange from gills to a lung-based respiratory system. During this shift the gill-producing branchial arches are modified into an embryonic complex of transient pharyngeal arches that is remodeled during development to produce the lower face, ear, neck, and great arteries. Mimicking its water-dwelling ancestor, the modern vertebrate embryo develops an aortic arch artery within each pharyngeal arch, thus the patterning of the early aortic arch arteries is, of necessity, tied to the development of pharynx. The embryonic heart, developing ventral to the pharynx, is connected with paired dorsal aortae by the aortic arch arteries originating from the aortic sac of the distal cardiac outflow tract

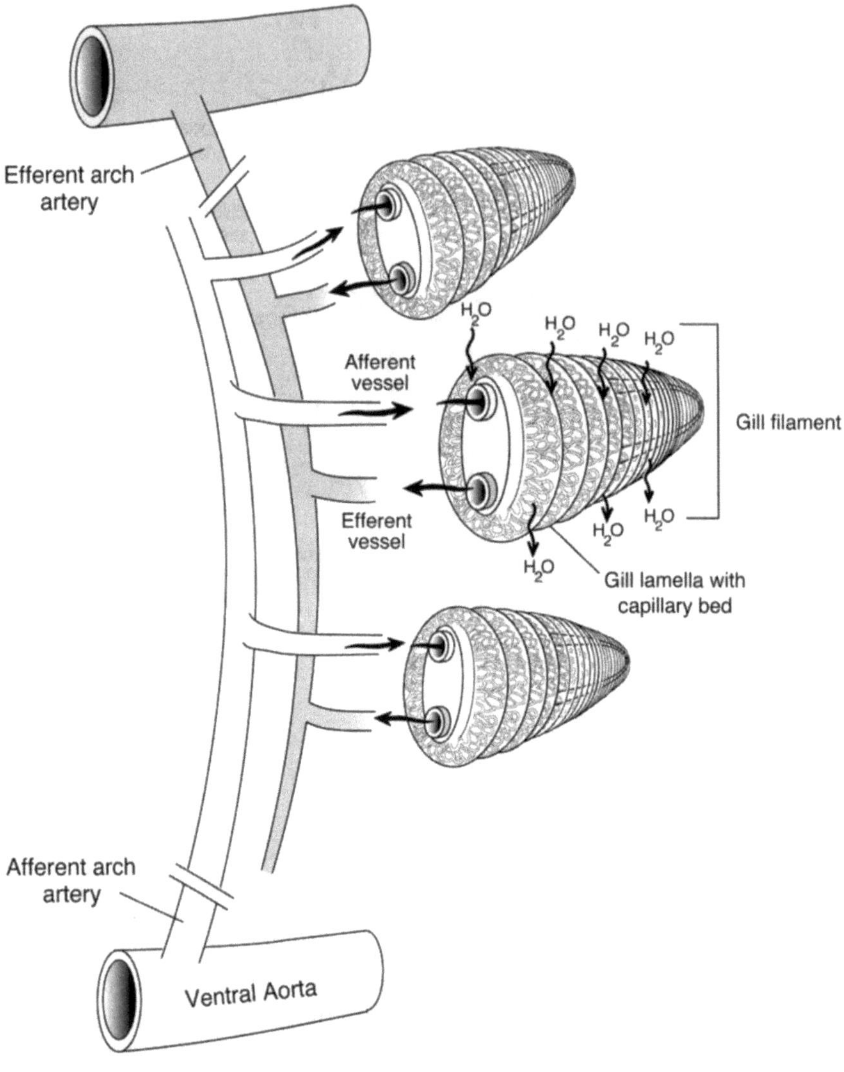

FIGURE 3. Each branchial arch in bony fish has an afferent and efferent arch artery. The afferent branchial arch artery branches from the ventral aorta and carries unoxygenated blood to the gill filaments where gases are exchanged as water passes over the capillary-filled gill lamella. Oxygenated blood is transported to the dorsal aorta after it is collected from the gill filaments by the efferent branchial arch arteries.

(Fig. 4). Subsequently, as the pharynx changes its morphology and the heart descends into the thoracic cavity, the original pharyngeal arterial pattern is transformed into the adult arterial configuration (Congdon 1922). In most vertebrate embryos, except fish and a few amphibians, there are 5 pairs of transient pharyngeal arches (branchial arches that persist as gills in gill-bearing vertebrates), numbering 1, 2, 3, 4, and 6. Each pair of pharyngeal arches, except the 6th, is demarcated caudally by a pair of pharyngeal pouches (Romer 1963). They appear sequentially

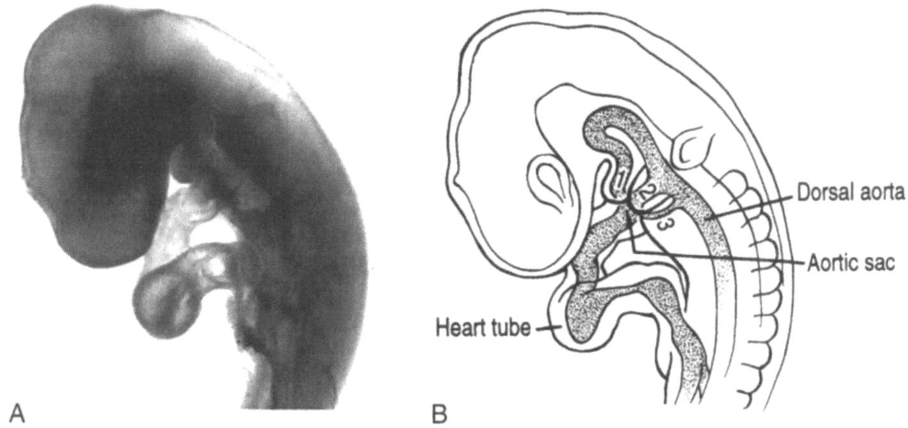

FIGURE 4. Stage 15/16 chick embryo, viewed from the left side. A. The beating cardiac loop develops ventral to the pharyngeal area until the anterior body wall forms and forces the heart into the thorax. The heart loops to the embryo's right such that the cardiac ouflow tract is away from the viewer. On the embryo's left side, nearest the viewer, the inflow part of the heart loop exits the ventral body wall. B. Aortic arch arteries (1, 2, and 3) connect the aortic sac at the distal end of the heart tube with the dorsal aorta. The first two pharyngeal arches have formed and the third is forming. The 3rd arch artery, not yet a robust artery, is small in comparison to the first two arch arteries since it has just lumenized.

in a cranial to caudal manner, but not all pairs of arch arteries are present at the same time. The 1st and 2nd pairs of arteries do not persist, but rather regress into capillaries as the 3rd, 4th, and 6th arch arteries appear (Fig. 5). The 5th arch artery appears transiently and is not a true arch artery because it connects the base of the 4th arch artery with the middle of the 6th arch artery, and is thus not an independent arch artery as are the other 5 arch arteries. The arrangement of the pharyngeal arterial basket is similar in the human and chick, with one exception. In the chick embryo, the 5th aortic arch artery appears briefly (Pexieder 1969; Bockman et al 1987; Locy 1995), but its presence has been debated in humans (Congdon 1922). In the human and chick, the proximal part of the 6th arch artery is formed from a primitive pulmonary artery that condenses from capillaries of the splanchnic plexus and becomes continuous with the aortic sac caudal to the base of the 4th arch artery before the appearance of the 6th arch artery (Fig. 6A) (Kastschenko 1887; Congdon 1922; Buell 1922; Phillips et al 1988). The 6th arch artery is completed when the primitive pulmonary artery is connected to the dorsal aorta by the ductus arteriousus, the distal segment of the 6th arch artery. Thus the true 6th arch artery is, in actuality, only the ductus arteriosus or distal part of what has traditionally been referred to as the sixth arch artery (Fig. 6B) (Bremer 1912; Kutsche and Van Mierop).

As the heart descends into the thorax, and the embryo's neck lengthens, the pharyngeal basket loses its symmetrical arrangement (Langman 1975) and lengthens (Pexieder 1969) in a dorsoventral plane. The aorticopulmonary (AP) septum, derived from neural crest cells, forms in the mesenchyme dorsal to the roof of the aortic sac between the 4th and 6th pairs of arch arteries (Fig. 7). The growth of the AP septum toward the cardiac outflow tract effectively divides the aortic sac into

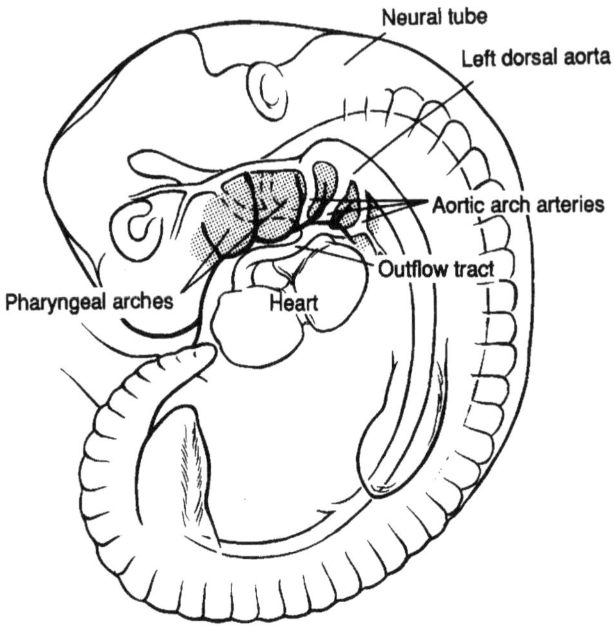

FIGURE 5. Human embryo, viewed from the left side. The 3 caudal pharyngeal arch arteries (3, 4, and 6) have formed in the 3rd, 4th, and 6th pharyngeal arches, while the first two arch arteries have become capillary beds in the 1st and 2nd pharyngeal arches. Dilations and constrictions have occurred in the heart tube demarcating the single atrium and the early ventricles of the heart. The aortic arch arteries branch from the aortic sac (distal cardiac outflow tract), which exits the primitive right ventricle. The narrowed atrioventricular canal connects the atrium with the primitive left ventricle.

two arterial channels: one systemic, the other pulmonary. Blood flowing through the systemic channel reaches the paired dorsal aortae via the 3rd and 4th arch arteries. The pulmonary channel is connected with the dorsal aorta by the 6th arch arteries, thus the pulmonary blood flow is primarily to the body at this stage of development. A small primitive pulmonary artery branches from the pulmonary trunk and is continuous with a vascular plexus forming in the developing lung buds (Waldo and Kirby 1993a); however, blood flow is minimal through the nascent pulmonary artery until much later in development (Romer 1963). In the human embryo, the distal part of the right 6th arch artery is obliterated early in development, but on the left side it persists to become the ductus arteriosus. At birth, the lungs inflate, decreasing the resistance to flow, which causes blood to be preferentially rerouted to the lungs. This and several other factors contribute to permanent closure of the ductus when blood flow is irrevocably committed to the lungs (Romer 1963). In the chick, both ductuses persist to hatching, but start closing a few days earlier when the chick initiates breathing (pipping) inside the egg.

In humans and chicks, the dorsal aorta between the 3rd and 4th arch arteries (the carotid duct) involutes and disappears (Congdon 1922; Hughes 1943). The distal parts of the 3rd arch arteries are released from the pharyngeal basket. This process allows the 3rd arch artery and its segment of the cranial dorsal aorta to expand cephalad with the lengthening neck, thereby committing its blood flow to the head, while allowing the remainder of the pharyngeal basket to descend caudally with the

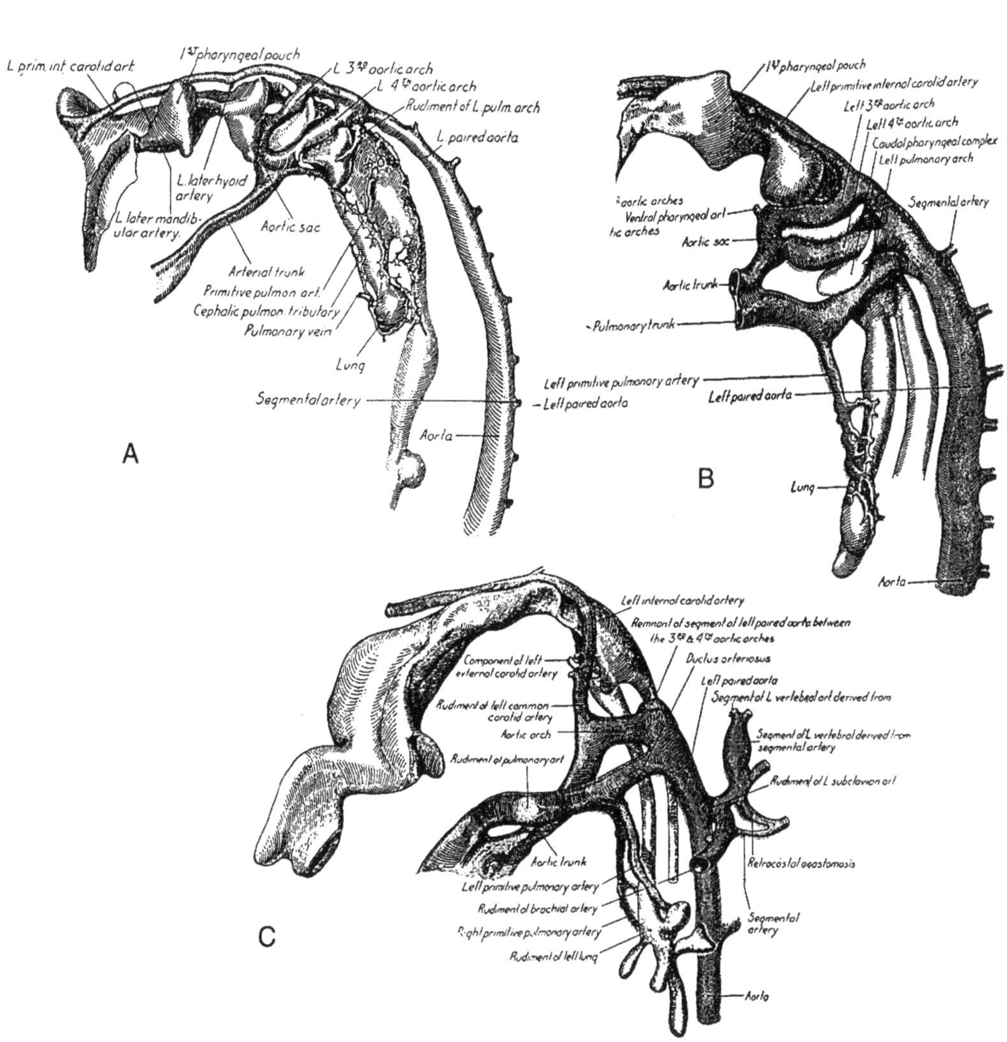

FIGURE 6. The configuration of the aortic arch arteries of the human embryo is viewed from the left side. The relationship of the arch arteries to the pharyngeal pouches is illustrated. **A.** 5-mm embryo. Aortic arch arteries 1 and 2 have become capillary beds. Arch arteries 3 and 4 are formed, and 6 (the pulmonary arch) is forming. The primitive pulmonary artery branches from the posterior part of the aortic sac at the base of the 4th arch artery and is continuous with forming capillary beds in the lung buds. **B.** 11-mm embryo. The 6th arch artery is completed as the ductus arteriosus, or the distal part of the 6th arch artery, joins the pulmonary artery with the dorsal aorta. On the right side (not shown) the right ductus arteriosus is already regressing. **C.** 14-mm embryo. As aorticopulmonary septation occurs, and the arches lengthen, the symmetrical pattern of the paired aortic arch arteries is lost in a transition from their early pattern toward the adult configuration. (Drawings reprinted from Congdon 1922.)

heart into the thorax (Figs. 6c and 8). As the heart descends, the paired dorsal aortae become shortened caudal to the 6th arches. In the human, each subclavian artery will develop from the 7th intersegmental artery that branches from the paired dorsal aortae at about this time caudal to the 6th arch arteries (Netter 1978) (Fig. 8). A primary subclavian derives from the 18th intersegmental artery in the chick (Fig. 9) (Hughes 1934; Lillie 1952).

After septation of the outflow tract, changes in the configuration of the 4th arch

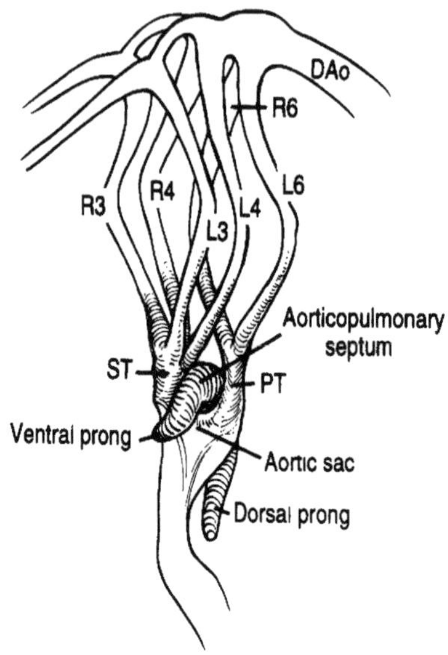

FIGURE 7. The arterial pharyngeal basket of a stage 26 ink-injected and cleared chick embryo has been illustrated from a left anterior view. The aorticopulmonary septum bridges the roof of the aortic sac causing it to sink inward toward the heart, thereby dividing the sac into two trunks: systemic (ST) and pulmonary (PT). The bridge of the aorticopulmonary septum is connected to a long dorsal prong that penetrates the dorsal outflow cushion (not shown) and a short ventral prong that penetrates part of the ventral outflow cushion. R3, L3, right and left third arch artery; R4, L4, right and left fourth arch artery; R6, L6, right and left sixth arch artery; DAo, dorsal aorta.

arteries occur. One involutes or becomes modified, leaving the contralateral artery to become the dominant aorta. In humans the left 4th arch artery persists to become a segment of the arch of the aorta as the right 4th arch artery and the dorsal aorta on the right side undergo extensive remodeling (Congdon 1922) (Figs. 6 and 8). The right 4th arch artery is transformed into the proximal part of the right subclavian, and the more distal segment of the right subclavian is formed by the right translocated 7th intersegmental artery. The left subclavian artery is formed completely from the left intersegmental artery, which is translocated to the aortic arch. In the chick, the left 4th arch artery normally disappers, leaving the right 4th arch artery and the right dorsal aorta to take part in formation of the aorta and its arch (Fig. 9) (Romanoff 1960; Pexieder 1969; Bockman et al 1987). The primary subclavians have moved cranially and join an arterial plexus derived from the ventral aorta near its connection with the 3rd arch artery. Degeneration of both the ventral aorta and the primary subclavian occurs, resulting in the formation of a secondary subclavian artery from the capillary plexus. This secondary subclavian, now originating from the 3rd arch artery at its base, becomes the definitive artery feeding the wing (Sabin 1905; Bakst and Chaffe 1928; Lillie 1952).

The 3rd arch arteries persist in both human and chick, but their final configuration differs. In the human, the 3rd arch artery, along with its cranial extension, the original cranial part of the dorsal aorta, becomes the common carotid and proximal internal carotid artery (Congdon 1922; Barry 1951). On the right side, however, part of the aortic sac is altered to form the brachiocephalic artery, which connects the right common carotid and subclavian arteries with the aortic arch. The left common carotid artery branches directly from the aorta (Fig. 8). In the chick, the 3rd arch arteries each give origin to a right or left brachiocephalic artery, which connects the subclavian and common carotid artery with the aorta (Fig. 9) (Romanoff 1960).

EARLY VASCULAR DEVELOPMENT

A great deal of our knowledge of embryonic vascular development derives from classical descriptive and experimental studies (Kastschenko 1887; Evans 1909; Fedorow 1910; Bremer 1912; Sabin 1917, 1920; Buell 1922; Congdon and Wang 1926; Pexieder 1969). Advances in immunohistochemistry and molecular biology have recently provided insights into human and nonhuman developmental processes that have broadened our understanding considerably. Through the development of monoclonal antibodies to quail endothelium and endothelial precursors 10 years ago (Dieterlen-Lievre 1984; Pardanaud et al 1987), we have been able to visualize the earliest formation of the cardiovascular system in quail embryos. From these experiments we have learned that early blood vessels are formed from endothelial precursors that assemble to form lumenized channels lined by endothelial cells. The source of these endothelial precursors, or angioblasts, has been the subject of controversy and much research. The proposal of His (1900) that all vessels were formed from extraembryonic angioblasts was questioned by Sabin in 1917, who noticed that endothelial vesicles formed in the embryo in splanchnic mesoderm, especially in the mesoderm–endoderm interface (Van Mierop 1979a). It was later demonstrated through transplantation experiments using [^{3}H] thymidine-labeled mesoderm, or species-specific markers in quail/chick chimeras, that blood vessels could be formed from mesoderm transplanted from various parts of the embryo (Reagan 1915; Rosenquist 1970; Noden 1991). Although subsequent studies using QH-1 (recognizing a perinuclear antigen specific for endothelial cells) enabled researchers to visualize for the first time the formation of the vascular system through the assembly of endothelial precursors into capillaries (Pardanaud et al 1987; Coffin and Poole 1988), the source of the precursors still remained controversial. Data from transplantation experiments by Noden (1991), using quail/chick chimeras, suggested that the origins of embryonic blood vessels are multiple. He proposed that early blood vessels form and grow by all of three different processes, including vasculogenesis (formation of a vessel from local endothelial precursors or from precursors that have migrated into the embryo from the yolk) (Pardanaud et al 1987; Risau and Lemmon 1988; Coffin and Poole 1988), angiogenesis (the formation of a new vessel from a preexisting vessel by budding or branching) (Folkman 1985), and the incorporation of local and wandering angioblasts (Noden 1991). That many of the earliest endothelial precursors seem to form in the interface between endoderm and mesoderm suggests that vasculogenesis may occur as a result of inductive interactions between the endoderm and the mesoderm (Pardanaud et al 1989). Angiogenesis has been more associated with organs derived from the ectoderm.

The aortic arch arteries, dorsal aortae, and heart tube are formed from endothelial precursors that assemble in the splanchnic mesoderm to form a capillary plexus on either side of the 1-somite embryo (Fig. 10). Many of these precursors are associated with the interface of the endoderm and mesoderm. As the splanchnic mesoderm is translocated ventrally because of growth of the foregut and the formation of the head fold, a horseshoe-shaped capillary plexus, the splanchnic plexus, is formed ventral to and on both sides of the embryo by the 3- or 4-somite stage (Coffin and Poole 1988; DeRuiter et al 1993). The heart tube, aortic arch arteries, and the vitelline vessels are all formed from this plexus, as are the paired dorsal aortae that develop dorsal to the developing gut. By joining and becoming continuous with the paired dorsal aortae, the 1st arch arteries connect the heart to systemic arteries (Fig. 11). The 2nd aortic arch arteries, as well as all the remaining arch arteries, are formed from cords of endothelial precursors that grow against the

---

FIGURE 8. Schematic summary of the transformation of the symmetrical early human pharyngeal arterial basket into the configuration of the great arteries at birth. The point of view has been moved ventrally. A. The pattern of the paired arch arteries is symmetrical as they branch from the truncoaortic sac (yellow) and join the dorsal aorta (DAo). The 1st and 2nd arch arteries have disappeared, leaving the 3rd (green), 4th (red), and 6th arch arteries (blue). The dorsal aorta between the 3rd and 4th arch arteries forms the carotid duct. The 7th intersegmental arteries (violet) branch from the dorsal aorta cranial to the aortic bifurcation. Adjoining each 7th intersegmental is a capillary plexus (orange) that will give rise to the future vertebral artery. **b** and **c**. Transition stages between the early pharyngeal arterial pattern and the final configuration of the great arteries. The carotid duct and the 8th segment of the right dorsal aorta involute and disappear. The right ductus arteriosus narrows and disappears, and the left ductus and the primitive pulmonary arteries enlarge. The dorsal aorta on the left side enlarges along with the 4th arch artery whereas the dorsal aorta on the right remains smaller in diameter. The 7th intersegmental arteries and the forming vertebral arteries are transported cranially. The aortic sac elongates causing the 4th arch arteries to shorten and become transported cranially. **d**. The configuration of the great arteries at birth. A, aorta; AA3, aortic arch artery 3; AA4, aortic arch artery 4; AA6, aortic arch artery 6; BC, brachiocephalic artery; DA, ductus arteriosus; DAo, dorsal aorta; DC, carotid duct; I (7th), 7th intersegmental artery; LCC, left common carotid artery; LPA, left pulmonary artery; LSC, left subclavian artery; LVC, left vertebral artery; P, pulmonary trunk; PA, pulmonary artery; RCC, right common carotid artery; RPA, right pulmonary artery; RSC, right subclavian artery; RVA, right vertebral artery; TAS, truncoaortic sac; VA, vertebral artery.

FIGURE 9. Development of the aortic arch arteries in the chick and their transformation into the great arteries at hatching. **a–c**. Schematic representations of ventral views summarizing the transformation of the arch arteries into the great arteries. Initially, the configuration of the pharyngeal arterial basket is similar to the human configuration. Arch arteries 1 and 2 have disappeared leaving the 3rd (green), 4th (red), and 6th (blue) arch arteries. The left 4th arch artery and the carotid duct involute and disappear; both ductuses arteriosus persist. The right 4th aortic arch artery and dorsal aorta enlarge. The primary subclavian arteries are formed initially, and replaced by the secondary subclavian arteries. The aortic sac elongates to form part of the aortic trunk. The primitive pulmonary arteries, at first minute, enlarge. **d–f**. Schematic drawings from the left side illustrating the configuration of the aortic arch arteries in chick embryos, at incubation days 5.5 (stage 26), 6.5 (stage 29), and 7.5 (stage 32). At stage 26 the aortic sac is divided to form a systemic (ST) and pulmonary trunk (PT). The pulmonary trunk is dorsal and the systemic trunk is ventral. The configuration of the aortic arch arteries is symmetrical. By stage 29, aorticopulmonary septation is well underway and the arch arteries are elongating. The relationship of the aorta to the pulmonary trunk is changing with the pulmonary trunk moving ventrally and the aorta rotating dorsally so that they have become side-by-side. The symmetrical pattern of the arch arteries is lost as the left 4th arch artery involutes. At stage 32, aorticopulmonary septation is just about completed and the aorta and pulmonary trunk have rotated such that the aorta is located dorsally and the pulmonary trunk ventrally. A, aorta; AA3, aortic arch artery 3; AA4, aortic arch artery 4; AA6, aortic arch artery 6; DA, ductus arteriosus; DAo, dorsal aorta; DC, carotid duct; I (18th), 18th intersegmental artery; LBC, left brachiocephalic artery; LCC, left common carotid artery; LSC, left subclavian artery; P, pulmonary trunk; PA, pulmonary artery; PSC, primary subclavian artery; RCC, right common carotid artery; RBC, right brachiocephalic; RPA, right pulmonary artery; RSC, right subclavian artery; SSC, secondary subclavian artery; TAS, truncoartic sac.

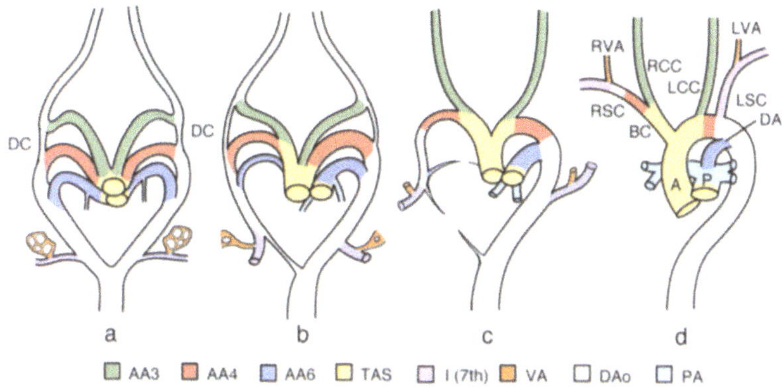

FIGURE 8.

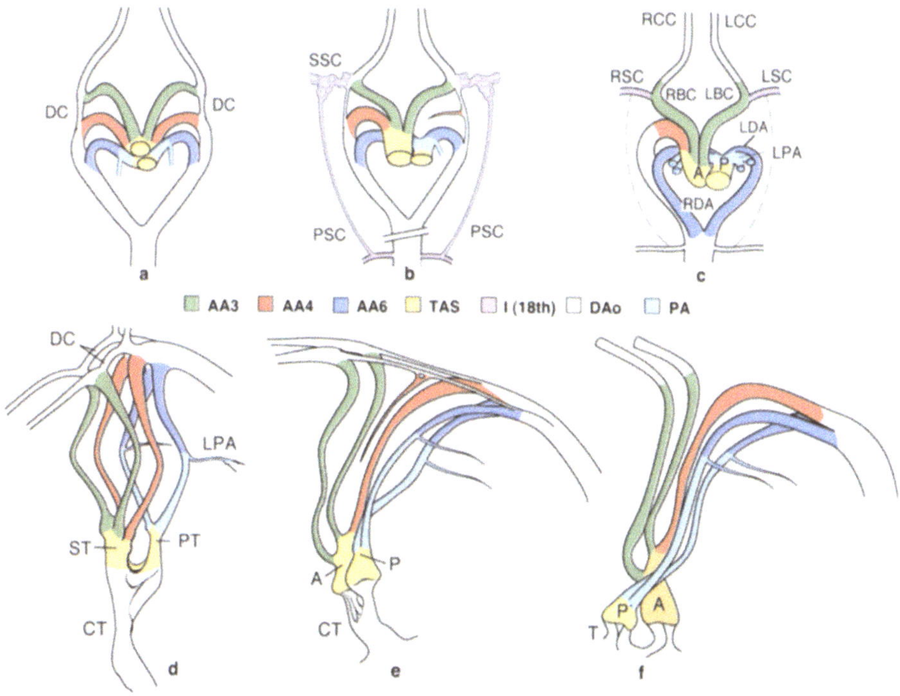

FIGURE 9.

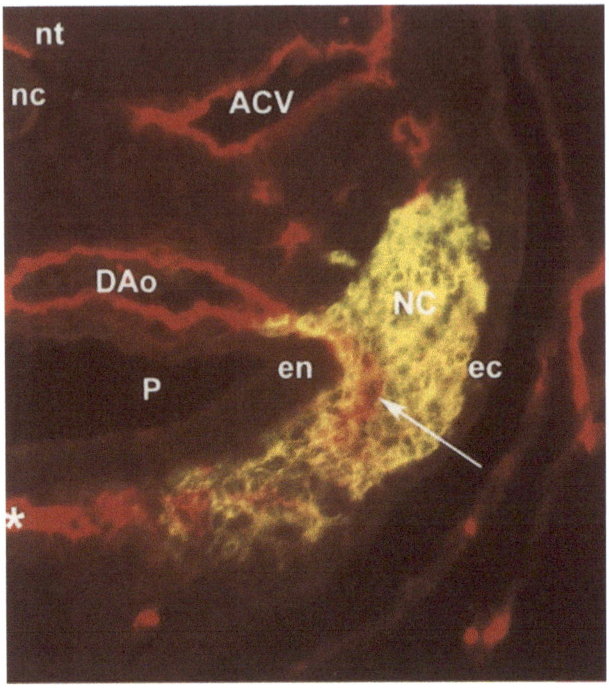

FIGURE 13.

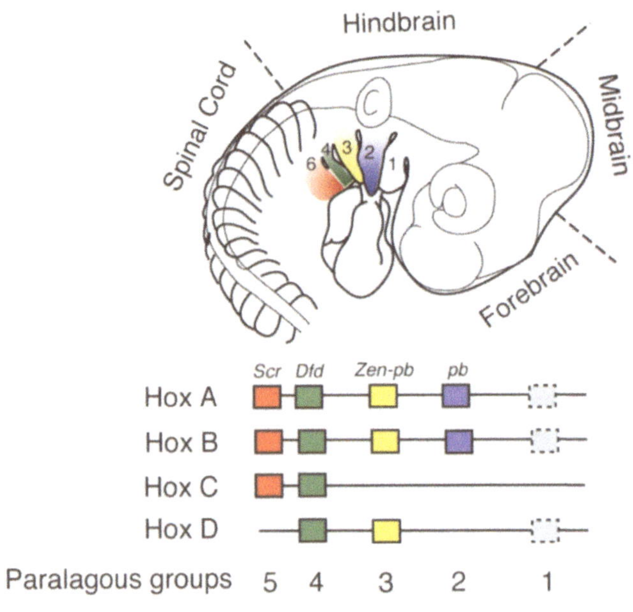

FIGURE 17.

pharyngeal endoderm in the endoderm–mesoderm interface (Fig. 12) (Coffin and Poole 1988; DeRuiter et al 1993). The pattern formed by the cords of endothelial precursors heralds the pattern of the future configuration of the pharyngeal arterial basket by the 3- to 7-somite stage (DeRuiter et al 1993). As each pair of endothelial cords lumenizes, the nascent endothelial tubes become connected distally with the dorsal aorta and proximally with the aortic sac to form an aortic arch artery. Lumenization begins at the proximal and distal ends of the aortic arch arteries, which caused the mistaken impression in classic studies that buds grew from the aortic sac and dorsal aorta and joined to form the arch artery. Patency of the last pair of aortic arch vessels is completed in the chick by stage 23 (Bockman et al 1987). By that time, the 1st and 2nd aortic arch arteries have regressed into capillary beds and are being remodeled into new vessels, and the 3 caudal pairs of arch arteries that will persist have begun to elongate and acquire a tunica media as they begin their transformation into the adult configuration.

EXPERIMENTAL STUDIES

Rychter (1962) reviewed the experiments altering aortic arch patterning by direct manipulation of the developing arch artery. Hinrichs (1931 as cited by Rychter, 1962) used localized UV irradiation to suppress all the right-sided aortic arch arteries. Mannhoff and Johnson (1951 as cited by Rychter, 1962) caused microcoagulation of the right 6th aortic arch artery to cause stenosis of the vessel. Using a metal filament Stéphan (1952 as cited by Rychter, 1962) suppressed one or more aortic arches on one or both sides. Vogel and McClenhan (1951 as cited by Rychter, 1962) occluded the carotid arteries of 6-day incubation chick by electrocauterization, resulting in carotid stenosis with anencephaly. The results from these studies were inconclusive and thus Rychter (1962) undertook to suppress development of virtually every possible combination of aortic arches 3, 4, and 6 mechanically using a microclip. If the clips were applied before the formation of the arch artery or during early development, they evoked agenesis of that aortic arch artery. This coincided with persistence of vessels that normally undergo regression. As might be expected, suppression and persistence of various combinations of arches altered

---

FIGURE 13. A stage 14 quail embryo labeled with QH-1, an antibody to quail endothelium and endothelial precursors (red), and HNK-1, an antibody to migrating neural crest cells (green). The embryo has been sectioned transversely through the pharyngeal area of the quail embryo to demonstrate the cord of endothelial precursors that will become the 3rd arch artery. Neural crest cells (NC) have migrated from the neural tube (nt) into the circumpharyngeal area and into the prospective 3rd pharyngeal arch area. As the crest cells migrate into the pharyngeal arch they separate the lumenizing endothelial cord (white arrow) away from the pharyngeal endoderm (en). More ventrally, where the neural crest cells have not yet migrated, the endothelial precursors still remain against the pharynx (*). ACV, anterior cardinal vein; DAo, dorsal aorta; ec, ectoderm, P, pharynx.

FIGURE 17. Diagram showing the anterior expression boundaries of *Hox* genes in paralogous groups 1–4. The anterior limit of expression of paralogous group 2 is pharyngeal arch 2, that of paralogous groups 3 and 4 are pharyngeal arches 3 and 4, and paralogous group 5 has its anterior limit of expression at the arch 4/6 boundary. Thus, paralogous groups 3, 4, and 5 are most likely to be involved in patterning of the great arteries because they are derived from arches 3, 4, and 6. (from Kirby et al. 1996.)

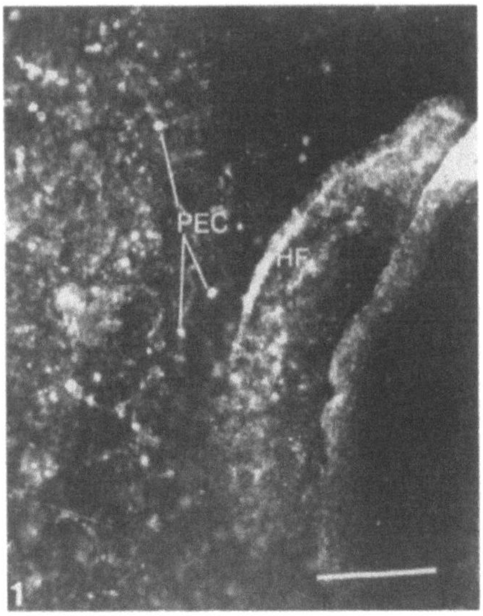

A

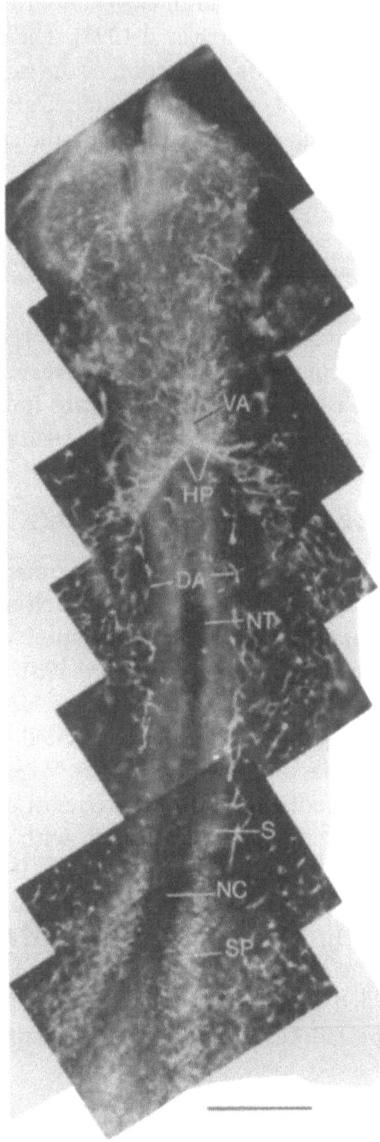

B

FIGURE 10. Developing embryonic vasculature in the quail embryo visualized using the antibody QH-1, a monoclonal antibody to quail endothelial precursor cells and quail endothelium. **A.** In the 1-somite embryo QH-1 positive endothelial precursors gather to form angiogenic islands that will become the dorsal aorta. PEC, presumptive endothelial cells; HF, head fold. **B.** A composite of a 4-somite embryo illustrates the developing cardiac primordia (HP), which join at the anterior intestinal portal to form the future heart tube (VA). The first pair of aortic arch arteries develop cranial to this area. The dorsal aorta (DA), not yet formed, consists of islands of angioblastic cells that will join to form the paired dorsal aortae. NT, neural tube; S, somite; SP, segmental plate; NC, notochord. (from Coffin and Poole 1988.)

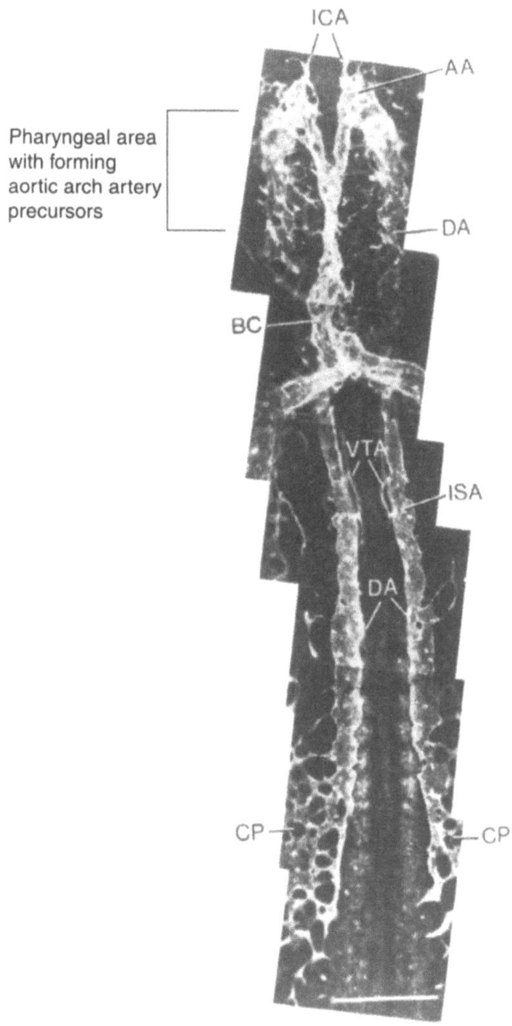

FIGURE 11. The forming vasculature of the 12-somite quail is labeled with the QH-1 antibody. The paired 1st-aortic arch arteries (AA) have formed and link the heart tube (BC) with the paired dorsal aortae (DA). Between the heart tube and the 1st arch arteries strands of endothelial precursors demarcate the future aortic arch arteries. CP, capillary plexuses; ICA, internal carotid artery; ISA, intersomitic arteries; VTA, vertebral arties. (from Coffin and Poole 1988.)

the final patterning of the arch derivatives in various abnormal (and largely unpredictable) patterns. It has been convenient to classify the result of these experiments as caused by altered hemodynamic patterns. If the hemodynamics of the early cardiovascular system were completely understood, these patterns might be predictable. Although it is known that there is a pressure gradient across the aortic arches early in development in chick embryos (Clark 1995), hemodynamic attributes of the aortic arch arteries are not well characterized, and so it has been more

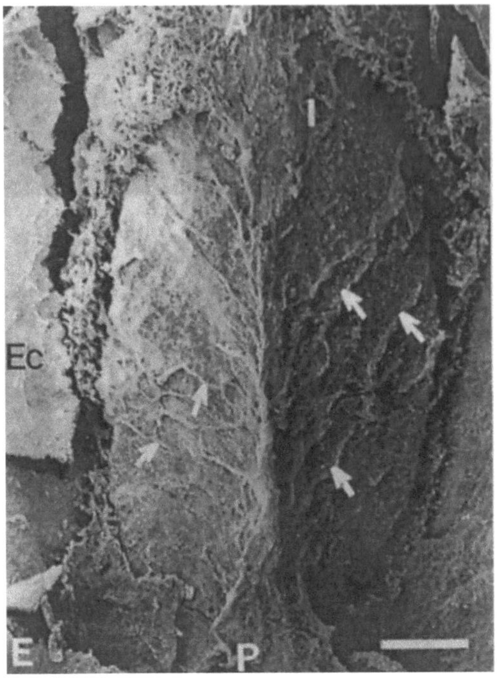

FIGURE 12. A scanning electron micrograph of the ventral surface of the pharynx in an 8-somite quail embryo in which the promyocardium and the lumenized endocardium have been dissected, illustrating the cords of endothelial precursors (white arrows) which will provide endothelial cells for constructing the aortic arch arteries, growing against the pharynx. A, anterior; Ec, ectoderm; H, head mesenchyme; I, 1st pair of aortic arch arteries; P, posterior. (from DeRuiter et al 1993.)

informative to learn about the developing aortic arch arteries using alternate approaches.

Experimental work with chick-quail chimeras has established that the tunica media of the aortic arch arteries is formed from neural crest-derived ectomesenchyme rather than mesodermally derived mesenchyme (Le Lièvre and Le Douarin 1975 Noden 1978; Kirby et al 1983; Miyagawa-Tomita et al 1991). The 3 caudal pharyngeal arches are populated by this ectomesenchyme before lumenization of the arch arteries (Kuratani and Kirby 1991). The ectomesenchyme supplements a core of mesodermally derived mesenchyme already present in each pharyngeal arch (Johnston 1966; Weston 1970). As the cords of endothelial precursors begin to lumenize to form arch arteries, they are separated from the pharyngeal endoderm by the ectomesenchyme (Fig. 13) (Waldo et al 1996). Subsequently the ectomesencymal cells in each pharyngeal arch gradually become arranged in concentric layers around the endothelial lumen. Later in development, the layers of ectomesenchymal cells first begin to develop reticular fibers, then elastin fibers followed by smooth muscle cell differentiation, and finally collagen fibers appear (Hughes 1943; Le Lièvre and Le Douarin 1975). Elastogenesis appears initially near the heart and proceeds distally along the aortic arch arteries (Hughes 1943; Rosenquist et al 1988). Smooth muscle actin is expressed transiently in the periendothelial part of the wall of the aortic arch arteries early in development. Much later in development, subsequent to differentiation of the smooth muscle cells, the entire thickness of the tunica media of the great arteries reexpresses smooth muscle-actin. As with elastogenesis, this process is initiated near the heart and progresses distally, starting with the adventitial perimeter and progressing toward the arterial lumen (Beall and Rosenquist 1990).

Although the early patterning of the pharyngeal arterial basket is similar in avians and humans, the final configuration of the great arteries varies for each species, depending, in part, on which arch arteries persist or go away. Experiments by Noden (1987, 1988) have suggested that blood vessels are patterned by interactions between the endothelium, the local mesenchyme, and the extracellular matrix. Experimental data have shown that endothelial precursors in transplanted mesoderm will migrate into craniofacial mesenchyme to take part in the patterning and histodifferentiation of vessels unique to the region they have migrated into, suggesting that endothelial cells receive messages from the surrounding environment, rather than receiving intrinsic cues (Noden 1987, 1988). From these data it could be hypothesized that the mesenchyme of the pharyngeal arches affects the patterning of the arch arteries, their histodifferentiation, and in part, their transformation into the adult configuration. The significance of this endothelial–mesenchymal interaction in the pharyngeal arches has been supported by neural crest ablations in chick and quail, and by antisense experiments in chick (see below).

The ectomesenchyme that migrates into pharyngeal arches 3, 4, and 6 is derived from neural crest cells that leave the hindbrain neural tube between the mid-otic placode and the posterior limit of somite 3 (rhombomeres 6, 7, and 8) (Fig. 14). These crest cells are called "cardiac neural crest" because a subpopulation of ectomesenchyme migrating to the 3 caudal pharyngeal arches continues into the heart to participate in aorticopulmonary septation (Fig. 15) (Kirby et al 1985). If the cardiac neural crest is ablated before leaving the neural tube, absence of the ectomesenchyme occurs, leaving only a core of mesodermally derived mesenchyme in the 3 caudal pharyngeal arches (Bockman et al 1989). This core of mesenchyme seems incapable of supporting sustained growth by the aortic arch arteries because anomalies of the great arteries occur in unpredictable patterns (Fig. 16). Some of the most common anomalies seen in neural crest-ablated chick embryos include ectopic or variable absences of the brachiocephalic arteries, interruption of the aorta, and absence of the ductus arteriosus (Nishibatake et al 1987). Neural crest ablation studies by Bockman and associates (Bockman et al 1987, 1989) demonstrated that the loss of ectomesenchyme can cause defects in aortic arch arteries even before the time that outflow septation occurs. Recently, a neural crest ablation experiment compared the developing 3rd aortic arch artery in embryos with and without cardiac neural crest (Waldo et al 1996), using QH-1 antibody to label the endothelium and endothelial precursors (Dieterlen-Lievre 1984; Pardanaud et al 1987), and HNK-1 to label migrating neural crest cells (Vincent et al 1983; Loring and Erickson 1987). It was shown that the endothelial precursor cords destined to form an arch artery lumenize normally but fail to become separated from the endoderm of the pharynx in the absence of ectomesenchyme. Development of the artery proceeded normally until blood flow was initiated, at which point the vessel became progressively more misshapen and by stage 18 became bilaterally asymmetrical. In subsequent stages unpredictable disappearance of arch arteries follows (Bockman et al 1987, 1989). These results suggest that the formation of an arch artery is independent of the presence of ectomesenchyme. However, the stability of the arch artery and its persistence is dependent on interactions between the endothelium and the neural crest-derived ectomesenchyme be-

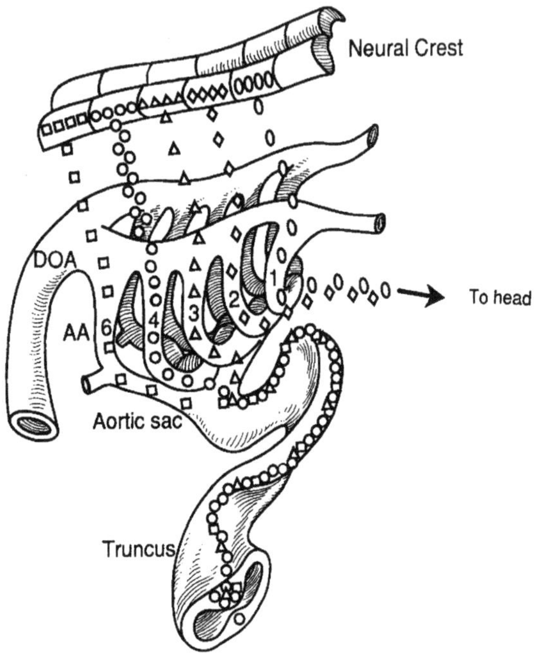

FIGURE 14. The neural crest cells that migrate to the pharyngeal arches are derived from specific rhombomeres of the hindbrain. Some of the cardiac neural crest cells that migrate to the 3 posterior pharyngeal arches (arches 3, 4, and 6) continue on into the cardiac outflow tract to form the aorticopulmonary septum. A majority of the cells that form the aorticopulmonary septum migrate through the 4th pharyngeal arches. The neural crest cells that migrate through the 1st and 2nd pharyngeal arches form many of the structures in the head. (from Kirby and Waldo 1990.)

cause the core of mesodermally derived mesenchyme remaining in the pharyngeal arches after crest ablation is incompetent to sustain continued growth of the arch arteries after blood flow is initiated.

The ectomesenchyme that migrates to the pharyngeal arches from the neural tube, not only contributes to the tunica media of the aortic arch arteries, but also to the connective tissue, cartilage, nerves, and glandular tissues derived from each pharyngeal arch (Horstadius 1950; Le Douarin 1982). It is believed that these cells may receive patterning instructions in the hindbrain, before their migration from the neural tube, and that these patterning instructions are carried into the pharyngeal arches by the migrating cells. The most likely candidate genes with segmental expression in the caudal hindbrain are *Hox* genes. Neural crest cells migrating to the persisting aortic arches, that is 3, 4, and 6, are derived from rhombomeres 6, 7, and 8. The anterior boundaries of expression of *Hox* genes in paralogous groups 3, 4, and 5 correspond exactly with the anterior boundaries of these rhombomeres, respectively, making these groups the most likely to be involved in patterning of the persisting aortic arch arteries (Fig. 17) (Hunt et al 1991). The function of the *Hox* proteins in paralogous groups 3, 4, and 5 has been suppressed in the neural crest-derived cells migrating to the 3 caudal pharyngeal arches of chick embryos by applying antisense oligonucleotides to the premigratory cardiac neural crest. Suppression of group 3 *Hox* proteins caused aortic arch 3 to regress in a manner similar

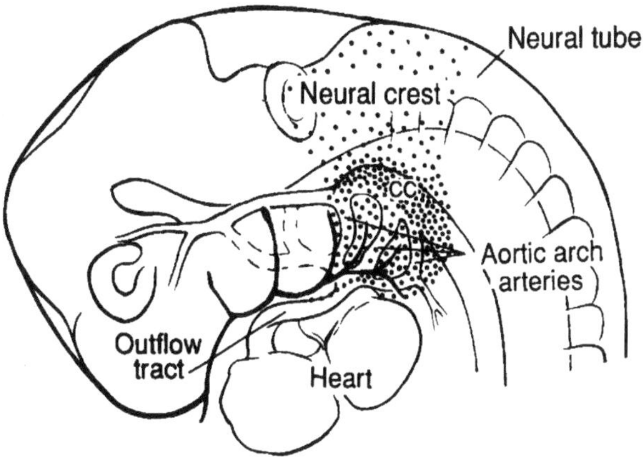

FIGURE 15. From data derived from chick embryos, the migratory pathway of the human cardiac neural crest cells would probably look similar to this diagram of the human embryo. The cardiac neural crest cells derived from the neural tube between the mid-otic placode and the posterior limit of somite 3 migrate through pharyngeal arches 3, 4, and 6 and into the cardiac outflow tract. As the neural crest cells migrate to the pharyngeal arches, they pause briefly in the circumpharyngeal area (CC) before descending into the arches. Some of the neural crest cells will remain in the pharyngeal arches to form the smooth muscle wall of the arch arteries.

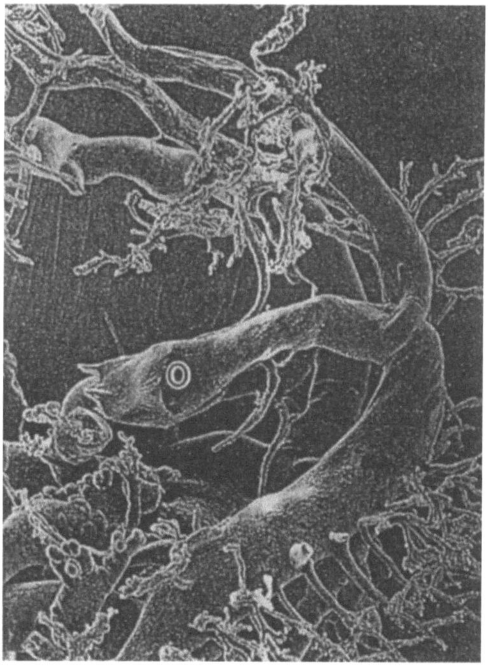

FIGURE 16. Scanning electron micrograph of a Mercox cast of a day 4 chick embryo in which the cardiac neural crest was ablated before its migration from the neural tube to the pharyngeal arches. Viewed from the left with the head toward the top of the micrograph. The symmetrical pattern of the pharyngeal aortic arch arteries normally seen at this stage is gone, leaving only one vessel rather than three pairs of vessels to connect the heart with the dorsal aorta and carotid arteries. (from Bockman et al 1989.) O, outflow tract.

to aortic arch 2. Similar suppression of group 4 *Hox* proteins produced no aortic arch phenotype, whereas inactivation of group 5 *Hox* proteins caused the appearance of an additional pharyngeal arch containing a novel and completely independent aortic arch artery. Because respecification of arch 4 to arch 3 should not be associated with an aortic arch phenotype, each of the phenotypes produced by inactivation of paralogous group 3, 4, or 5 *Hox* proteins is consistent with a shift of the phenotype of the arch to that of a more anterior arch. This provides the first evidence that aortic arch identity is under the control of *Hox* genes (Kirby et al 1997). The altered aortic arch phenotypes were not associated with heart defects.

Little is known about molecular mechanisms that regulate blood vessel differentiation (Schlaeger et al 1995). Recent experiments have identified some of the factors that influence endothelial cell growth and patterning. The cytokines that are known to stimulate angiogenic responses are vascular endothelial growth factor (VEGF), platelet-derived growth factor (PDGF), and insulin-like growth factor-1 (IGF-1) (Nicosia et al 1994). Both PDGF and IGF-1 appear to have more influence on vessel matrix and wall development than on endothelial development. The sites and times of expression of VEGF, also called vascular permeability factor (VPF) because of its ability to make blood vessels leaky, suggest a direct role for this cytokine during vasculogenesis and angiogenesis (Jakeman et al 1993; Nicosia et al 1994). Three tyrosine kinase receptors are known to be responsive to VEGF: *Flt-1* (*Fms*-like tyrosine kinase-1), and *Flk-1* and *Flk-4*, (Millauer et al 1993; Nicosia et al 1994; Seetharam et al 1995; Borg et al 1995). These receptors are coexpressed in endothelial cells, and *Flt-1* is known to mediate strong activation of the mitogen-activated protein (MAP) kinases (Seetharam et al 1995). Embryos lacking the ability to make *Flt-1* protein form endothelial cells in embryonic and extraembryonic tissues, but the cells are assembled into abnormal vascular channels and the animals die at midsomite stages (Fong et al 1995). On the other hand, *Flk-1* is expressed in yolk sac blood island progenitors and marks putative common endothelial and hematopoietic precursors. Absence of *Flk-1* expression is associated with absence of blood island differentiation and early embryonic death (Shalaby et al 1995). Thus *Flt-1* may regulate cell–cell or cell–matrix interactions of the endothelial cell rather than its ability to proliferate or differentiate whereas it is likely that *Flk-1* is associated with proliferation or differentiation of endothelial cells. *Tie-1* is another tyrosine kinase receptor that is expressed uniquely in endothelial cells, but its ligand is not known. Embryos deficient in *Tie-1* fail to establish structural integrity of vascular endothelial cells, resulting in edema and localized hemorrhage (Sato et al 1995). *Tie-2* is also expressed in endothelial cell precursors, and animals that are unable to make *Tie-2* protein fail to establish vascular endothelial networks in early development (Sato et al 1995). PECAM-1 (platelet-endothelial cell adhesion molecule-1) is a member of the immunoglobulin family that is expressed by endothelial cells and appears to mediate cell–cell adhesion (Baldwin and Buck 1994).

Fibroblast growth factor (FGF) is secreted by mature aortic endothelial cells but there is some question as to whether FGF plays a role in embryonic angiogenesis and vasculogenesis (Vlodavsky et al 1987). FGF is known to be a mitogen in angiogenesis during would healing and tumor growth. Smooth muscle cell growth appears to be regulated by FGF-2 and PDGF. FGF-2 is known to promote smooth muscle differentiation of neural crest cells (Murphy et al 1994).

Vascular cell adhesion molecule (VCAM-1) is a transmembrane protein that belongs to the immunoglobulin superfamily. VCAM-1 function is primarily associated with interactions of white cells with endothelial cells. It is expressed in developing myocardium particularly in regions of atrioventricular and outflow septation and in the yolk sac at sites of hematopoiesis. Targeted disruption of VCAM-1 causes a reduction of the compact layer of the ventricular myocardium and intraventricular septum. Most significantly though, the hearts lack an epicardium (Kwee et al 1995).

FORMATION OF THE AORTA AND PULMONARY TRUNKS

As a result of septation of the distal cardiac outflow tract, including the aortic sac, the truncoaortic sac is divided into aortic and pulmonary channels, which will become the aortic and pulmonary roots, and the proximal parts of the ascending aorta and the pulmonary trunk (Van Mierop 1979a). Thus in humans, although the persisting left fourth arch artery is usually described as the definitive aorta, in reality it forms, along with the caudal portion of the left dorsal aorta, a small segment of the arch of the adult aorta (Congdon 1992; Barry 1951; Skandalakis et al 1994). The descending portion of the thoracic aorta originates from the unpaired embryonic aorta (Barry 1951). In the chick, the ascending aorta and its arch are derived from the right 4 arch artery, which is continuous with the truncoaortic sac ventrally, and from a new segment of the right dorsal aorta created by a secondary division of the single dorsal aorta (Hughes 1943; Romanoff 1960).

The human pulmonary trunk is formed from a small part of the aortic sac and through fusion of the most proximal parts of the 6 arch arteries. As this occurs, the proximal part of the left 6 arch artery is absorbed and becomes the bifurcation of the pulmonary trunk. The left pulmonary artery derives from the primitive pulmonary artery. The definitive right pulmonary artery corresponds to the right proximal 6 arch artery and the primitive pulmonary artery (Congdon 1922; Skidmore 1975; Skandalakis et al 1994). As in humans, the pulmonary trunk of the chick is partially derived from the truncoaortic sac. It is unclear whether the proximal 6 arch arteries are absorbed into, or are fused to form part of, the pulmonary trunk. The definitive right and left pulmonary arteries that branch from the pulmonary trunk are formed from the proximal part of the 6th arch artery and the primitive pulmonary artery on each side of the embryo (Waldo and Kirby 1993b).

Septation of the truncoaortic sac occurs as a result of the formation of the AP septum from condensed ectomesenchyme derived from cardiac neural crest cells (Kirby et al 1983). Although we have followed recent convention in referring to this as the AP septum, the septum has three components: a true aorticopulmonary septal component in the aortic sac dividing the base of the aorta and pulmonary trunk, a truncal component dividing the semilunar valves, and a conal component dividing the intracardiac portion of the outflow tract proximal to the valves. This distinction becomes important in considering AP window, which is a defect in the distal portion of the outflow septum that does not involve the more proximal portions of the septum. Experimental studies have shown that complete ablation of cardiac neural crest cells results in persistent truncus arteriosus in which a single arterial trunk overrides the ventricular septum or originates directly from the right ventricle. Partial ablation of the cardiac neural crest results in variable defects, including dextroposed aorta, overriding aorta, tetralogy of Fallot, and double-outlet right ventricle (Kirby et al 1985; Nishibatake et al 1987). All may be accompanied by variable anomalies of the great arteries as previously described. Three percent to ten percent of cases of persistent truncus arteriosus and dextroposed aorta defects occur with inflow anomalies, such as tricuspid atresia, straddling tricuspid valve, and double-inlet left ventricle (Nishibatake et al 1987). AP window has never been seen after neural crest ablation and is assumed to have an origin distinct from global neural crest dysfunction (Kutsche and Van Mierop 1987).

MALFORMATIONS OF THE AORTIC ARCH COMPLEX

General

The formation of arterial or vascular rings has been and continues as a major method to understand many malformations of the aortic arch system (Fig. 18). Stewart and coworkers (1964) proposed that formation of the normal aortic arch system depends on regression of the 8th segment of the right dorsal aortic root (the portion of the dorsal aorta between the origins of the 7th and 8th intersegmental arteries). In addition, regression of the carotid duct (ductus caroticus), the segment of the dorsal aorta between the 3rd and 4th aortic arch arteries, must occur bilaterally to commit the blood flow in the 3rd arch artery to the head. Abnormal sites of regression are usually in four specific locations: the right or left arches or the right or left 8th dorsal aortic segment (Stewart et al 1964). Regressions can also occur in either of the distal 6th arch arteries. The regressions can be unilateral or bilateral

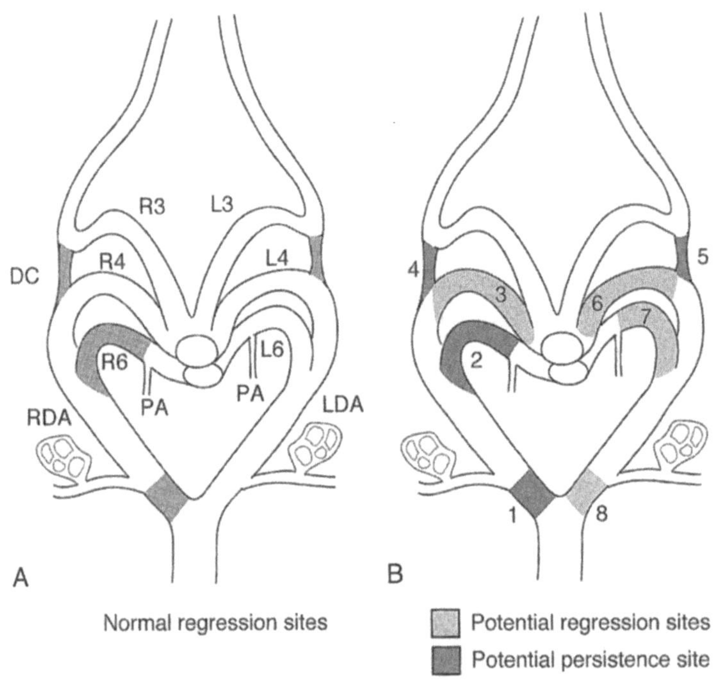

FIGURE 18. The drawing on the left illustrates the normal sites of vessel regression to produce normally patterned great arteries and the drawing on the right shows the potential sites of regression that are seen in human malformations involving abnormal patterning of the great arteries. R3, L3, right and left third arch artery; R4, L4, right and left fourth arch artery; R6, L6, right and left sixth arch artery; PA, pulmonary artery; DC, carotid duct; RDA, LDA, right and left dorsal aorta.

(Fig. 18). Stewart and colleagues (1964) classify improper regressions of these four sites into four groups: (1) double aortic arch in which there is complete double aortic arch with no interruption, (2) left aortic arch, (3) right aortic arch, and (4) rare malformations in which there are combinations of interruptions at all four sites. The most common vascular rings or slings are double arch, left arch with brachiocephalic artery compression of the trachea, left arch with right descending aorta, and right arch (Moes and Freedom 1992).

Abnormalities of Aortic Arch Artery 3 Derivatives

Aortic arch 3 is not generally subject to regressions, perhaps because of hemodynamic load. However, it can have an aberrant origin and the subclavian contralateral to the aortic arch has a high incidence of abnormal origin. Aberrant brachiocephalic artery (Skandalakis et al 1994) is characterized by origin of the left common carotid from the brachiocephalic trunk. In this case there can be independent origin of the left vertebral artery from the aortic arch.

Cervical aortic arch complex has three components: (1) the apex of the arch is in the neck; (2) there is a separate origin of the carotid contralateral to the arch with anomalous origin of the subclavian artery contralateral to the arch from the descending aorta; and (3) a retroesophageal descending thoracic aorta crosses contralateral to the side of the aortic arch (Sissman 1983). This complex is found with equal frequency in left- and right-sided arches. Because it most often occurs with malformations of branches of arch 3, it may be caused by a persistence of the embryonic 3 aortic arch rather than the 4th as the definitive aortic arch. In this case the carotid duct would fail to regress, leaving arch 3 connected to the descending aorta rather than being committed to the head.

Abnormalities of Aortic Arch Artery 4 Derivatives

The ascending aorta arises form the base of the left ventricle behind the left sternal margin opposite the 3rd costal cartilage. The dilated origin of the aorta is referred to as the aortic bulb because of its radiographic appearance. The arch of the aorta begins behind the 2nd rib cartilage and traverses posteriorly behind the lower part of the sternal manubrium to join the thoracic aorta at the left of the vertebral column about the level of the 4th thoracic vertebra. According to Weinberg (1995), the aortic arch is derived from the aortic portion of the truncus (aortic semilunar valve), the left branch of the truncoaortic sac (ascending aorta), the left 4th aortic arch (aortic arch proper), the left dorsal aorta between the left 4th and 6th arch arteries (aorta between the left carotid and ligamentum arteriosus), and the left dorsal aorta distal to arch artery 6 (thoracic aorta just distal to the ligamentum arteriosus).

Great variations can be found in the origins of the vessels arising from the aortic arch (McVay 1984). The most common anomaly is mirror image right aortic arch. Right-sided aortic arch occurs in 13% to 34% of patients with tetralogy of Fallot and about 8% with transposition of the great arteries (Weinberg 1995). Double aortic arch results from failure of regression of the embryonic right 8th dorsal aortic segment (Fig. 18, potential persistence site 1). It was first described in 1737 by Hommel (cited by Stewart et al 1964). In double aortic arch, both left and right aortic arches arise by branching from the ascending aorta (Sissman 1983). These unite posteriorly to form a single descending aorta, which can lie on either left or unite posteriorly to form a single descending aorta, which can lie on either left or right sides of the vertebral column. In true double aortic arch, three major trunks arise from each side of the arch: subclavian, internal carotid, and external carotid (McVay 1984). Abnormal regression of the right 4th arch with persistent patency of the right 8th dorsal aortic segment results in an aberrant right subclavian in which the right subclavian arises distal to the left subclavian and courses behind the esophagus, producing a retroesophageal subclavian (Fig. 18, sites 1 and 3). This is the second most common anomaly of the aortic arch system with an incidence of 0.9% in the general population (Weinberg 1995). It is frequently seen in conjunction with tetralogy of Fallot and coarctation of the aorta (Sissman 1983), and it occurs in high frequency (38%) in Down's patients with congenital heart disease (Weinberg 1995). Because it is found with cardiac malformations in the neural crest spectrum, it may be related to abnormal function of arch 4 neural crest.

An aortic arch with a double lumen can occur. In this case the arch between the origins of the brachiocephalic artery and left subclavian has two separate lumina (Sissman 1983). This has been thought to be caused by persistence of a 5th arch. Interestingly, molecular studies eliminating the expression of paralogous group 5 *Hox* genes in chick cardiac neural crest causes a similar condition. In this case the animals developed an extra arch 4-like artery that persisted as a bifid aorta (Kirby et al 1995).

Circumflex retroesophageal aortic arch occurs when the left aortic arch turns medially to cross the midline behind the esophagus and descends on the right of the thoracic vertebrae (Sissman 1983). A right aortic arch can also cross the midline and descend on the left side of the thoracic vertebrae.

In right-sided aortic arch, the ascending aorta and aortic arch pass anterior to the right mainstem bronchus and then posterior to the right of the trachea and esophagus (Fig. 18, sites 6 and 8) (Sissman 1983). If this condition occurs with no retroesophageal component, that is as a mirror-image of normal, it is usually associated with intracardiac defects. If the right aortic arch extends to the left behind the esophagus, there is an extension with a diverticulum from which an aberrant left subclavian arises associated with a left ductus. This is a retroesophageal component that is not a circumflex aortic arch and is not usually associated with intracardiac defects.

Coarctation of the aorta is a constriction of the aorta located at the junction of the thoracic aorta and aortic arch just distal to the left subclavian (Gersony 1983). The "adult" type of coarctation is located just distal to the ligamentum arteriosum and predominates over the preductal variety in frequency of occurrence (McVay 1984). It is frequently associated with intracardiac lesions although isolated coarctation is the 5th or 6th most common of congenital cardiovascular defects. The classification of coarctation is based on the presence or absence of severe isthmic narrowing as opposed to discrete obstruction and major associated lesions. In long segment isthmic narrowing the blood to the lower body is provided via the ductus arteriosus. The evolution of coarctation of the aorta is thought to be an active process resulting in an increasing degree of obstruction and low pressure gradient with time.

Hemodynamic theory holds that interruption of the aortic arch causes severe isthmic narrowing leading to discrete coarctation. This can be caused by any cardiac abnormality that decreases antegrade aortic flow and increases pulmonary artery and ductal flow. A contraductal shelflike structure divides the ductal flow between the left subclavian and descending aorta. In pseudocoarctation of the aorta, the distal portion of the aortic arch and proximal portion of the upper descending aorta are abnormally elongated, tortuous, and kinked, having the appearance of a number 3 from the left side (Sissman 1983; Skandalakis et al 1994). This is associated with lesions of the aortic valve.

Complete interruption of the aorta is associated with abnormal regression of aortic arch 4 (Fig. 18, sites 6 and 8) (Sissman 1983; Skandalakis et al 1994). In this condition the continuity of the aorta is interrupted. Interruption is classified into 3 types: A, B, and C. In type A the interruption is distal to the left subclavian. In type B the interruption is between the left carotid and left subclavian. In type C it is proximal to the origin of the left carotid. In subclassifications A2 and B2 the right subclavian arises anomalously from the distal aortic segment. Type B is the most common. Almost all accompany intracardiac defects and patent ductus arteriosus. They can occur with ventricular septal defect, subaortic stenosis, bicuspid aortic valve, persistent truncus arteriosus, and AP window.

Abnormalities of Aortic Arch Artery 6 Derivatives

The ductus arteriosus is the distal portion of the left 6th aortic arch that connects the left pulmonary artery with the descending aorta (Heymann 1983). It is 5 to 10 mm distal to the origin of the left subclavian. The ductus has a length of only 4 mm with a diameter of 10 mm, similar to that of the descending aorta. The tunica media of the ductus consists of dense layers of smooth muscle arranged spirally leftward and rightward. The tunica intima is thicker than that of the adjoining arteries and has an increased amount of mucoid substance. Small thin-walled vessels can be found in the subendothelial region. Development of bilateral ductus followed by regression of the right ductus is inferred in man because of two pieces of information: right-sided or bilateral ductus does occur occasionally in human malformations (Stewart et al 1964), and in mice the ductus arteriosus can be observed in timed series to develop bilaterally with subsequent regression on the right side (personal observation), leaving a single left-sided ductus. By the 6th week of gestation the ductus arteriosus carries the major portion of the right ventricular output. Postnatal closure of the ductus involves contraction of the smooth muscles of the tunica media, which causes shortening and increased wall thickness. This leads to protrusion of the intima into the lumen effecting a functional closure. By 2 to 3 weeks postnatally, there is dusruption and proliferation of the subintimal layers with small hemorrhages and necrosis leading to connective tissue formation and fibrosis.

Congenital defects of the ductus include persistent patency (Heymann 1983). Maintenance of patency during fetal life is dependent on prostaglandins and to some extent on arterial oxygen tension. After parturition prostaglandin inhibitors in the inflated lungs work to decrease the circulating levels of prostaglandins. In addition the smooth muscle in the tunica media is sensitive to oxygen and contracts with increased arterial oxygen tension. It is not known what causes the ductus to remain patent when it is an isolated defect. If the arch of the aorta is right-sided the ductus arteriosus may be on the right connecting the right pulmonary artery and right aortic arch distal to the right subclavian. More commonly it is on the left joining the left pulmonary and proximal left subclavian. More commonly it is on the left joining the left pulmonary and proximal left subclavian. It is rarely bilateral (although we have pointed out that the normal ductus arteriosus in birds is bilateral). Ductus arteriosus sling is a 4-mm vessel branching from the right pulmonary artery between the trachea and esophagus to join the aorta opposite the origin of an anomalous right subclavian artery (Sissman 1983).

The pulmonary artery can have an anomalous origin. The bilateral pulmonary arteries develop originally as branches from the base of their respective 4th arch arteries and are subsequently shifted to the 6th arches when the ductus arteriosus forms. In anomalous left pulmonary artery (vascular sling), the normal left pulmonary artery is not present. The vessel functioning as the left pulmonary artery arises from the main or right pulmonary artery and courses right, then dorsally, then left encircling the right bronchus just distal to the carina (Sissman 1983). It passes left between the trachea and esophagus and enters the left lung (Stewart et al 1964). Associated anomalies can include patent ductus arteriosus, atrial septal defect, left superior vena cava, and tracheal abnormalities. A pulmonary artery can originate from the ascending aorta, usually about 1 cm above the aortic semilunar valve from the side or posteriorly (Sissman 1983). This can be associated with patent ductus arteriosus, ventricular septal defect, or tetralogy of Fallot. These defects may represent abnormal regression of the proximal left 6th arch (Sissman 1983; Morrow and Huhta 1990), which almost always occurs on the side opposite the aortic arch.

Aortic Sac

Hypoplastic left heart syndrome, also called aortic atresia, occurs with underdevelopment of the left atrium, mitral valve, left ventricle, aorta, and aortic valve (Freedom 1983). The left ventricle is normal in only 2% to 7% of patients with aortic atresia. All have a ventricular septal defect and perforate mitral valve.

Aortic stenosis can occur in four forms: valvular aortic stenosis; subaortic stenosis; narrowing of the supravalvular ascending aorta; and idiopathic hypertrophic subaortic stenosis. Valvular aortic stenosis occurs in 3% to 6% of patients with congenital heart disease (Friedman and Benson 1983). It consists of thickening and increased rigidity of the valve tissue. Congenital bicuspid aortic valve is frequently associated with valvular aortic stenosis and is the most common congenital malformation of the heart. It occurs 4 times more frequently in males than in females.

Discrete subaortic stenosis is found in 8% to 10% of aortic stenoses and occurs 2 times more frequently in males than in females (Chitnis et al 1995). In this condition, a membranous diaphragm or fibrous ring encircles the left ventricular outflow beneath the base of the aortic valve. It is uncommon but possible to have valvular with subvalvular aortic stenosis in which there is a tunnel-like narrowing of the left ventricular outflow tract. Small ascending aorta with hypoplasia of the aortic valve ring and thickened valve leaflets are hallmarks of subaortic stenosis.

In supravalvular aortic stenosis, also called hypoplasia of the aorta, the ascending aorta is narrowed from the superior margins of the aortic sinuses just above the coronary orifices (Chitnis et al 1995). The valve, valve ring, and left ventricle are all normal. The degree and length of narrowing of the lumen vary. Supravalvular aortic stenosis occurs with idiopathic infantile hypercalcemia thought for years to be caused by deranged vitamin D metabolism, but possibly caused by abnormal development of calcitonin-producing cells in the thyroid gland that are derived from neural crest cells in the 6th pharyngeal arch. In Williams syndrome, supravalvular aortic stenosis is associated with mental retardation, "elfin facies", narrowed peripheral systemic and pulmonary arteries, inguinal hernia, strabismus,

TABLE 1. **Association of Arch Artery Defects With Neural Crest**

No Association	Probable Association
1 Double aortic arch	1 Interrupted aortic arch
5 Interrupted arch—type C	2 Supravalvular stenosis (hypoplasia)
6 Patent ductus arteriosus	3 Aortic arch with double lumen
7 AP window	4 Right-sided aortic arch
	5 Interrupted arch—type A
	6 Bilateral ductus arteriosus
	7 Supravalvular stenosis
	8 Retroesophageal subclavian

and abnormal dental development. This condition is now known to be linked with a defect in the elastin gene on chromosome 7 (Johnson et al 1995)

Pulmonary stenosis can occur in 25% to 30% of individuals with congenital heart disease. The stenosis may involve the right ventricular cavity or conus, the pulmonary valve and the pulmonary trunk, or the pulmonary arteries. Pulmonary stenosis is a key feature of tetralogy of Fallot. It is most likely caused by unequal division of the aortic sac by the most cranial part of the outflow septum (Emmanouilides and Baylen 1983).

Complete absence of the outflow septum results in persistent truncus arteriosus (clinically known as truncus arteriosus). This is an uncommon congenital malformation apparently caused by malfunction of cardiac neural crest. It is most frequently associated with other abnormalities involving cranial neural crest, such as craniofacial anomalies, and absence or hypoplasia of the glands derived from the pharyngeal arches. This constellation of abnormalities has recently been classified under the name CATCH-22 because it is frequently associated with a microdeletion in the region of human chromosome 22q11 (Johnson et al 1995). In the chick a similar constellation of abnormalities is caused by neural crest ablation (Kirby and Waldo 1995).

AP window (also called AP septal defect) is a rare anomaly in which an abnormal communication occurs between the aorta and pulmonary trunk somewhere between the semilunar valves and the bifurcation of the pulmonary trunk. Skandalakis and associates (1994) classify AP window into 3 types depending on the size and characteristics of the border of the defect. The lower border of the window is usually just distal to the coronary artery ostia. This and several other malformations of the aortic arch artery system have no known association with neural crest (Table 1).

REFERENCES

Bakst HJ, Chaffe FH. 1928. The origin of the definitive subclavian artery in the chick embryo. Anat Rec 38:129–40.

Baldwin HS, Buck CA. 1994. Integrins and other cell adhesion molecules in cardiac development. Dev Biol 121:220–36.

Barry A. 1951. Aortic arch derivatives in the human adult. Anat Rec 111:221–28.

Beall AC, Rosenquist TH. 1990. Smooth muscle cells of neural crest origin form the aorticopulmonary septum in the avian embryo. Anat Rec 226:360–36.

Bockman DE, Redmond ME, Waldo K, Davis H, Kirby ML. 1987. Effect of neural crest ablation on development of the heart and arch arteries in the chick. Am J Anat 180:332–41.

Bochman DE, Redmond ME, Kirby ML. 1989. Alteration of early vascular development after ablation of cranial neural crest. Anat Rec 225:209–17.

Borg JP, DeLapeyrière O, Noguchi T, Rottapel R, Dubreuil P, Birnbaum D. 1995. Biochemical characterization of two isoforms of FLT4, a VEGF receptor-related tyrosine kinase. Oncogene 10:973–84.

Bremer JL. 1912. Aorta and aortic arches in rabbits. Am J Anat 13:111–28.

Buell CE. 1922. Origin of the pulmonary vessels in the chick. Carnegie Inst Contr Embryol 14:11–28.

Chitnis A, Henrique D, Lewis J, Ish-Horowicz D, Kintner C. 1995. Primary neurogenesis in *Xenopus* embryos regulated by a homologue of the *Drosophila* neurogenic gene *Delta*. Nature (Land) 375:761–66.

Clark EB. 1995. Growth, morphogenesis, and function. The dynamics of cardiac development. In: Moller JH, Neal WA, editors Fetal, neonatal, and infant cardiac disease Norwalk, CT: Appleton & Lange. p 3–24.

Coffin DJ, Poole TJ. 1998. Embryonic vascular development: immunohistochemical identification of the origin and subsequent morphogenesis of the major vessel primordia in quail embryos. Development (Camb) 102:735–48.

Congdon ED. 1992. Transformation of the aortic-arch system during the development of the human embryo. Carnegie Inst Contr Embryol 14:47–10.

Congdon ED, Wang HD. 1926. The mechanical processes concerned in the formation of the different types of aortic arches in the chick and the pig and in the divergent early development of their pulmonary arches. Am J Anat 37:499–520.

DeRuiter MC, Poelmann RE, Mentink MMT, Vaniperen L, Gittenberger- Groot AC. 1993 Early formation of the vascular system in quail embryos. Anat Rec 235:261–74.

Dieterlen-Lievre F. 1984. Emergence of intraembryonic blood stem cells in avian chimeras by means of monoclonal antibodies. Dev Comp Immunol 3: 75–80.

Dohrn A. 1885. Studien zur urgeschichte des wirbelthierkorpers. VII. Entstehung und differenzierung des zungenbeins und kieferapparates der selachier. Mitt Zool Stat Neapel 6:1–48.

Emmanouilides GC, Baylen BG. 1983. Pulmonary stenosis. In: Adams FH, and Emmanouilides GC, editors. Moss heart disease in infants, children, and adolescents. 3rd ed. Baltimore, MD: Williams & Wilkins. p 234–62.

Evans HM. 1909. On the development of the aortae, cardinal and umbilical veins and other blood vessels of vertebrate embryos from capillaries. Anat Rec 3:498–518.

Fedorow V. 1910. Uber die entwickelung der lungenvene. Anat Hefte. 1 bd 40:529–607.

Folkman J. 1985. Toward an understanding of angiogenesis: search and discovery. In: Garber, Edward D., editor, Perspectives in biology and medicine. 29th ed. Chicago, IL: University of Chicago Press. p 10–36.

Fong GH, Rossant J, et al. 1995. Role of the Flt-1 receptor tyrosine kinase in regulating the assembly of vascular endothelium. Nature (Lond) 376:66–70.

Freedom RM. 1983. Hypoplastic left heart syndrome. In: Adams FH, Emmanouilides GC, editors. Moss' heart disease in infants, children, and adolescents. 3rd ed. Baltimore, MD: Williams & Wilkins. p 411–22.

Friedman WF, and Benson LN. 1983. Aortic stenosis. In: Adams FH, Emmanouilides GC, editors. Moss' heart disease in infants, children, and adolescents. 3rd ed. Baltimore, MD: Williams & Wilkins. p 171–88.

Gersony WM. 1983. Coarctation of the aorta. In: Adams FH, Emmanouilides GC, editors. Moss' heart disease in infants, children, and adolescents. 3rd ed. Baltimore: Williams & Wilkins. p 188–99.

Getty R. 1975. Sisson and Grossman's The Anatomy of the Domestic Animals. Philadelphia: W.B. Saunders.

Gray H. 1973. Anatomy of the Human Body. 29th ed. Philadelphia: Lea & Febiger.

Heymann MA. 1983. Patent ductus arteriosus. In: Adams FH, Emmanouilides GC, editor.

MD Heart disease in infants, children, and adolescents. 3rd ed. Baltimore, MD: Williams & Wilkins. 158–71.
Hiss W. 1900. Lecithoblat un angioblast: Abhandelr math phys KK sachs gessellschaft wissenchaft. Abhandl. Math.-Phys. KI. K. sachs Ges. 25:171–328.
Horstadius, S. (1950) The Neural Crest. Its Properties and Derivatives in the Light of Experimental Research. London: Oxford University Press.
Hughes, A.F.W. (1934) On the development of the blood vessels in the head of the chick. Phil. Trans. R. Soc. Lon: B Biol Sci 224:75–129.
Hughes, A.F.W. (1943) The histogenesis of the arteries of the chick embryo. J. Anat. 77:266–287.
Hunt, P., Whiting, J., Muchamore, I., Marshall, H. and Krumlauf, R. (1991) Homeobox genes and models for patterning the hindbrain and branchial arches. Development (Camb) 112 (Suppl. 1):187–196.
Jakeman, L.B., Armanini, M., Phillips, H.S. and Ferrara, N. (1993) Developmental expression of binding sites and messenger ribonucleic acid for vascular endothelial growth factor suggests a role for this protein in vasculogenesis and angiogenesis. Endocrinology 133:848–59.
Johnson, M.C., Payne, R.M., Grant, J.W. and Strauss, A.W. (1995) The genetic basis of paediatric heart disease. Ann Med. 27:289–300.
Johnston, M.C. (1966) A radioautographic study of the migration and fate of cranial neural crest cells in the chick embryo. Anat. Rec. 156:143–156.
Kastschenko, N. (1887) Das schlundspaltgebiet des huhnchens. Arch. Anat. Physiol. Anat. Abst. 258–300.
Kirby, M.L., Gale, T.F. and Stewart, D.E. (1983) Neural crest cells contribute to aorticopulmonary septation. Science 220:1059-1061.
Kirby, M.L., Turnage, K.L. and Hays, B.M. (1985) Characterization of conotruncal malformations following ablation of "cardiac" neural crest. Anat. Rec. 213:87–93.
Kirby, M.L., Hunt, P. and Thorogood, P. (1997) Normal development of the cardiac outflow tract is not dependent on normal patterning of the aortic arch arteries. Dev. Dyn. 208:34–47.
Kirby ML, Waldo KL. 1995. Neural crest and cardiovascular patterning. Circ Res 77:211–5.
Kuratani SC, Kirby ML. 1991. Initial migration and distribution of the cardiac neural crest in the avian embryo: an introduction to the concept of the circumpharyngeal crest. Am. J. Anat. 191:215–27.
Kutsche LM, Van Mierop LHS. 1987. Anatomy and pathogenesis of aorticopulmonary septal defect. Am. J. Cardiol. 59:443–7.
Kutsche LM, Van Mierop LHS. 1988. Anomalous origin of a pulmonary artery from the ascending aorta: associated anomalies and pathogenesis. Am. J. Cardiol. 61 (10):850–856.
Kwee L, Baldwin HS, Shen HM, Stewart CL, Buck C, Buck CA, Labow MA. 1995. Defective development of the embryonic and extraembryonic circulatory systems in vascular cell adhesion molecule (VCAM-1) deficient mice. Development (Camb) 121:489–503.
Langman J. 1975. Medical Embryology. Baltimore, MD: Williams & Wilkins.
Le Douarin N. 1982. The Neural Crest. Cambridge: Cambridge University Press.
Lehman, H. 1905. On the embryonic history of the aortic arches in mammals. Anat. Anz. 26:406–424.
Le Lièvre CS, Le Douarin NM. 1975. Mesenchymal derivatives of the neural crest. Analysis of chimaeric quail and chick embryos. J. Embryol. Exp. Morphol. 34:125–54.
Lillie FR. 1952. Development of the Chick. New York: H. Half & Co.
Locy WA. 1995. The fifth and sixth aortic arches in chick embryo, with comments on the conditions of the same vessels in other vertebrates. Anat. Anz. 29:287–300.
Loring JF, Erickson CA. 1987. Neural crest cell migratory pathways in the trunk of the chick embryo. Dev. Biol. 121:220–36.
McVay C. 1984. Anson & McVay Surgical Anatomy. Philadelphia: W.B. Saunders.

Millauer B, Wizigmann-Voos S, Schnürch H, Martinez R, Moller NPH, Risau W, Ullrich A. 1993. High affinity VEGF binding and developmental expression suggest Flk-1 as a major regulator of vasculogenesis and angiogenesis. Cell 72:835–46.

Miyagawa-Tomita S, Waldo K, Tomita H, Kirby ML. 1991. Temporospatial study of the migration and distribution of cardiac neural crest in quail-chick chimeras. Am. J. Anat. 192, 79–88.

Moes CAF, Freedom RM. 1992. Rings, slings, and other things: vascular structures contributing to a neonatal "noose". In: Freedom RM, Benson LN, Smallhorn JF, editors. Neonatal heart disease. London: Springer-Verlag. p 731–49.

Morrow WR, Huhta JC. 1990. Aortic arch and pulmonary artery anomalies. In: Garson A, Bicker JT, McNamara DG, editors. The science and practice of pediatric cardiology. Philadelphia: Lea & Febiger. p 1421–52.

Murphy M, Reid K, et al. 1994. FGF2 regulates proliferation of neural crest cells, with subsequent neuronal differentiation regulated by LIF or related factors. Development (Camb) 120: 3519–28.

Netter FH. 1978. Embryology. In: Yonkman, Frederick F., editor, Heart, New York: CIBA p 111–30.

Nicosia RF, Nicosia SV, Smith M. 1994. Vascular endothelial growth factor, platelet-derived growth factor, and insulin-like growth factor-1 promote rat aortic angiogenesis in vitro. Am J Pathol 145: 1023–9.

Nishibatake M, Kirby ML, van Mierop LH. 1987. Pathogenesis of persistent truncus arteriosus and dextroposed aorta in the chick embryo after neural crest ablation. Circulation. 75: 255–64.

Noden DM. 1978. The control of avian cephalic neural crest cytodifferentiation. I. Skeletal and connective tissues. Dev Biol 67: 296–312.

Noden DM. 1987. Interactions between cephalic neural crest and mesodermal populations. In: Maderson, Paul, editor, Developmental and evolutionary aspects of the neural crest. New York: John Wiley & Sons. p 88–119.

Noden DM. 1988. Interactions and fates of avian craniofacial mesenchyme. Development (Camb) 103 (Suppl):121–40.

Noden DM. 1991. Cell movements and control of patterned tissue assembly during craniofacial development. J Craniofac Genet Dev Biol 11: 192–213.

Padget DH. 1948. Development of cranial arteries in human embryo. Contrib Embryol Carnegie Inst Wash 207: 205–12.

Pardanaud L, Altmann C, Kitos P, Dieterlen-Lievre F, Buck CA. 1987. Vasculogenesis in the early quail blastodisc as studied with a monoclonal antibody recognizing endothelial cells. Development (Camb) 100: 339–49.

Pardanaud L, Yassine F, Dieterlen-Lievre F. 1989. Relationship between vasculogenesis, angiogenesis and haemopoiesis during avian ontogeny. Development (Camb) 105: 473–485.

Pexieder T. 1969. Some quantitative aspects on the development of aortic arches in chick embryos between the 2nd and 8th day of incubation. Praha, Folia Morphol 17:273–90.

Phillips MTI, Waldo KL, Kirby ML. 1988. Neural crest ablation does not alter pulmonary vein development in the chick embryo. Anat Rec 223:292–98.

Reagan FP. 1915. Vascularization phenomena in fragments of embryonic bodies completely isolated from yolk-sac entoderm. Anat Rec 9:329–41.

Risau W, Lemmon V. 1988. Changes in the vascular extracellular matrix during embryonic vasculogenesis and angiogenesis. Dev Biol 125:441–50.

Romanoff AL. 1960. The Avian Embryo: Structural and Functional Development. New York: Macmillan.

Romer AS. 1963. The Vertebrate Body. Philadelphia: W.B. Saunders.

Rosenquist GC. 1970. Location and movements of cardiogenic cells in the chick embryo: the heart-forming portion of the primitive streak. Dev Biol 22:461–75.

Rosenquist TH, McCoy JR, Waldo KL, Kirby ML. 1988. Origin and propagation of elastogenesis in the developing cardiovascular system. Anat Rec 221:860–71.
Rychter Z. 1962. Experimental morphology of the aortic arches and the heart loop in chick embryos. Adv Morphog 2:333–71.
Sabin CG. 1905. The origin of the subclavian artery in the chick. Anat Anz 26:317–32.
Sabin FR. 1917. Origin and development of the primitive vessels of the chick and of the pig. Contrib Embryol Carnegie Inst Wash 6:63–124.
Sabin FR. 1920. Studies on the origin of the blood vessels and of red blood corpuscles as seen in the living blastoderm of chick during the second day of incubation. Carnegie Contrib Embryol 9:215–62.
Sato TN, Tozawa Y, Deutsch U, Wolburg-Buchholz K, Fujiwara Y, Gendron-Maguire M, Gridley T, Wolburg H, Risau W, Qin Y. 1995. Distinct roles of the receptor tyrosine kinases Tie-1 and Tie-2 in blood vessel formation. Nature (Land) 376:70–74.
Schlaeger TM, Qin Y, Fujiwara Y, Magram J, Sato TN. 1995. Vascular endothelial cell lineage-specific promoter in transgenic mice. Development 121:1089–98.
Seetharam L, Gotoh N, Maru Y, Neufeld G, Yamaguchi S, Shibuya M. 1995. A unique signal transduction from FLT tyrosine kinase, a receptor for vascular endothelial growth factor VEGF. Oncogene 10:135–47.
Shalaby F, Rossant J, Yamaguchi TP, Gertsenstein M, Wu X-F, Breitman ML, Schuh AC. 1995. Failure of blood-island formation and vasculogenesis in Flk-1- deficient mice. Nature 376:62–66.
Sissman NJ. 1983. Anomalies of the aortic arch complex. In: Adams FH, Emmanouilides GC, editors. Moss' heart disease in infants, children, and adolescents. 3rd ed. Baltimore, MD: Williams & Wilkins. p 199–215.
Skandalakis JE, Gray SW, Symbas P. 1994. The thoracic and abdominal aorta. In: Skandalakis JE, Editor. Embryology for surgeons. 2nd ed. Baltimore, MD: Williams & Wilkins. p 976–1030.
Skidmore FD. 1975. Development of the right outflow tract and pulmonary arterial supply. Ann. R. Coll. Surg. Engl. 57:186–97.
Stewart JR, Kincaid OW, Edwards JE, editors. 1964. An Atlas of Vascular Rings and Related Malformations of the Aortic Arch System. Springfield, IL: Charles C. Thomas.
Van Mierop LHS. 1979a. Morphological development of the heart. In: Berne RM, Sperelakis N, Geiger SR, editors. The cardiovascular system. Baltimore, MD: Waverly Press. p 1–28.
Van Mierop LHS. 1979b. Embryology of the univentricular heart. Herz 4:78–85.
Vincent M, Duband J-L, Thirey J-P. 1983. A cell surface determinant expressed early on migrating avian neural crest cells. Dev. Brain. Res. 9:235–8.
Vlodavsky I, Fridman R, et al. 1987. Aortic endothelial cells synthesize basic fibroblast growth factor which remains cell associated and platelet-derived growth factor-like protein which is secreted. J. Cell. Physiol 131:402–6.
Waldo KL, Kumiski D, Kirby ML. 1996. Cardiac neural crest is essential for the persistence rather than the formation of an arch artery. Dev. Dyn. 205:281–292.
Waldo KL, Kirby ML. 1993a. Cardiac neural crest contribution to the pulmonary artery and sixth aortic arch artery complex in chick embryos aged 6 to 18 days. Anat. Rec. 237:385–99.
Waldo KL, Kirby ML. 1993b. Cardiac neural crest contribution to the pulmonary artery and sixth aortic arch artery complex in chick embryos aged 6 to 18 days. Anat Rec 237:385–99.
Weinberg PM. 1995. Aortic arch anomalies. In: Emmanouilides GC, Riemenschneider TA, Allen HD, Gutgesell HP, editors. Moss and Adams heart disease in infants, children, and adolescents including the fetus and young adult. 5th ed. Baltimore, MD: Williams & Wilkins. p 810–37.
Weston, JA. 1970. The migration and differentiation of neural crest cells. Adv. Morphog 8:41–117.

CHAPTER 10

Primitive Cardiac Segment, Normal Heart, and Congenital Heart Diseases

María V. de la Cruz

From the new information acquired by means of the in vivo labeling techniques on the embryological constitution of the cardiac cavities (de la Cruz et al 1977, 1989, 1991) and the cardiac septa (de la Cruz et al 1982, 1983, 1997), we selected the anatomical structures of the normal heart that allow us to identify each of the cardiac cavities and to recognize the limits and the anatomical structures of the cardiac septa, which are important in the location of the congenital septal defects. This information also allows us to establish a regionalization of the congenital pathology at the ventricular level (de la Cruz et al 1991). This knowledge is of the utmost importance in the diagnosis of congenital cardiopathies, because it permits us to distinguish the cardiac cavities independently of their spatial positions and the connections among each other. The same is true for ventricular congenital pathology, in which one of the primitive cardiac segments that contributes to the definitive ventricle is absent, as occurs in double-outlet right ventricle, in which the anatomical left ventricle lacks its outlet. With respect to the septa, it is essential to know their boundaries to identify the different anatomical types of congenital septal defects.

We will divide this chapter into two sections: (1) The definitive cardiac cavities and the primitive cardiac segments, and (2) the definitive cardiac septa, their limits, and the congenital septal defects.

THE DEFINITIVE CARDIAC CAVITIES AND THE PRIMITIVE CARDIAC SEGMENTS

The definitive cardiac cavities are anatomical units, but not embryological units, because they are constituted by different primitive cardiac segments (de la Cruz et al 1977, 1989, 1991). Each of these embryonic segments of the cardiac tube gives origin to a specific anatomical region of a definitive cardiac cavity (de la Cruz et al 1977, 1989, 1991) (chapter III, Figs. 4 and 5; chapter IV, Figs. 5 and 7) (Fig. 1).

We will study separately the atria and the ventricles.

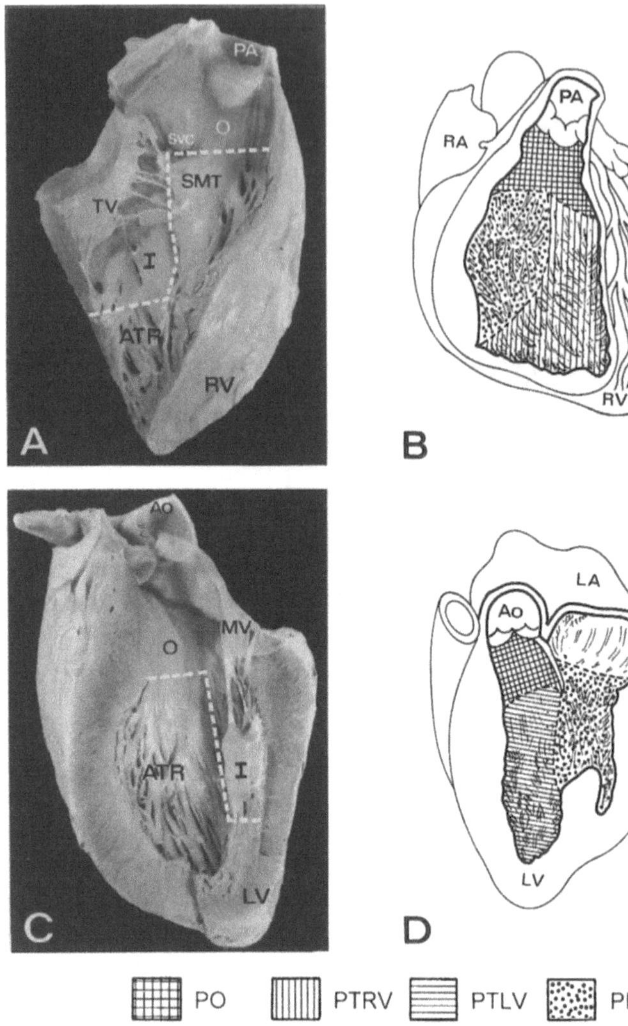

FIGURE 1. Photographs and diagrams of dissections of the right and left ventricular cavities in man showing the septal wall of each ventricle. The dotted line indicates the boundaries between the inlet region, the apical trabeculated region, and the outlet region. The diagrams of these dissections portray the embryological origin of each of the regions. **A.** Septal wall of the anatomical right ventricle. **B.** Diagram of the septal wall of the anatomical right ventricle. **C.** Septal wall of the anatomical left ventricle. **D.** Diagram of the septal wall of the anatomical left ventricle. I = inlet; ATR = apical trabeculated region; O = outlet; PA = pulmonary artery; TV = tricuspid valve; SVC = supraventricular crest; SMT = septomarginal trabeculation; RV = anatomical right ventricle; RA = anatomical right atrium; MV = mitral valve; Ao = aorta; LV = anatomical left ventricle; LA = anatomical left atrium; PO = primitive outlet; PI = primitive inlet; PTRV = primitive apical trabeculated region of the anatomical right ventricle; PTLV = primitive apical trabeculated region of the anatomical left ventricle.

Atria

It is indispensable in the diagnosis of the visceroatrial situs to distinguish the anatomical right atrium from the anatomical left atrium (Van Mierop et al 1972; Van Praagh and Van Praagh 1990). Furthermore, this is a very important parameter, together with the identification of the anatomical right ventricle and the anatomical left ventricle, in the diagnosis of atrioventricular concordance and discordance (Shinebourne et al 1976) (chapter VIII).

The definitive right atrium or anatomical right atrium is constituted by two primitive cardiac segments: (1) the primitive right atrium whose anatomical expression is the pectinate muscles (chapter VIII, Figs. 2C and 5A), and (2) the right horn of the sinus venosus, which gives origin to the sinus region of this atrium (chapter VIII, Figs. 2C and 5A). Although it has not been proven that the pectinate muscles originate from the primitive right atrium, the fact that the anatomical right atrium in the chick exhibits pectinate muscles but lacks a smooth region or sinus region, and also that the sinus venosus is connected to but not incorporated in to this atrium allows us to conclude that the pectinate muscles originate from the primitive right atrium (chapter VIII, Fig. 2, A and B).

The definitive left atrium or anatomical left atrium is constituted by two primitive cardiac segments: (1) the primitive left atrium whose anatomical expression is to form a smooth surface, and (2) the sinus venosus. Recent research in the chick embryo and the mouse have shown that the pulmonary veins incorporate into the left atrium through the sinus venosus (DeRuiter et al 1995). Fustheremore, we do not know the stage of development of the human embryo that shows the beginning of the connection of the pulmonary veins sinus with the left atrium (chapter VIII). Consequently, we may suppose that in man the pulmonary region of the sinus venosus (pulmonary veins) incorporates into the left atrium (chapter VIII). Because neither of the two primitive cardiac segments (sinus venosus and primitive left atrium) that constitute the anatomical left atrium give origin to pectinate muscles, the atrial wall is smooth; in addition there is no anatomical structure that indicates the boundary between the two primitive cardiac segments that form it (chapter VIII, Figs. 2D and 5A).

The appendage of the anatomical right atrium is morphologically different from that of the anatomical left atrium, but it is not a safe parameter to distinguish between the atria because in congenital cardiopathies with atrial dilatation, the shape of the atrial appendages is altered by the blood flow. The interatrial septum is not useful either to distinguish the anatomical right atrium from the anatomical left atrium in congenital cardiopathies because it may be absent. With respect to the identification of the anatomical left atrium, the drainage of the pulmonary veins is not useful, because there is a cardiopathy designated as total anomalous pulmonary venous connection.

Ventricles

Each of the ventricles is constituted by three embryological components or primitive cardiac segments (de la Cruz et al 1977, 1989, 1991). Each of these segments has a specific anatomical expression in the definitive ventricle (chapter III, Fig. 6) (Fig. 1). There are two primitive cardiac segments that are common for both ventricles: the primitive inlet, which by a septation process gives origin to the inlet of each ventricle (de la Cruz et al 1991) (chapter IV, Figs. 2 and 7; chapter VI, Fig. 2), and the primitive outlet, which also by a septation process gives origin to the outlet of each ventricle (de la Cruz et al 1977, 1989, 1991) (chapter VII). In addition, there is a specific primitive cardiac segment for each ventricle, which gives origin to the apical trabeculated region of the anatomical right ventricle and that of the apical trabeculated region of the anatomical left ventricle (de la Cruz et al 1989, 1991) (chapters III and V) (chapter III, Figs. 4–6).

Each of the embryological components (primitive cardiac segments) that constitute the definitive ventricles corresponds to the anatomical regions into which Goor and Lillehei (1975) divided the definitive ventricles: the inlet, the apical trabeculated region, and the outlet (Fig. 1).

Because the apical trabeculated region of each ventricle has its own primordium or primitive cardiac segment (de la Cruz et al 1989, 1991), its anatomical manifestation distinguishes the anatomical right ventricle from the anatomical left ventricle (chapters III and V). The anatomical right ventricle is characterized by its apical trabeculated region, which is richly trabeculated, and by the presence of septomarginal trabeculation (Fig. 2, A and B). The septomarginal trabeculation is a muscular structure located in the trabeculated region of the septal aspect of the anatomical right ventricle. It is Y-shaped; it is fused at its apical pad to the anterior papillary muscle by means of the moderator band whereas its basal end is divided into two limbs, one anterior (or superior) and the other posterior (or inferior) (Fig. 2, A and B). When there is no pathology of the outlet, the supraventricular crest is attached to the junction between these two limbs (Fig. 2, A and B). On the other hand, the anatomical left ventricle lacks a septomarginal trabeculation and its walls are scarcely trabeculated at its apical trabeculated region (Fig. 2C).

A ventricular inlet is characterized anatomically by the presence of an atrioventricular valve apparatus, the tricuspid on the right side and the mitral on the left side (chapter VI) (Fig. 1, A and C). If the primitive inlet does not become septated, a single atrioventricular valve apparatus is originated, which is neither tricuspid nor mitral, such as seen in the atrioventricular canal defect. Consequently, neither the tricuspid valve apparatus nor the mitral are parameters that permit absolute distinction between the anatomical right and the anatomical left ventricles. Furthermore, there may be different types and varieties of abnormal embryological development of the atrioventricular valve apparatus, whose anatomical manifestation corresponds to the group of specific congenital cardiopathies of the inlet, e.g., tricuspid atresia, straddling and overriding of the mitral or the tricuspid valve.

The outlet is the subarterial segment of each ventricule. Its boundaries are, for the anatomical right ventricle, the arterial valve and a tangential plane at the proximal border of the supraventricular crest (chapter VII) (Figs. 1A and 2A); in the anatomical left ventricle, its boundaries are defined by the arterial valve and a tangential plane at the free border of the anteroseptal leaflet of the mitral valve, which constitutes the mitroaortic continuity (chapter VII) (Fig. 1C). Because both outlets originate from the same primitive outlet, if the latter is not septated, it gives origin to a single outlet (de la Cruz et al 1977, 1991), as is the case in truncus arteriosus (sometimes called common truncus or persistent truncus). Consequently, the anatomical characteristics of the outlet are not parameters for the distinction between the ventricles.

The supraventricular crest, however, is a very important anatomical structure in the diagnosis of the specific pathology of the outlets. This crest is a muscular

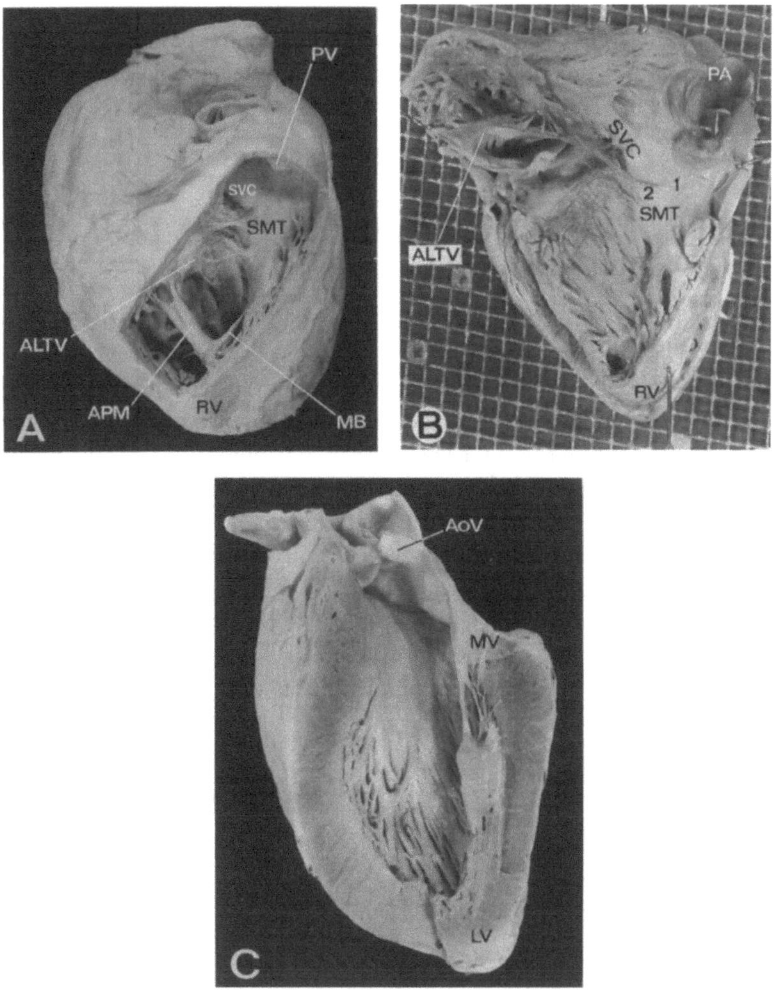

FIGURE 2. Photographs of dissections of the right and left ventricular cavities in man. **A** and **B.** Dissection of the anatomical right ventricle, exhibiting the septomarginal trabeculation (SMT) that characterizes this ventricle. Notice at the basal end of this trabecula, its anterior or superior limb (1) and its posterior or inferior limb (2), and at its apical end, the moderator band (MB), which unites it to the anterior papillary muscle (APM); also note the trabeculated aspect of this ventricle. **C.** Dissection of the anatomical left ventricle, showing that there is no septomarginal trabeculation and that its wall is poorly trabeculated. ALTV = anterior leaflet of the tricuspid valve; SVC = supraventricular crest; RV = anatomical right ventricle; LV = anatomical left ventricle; PV = pulmonary valve; PA = pulmonary artery; AoV = aortic valve; MV = mitral valve.

structure located at the base of the anatomical right ventricle and it constitutes one part of the wall of the right outlet that separates it from the tricuspid annulus (Fig. 2B). The supraventricular crest is inserted between the two limbs of the septomarginal trabeculation (Fig. 2B), and it extends up to the union of the free wall of the outlet of the right ventricle with the border of the tricuspid annulus (chapter VII, Fig. 1, A and C.) (Fig. 2B).

The same as with the inlets, there are several types and varieties of abnormal embryological development of the embryological structures that constitute the outlets and manifest themselves anatomically by a peculiar pathology of this region of the heart. Some examples are tetralogy of Fallot, the Taussig-Bing anomaly, and double-outlet right ventricle.

THE DEFINITIVE CARDIAC SEPTA, THEIR LIMITS, AND THE CONGENITAL SEPTAL DEFECTS

The in vivo labeling of the inferior (de la Cruz et al 1983) and superior cushions (de la Cruz et al 1982) of the atrioventricular canal and of the primitive interventricular septum (de la Cruz et al 1997), together with the atrial septum primum, indicates how the first septum develops in the heart. We have termed this structure the primitive cardiac septum (de la Cruz et al 1983) (chapters V–VIII) (chapter VI, Fig. 2). The tracing of in vivo labels into the mature heart has also rendered valuable information concerning the true contribution of each of these embryological structures to the cardiac septation (chapters V–VIII). From this information, we made a map that shows the topographic location of these embryological components in the interatrial septum, the atrioventricular septum, and the interventricular septum and indicates their anatomical manifestation (chapter V, Fig. 3). This knowledge is essential in the selection of the normal anatomical structures of the cardiac septa

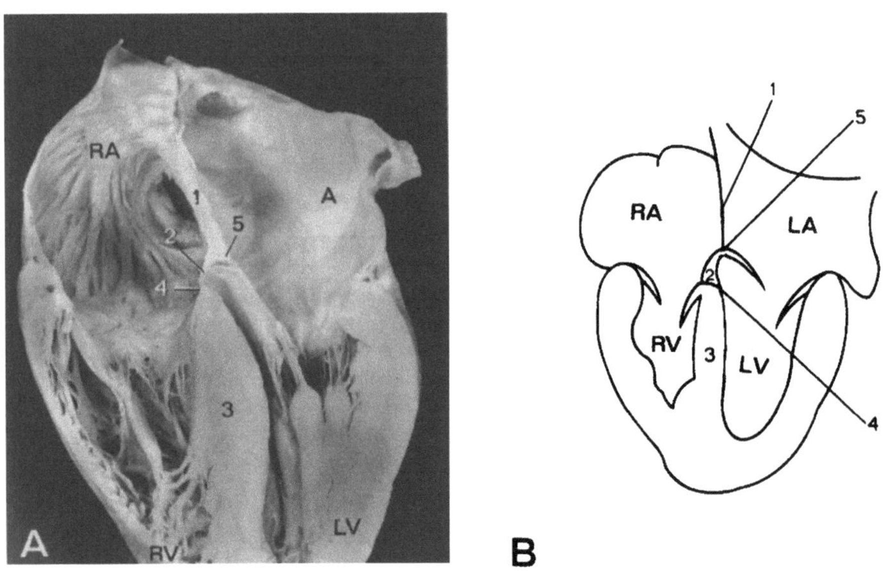

FIGURE 3. Photograph and diagram of a four-chamber section at the level of the membranous portion of the atrioventricular septum in a human heart showing the interatrial septum (1), the atrioventricular septum (2), and the interventricular septum (3); their anatomical boundaries; and the cardiac cavities that these septa separate. RA = anatomical right atrium; LA = anatomical left atrium; RV = anatomical right ventricle; LV = anatomical left ventricle; 1 = interatrial septum; 2 = atrioventricular septum; 3 = interventricular septum; 4 = septal insertion of the septal leaflet of the tricuspid valve; 5 = septal insertion of the anterior leaflet of the mitral valve.

that are important for the diagnosis of congenital cardiopathies in the field of septal defects.

Therefore, there are three definitive cardiac septa; the interatrial, the atrioventricular, and the interventricular. Each of them has its precise anatomical boundaries and they separate specific cardiac cavities (Fig. 3).

The boundaries between the interatrial septum and the atrioventricular septum are (1) in the left cavities, the septal insertion of the anterior leaflet of the mitral valve (Fig. 3) (chapter VIII, Fig. 7); and (2) in the right cavities, the projection of the insertion of this leaflet in the septal wall of the anatomical right atrium (Fig. 3) (chapter VIII, Fig. 7). Thus, the septal wall of the anatomical left atrium is exclusively formed by the interatrial septum, whereas the septal wall of the anatomical right atrium is partly interatrial septum and also atrioventriuclar septum in the region adjacent to the insertion site of the septal leaflet of the tricuspid valve, which corresponds to the ventricular limit of the atrioventricular septum (Fig. 3) (chapter VIII, Fig. 7B). Therefore, the septal defects located above the septal insertion of the anterior leaflet of the mitral valve are interatrial defects (Fig. 3) (chapter VIII, Fig. 7B).

The atrioventricular septum comprises the area between the septal insertion of the anterior leaflet of the mitral valve (limit with the anatomical left atrium) and the insertion of the septal leaflet of the tricuspid valve (limit with the anatomical right ventricle) (Fig. 3) (chapter VIII, Fig. 7B). Therefore, this septum separates the anatomical right atrium from the anatomical left ventricle and forms the region of the septal wall of the anatomical right atrium adjacent to the insertion of the septal leaflet of the tricuspid valve and the septal wall of the inlet of the anatomical left ventricle adjacent to the septal insertion of the anterior leaflet of the mitral valve (Fig. 3) (chapter VIII, Fig. 7). Consequently, the defects located between the septal insertion of the anterior leaflet of the mitral valve and the insertion of the septal leaflet of the tricuspid valve are atrioventricular defects and communicate the anatomical right atrium with the anatomical left ventricle (Fig. 3).

The anatomical limit between the interventricular septum and the atrioventricular septum corresponds to the insertion of the septal leaflet of the tricuspid valve (Fig. 3) (chapter VIII, Fig. 7). The interventricular septum is divided into thirds: the basal, the middle, and the apical (Figs. 3 and 4). The region adjacent to the insertion of the septal leaflet of the tricuspid valve or basal third of the interventricular septum is subdivided into two regions, a muscular region that separates the inlet of both ventricles and a membranous region that separates the inlet of the anatomical right ventricle from the outlet of the anatomical left ventricle (Fig. 4). One of the boundaries of the membranous region of this septum is the central fibrous body of the heart (Soto et al 1980); in addition, it is partially covered by the septal leaflet of the tricuspid valve and is adjacent to the posterior or inferior limb of the septomarginal trabeculation (Fig. 4). The septal defects located in the muscular basal third communicate both ventricular inlets with each other (Fig. 4), and those located in the membranous region communicate the inlet of the anatomical right ventricle with the outlet of the anatomical left ventricle (Soto et al 1980) (Fig. 4). The middle third and the apical third of the interventricular septum separate the apical trabeculated region of both ventricles, and the septal defects located in this area communicate both apical regions (Fig. 4). In the septal wall of the outlet of the anatomical right ventricle, there is a small area adjacent to the anterior or superior limb of the septomarginal trabeculation, in which a septal defect that communicates both outlets may be present (Soto et al 1980), because the greatest part of the so-called septal

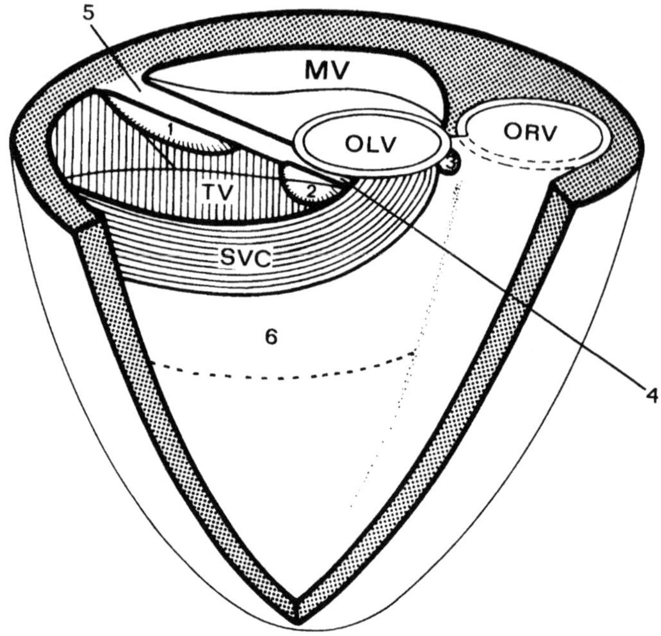

FIGURE 4. Diagram representing the basal third of the interventricular septum, showing the relationships between the inlet of both ventricles, the inlet of the right ventricle with the outlet of the left ventricle, and the outlet of both ventricles. TV = tricuspid valve; MV = mitral valve; OLV = outlet of the left ventricle; ORV = outlet of the right ventricle; SVC = supraventricular crest; 1 = interventricular septal defect located in the muscular basal third; 2 = interventricular septal defect located in the membranous region; 3 = interventricular septal defect located between the outlet of both ventricles; 4 = membranous region of the interventricular septum; 5 = muscular region of the interventricular septum; 6 = basal third of the interventricular septum.

wall of the outlet of the anatomical right ventricle is part of the free ventricular wall (Fig. 4) (Chapter VIII, Fig. 2, A and B).

CONCLUSIONS

The results of the in vivo labeling experiments have rendered new information about the embryological components of the cardiac cavities and their septa. By means of this knowledge, the anatomical structures of the normal heart that are important in the diagnosis of congenital cardiopathies were selected; the regionalization of these cardiopathies at the ventricular level is revealed.

1. The specific normal anatomical structures of each of the definitive cardiac cavities that permits the distinction between them in congenital cardiopathies at the atrial level are the pectinate muscles in the anatomical right atrium and their absence in the anatomical left atrium. At the ventricular level these structures are the septomarginal trabeculation and its apical region, which is richly trabeculated in the anatomical right ventricle, and the absence of the septomarginal trabeculation and the scantly trabeculated apical region in the anatomical

left ventricle. The differences between these cardiac cavities are given by their embryological constitution.

2. Each ventricle is constituted by three primordia or primitive cardiac segments: (1) the primitive inlet, whose anatomical expression is the atrioventricular valve apparatus and which by a septation process gives origin to the inlet of each ventricle; (2) the primitive outlet, which gives origin to the outlet of each ventricle; and (3) with respect to the apical trabeculated region of each ventricle, its own primordium. These facts determine that there is a regional pathology of the outlets and of the inlets and in addition that the differential anatomical characteristic of each ventricle is its apical trabeculated region.
3. There are four definitive cardiac cavities and three septa; the interatrial, the atrioventricular and the interventricular. The anatomical boundaries between each of these septa are important in the diagnosis of congenital septal defects. The anatomical boundary of the interatrial septum in the left cavities is the septal insertion of the anterior leaflet of the mitral valve, and in the anatomical right atrium, this corresponds to the projection of the insertion of this leaflet in the septal wall of this atrium. The defects located in this septum communicate both atria with each other. The atrioventricular septum comprises the area between the septal insertion of the anterior leaflet of the mitral valve and the septal leaflet of the tricuspid valve; this septum separates the anatomical right atrium from the anatomical left ventricle. The defects located in this septum communicate the right atrium with the anatomical left ventricle. The boundary of the interventricular septum corresponds to the insertion of the septal leaflet of the tricuspid valve. This septum separates both ventricles from each other. The basal third of the interventricular septum is adjacent to the insertion of the septal leaflet of the tricuspid valve; it has a muscular region between both inlets and a membranous region between the inlet of the anatomical right ventricle and the outlet of the anatomical left ventricle; one of its boundaries is the central fibrous body of the heart.

REFERENCES

de la Cruz MV, Castillo MM, Villavicencio L, Valencia A, Moreno-Rodriguez RA. 1997. Primitive interventricular septum, its primordium, and its contribution in the definitive interventricular septum: in vivo labelling study in the chick embryo heart. Anat Rec 247:512–20.

de la Cruz MV, Gímenez-Ribotta M, Saravalli O, Cayré R. 1983. The contribution of the inferior endocardial cushion of the atrioventricular canal to cardiac septation and to the development of the atrioventricular valves: study in the chick embryo. Am J Anat 166:63–72.

de la Cruz MV, Quero-Jiménez M, Arteaga M, Cayré R. 1982. Morphogénèse du septum interventriculaire. Coeur 13:443–8.

de la Cruz MV, Sánchez-Gómez C, Cayré R. 1991. The developmental components of the ventricles: their significance in congenital cardiac malformations. Cardiol Young 1:123–8.

de la Cruz MV, Sánchez-Gómez C, Arteaga M, Argüello C. 1977. Experimental study of the development of the truncus and the conus in the chick embryo. J Anat 123:661–86.

de la Cruz MV, Sánchez-Gómez C, Palomino MA. 1989. The primitive cardiac regions in the straight tube heart (stage 9−) and their anatomical expression in the mature heart: an experimental study in the chick embryo. J Anat 165:121–31.

DeRuiter MC, Gittenberg-de Groot AC, Wenink ACG, Poelmann RE, Mentink MMT.

1995. In normal development pulmonary veins are connected to the sinus venosus segment in the left atrium. Anat Rec 243:84–92.
Goor DA, Lillehei CW. 1975. Congenital malformations of the heart: The Anatomy of the Heart. In: Embryology, anatomy and operative considerations. New York: Grune and Stratton. p 1–37.
Shinebourne EA, Macartney FJ, Anderson RH. 1976. Sequential chamber localization—logical approach to diagnosis in congenital heart disease. Br Heart J 38:327–40.
Soto B, Becker AE, Moulaert AJ, Lie JT, Anderson RH. 1980. Classification of ventricular septal defects. Br Heart J 43:332–43.
Van Mierop LHS, Gessner IH, Schiebler GL. 1972. Asplenia and polysplenia syndrome. Birth Defects, Original Article Series. Vol. 8. 1:74–82.
Van Praagh R, Van Praagh S. 1990. Atrial isomerims in the heterotaxy syndromes with asplenia, or polysplenia, or normally formed spleen: an erroneous concept. Am J Cardiol 66:1504–6.

Index

MIX
Papier aus verantwortungsvollen Quellen
Paper from responsible sources
FSC® C105338

If you have any concerns about our products,
you can contact us on
ProductSafety@springernature.com

In case Publisher is established outside the EU,
the EU authorized representative is:
Springer Nature Customer Service Center GmbH
Europaplatz 3, 69115 Heidelberg, Germany

Printed by Libri Plureos GmbH
in Hamburg, Germany